A PRACTICAL APPROACH

to

EKG INTERPRETATION

By

RAJ K. ANAND
MD, FACC, FASLMS

Associate Professor Emeritus
Cardiovascular Medicine
University of Massachusetts Medical School

DEDICATED

TO MY WIFE

AND

TO MY STUDENTS

FOR INSPIRING ME OVER THE YEARS

PREFACE

During my 40 years of teaching experience, I have been repeatedly reminded of the difficulty which the students feel in comprehending the method to calculate the QRS axis. More importantly, they lack in their understanding of basic principles which form the very foundation of the approach to diagnosis of a rhythm in an electrocardiogram. These two areas have always been of great concern to me. Therefore, I have created a new method for calculating the QRS axis. This method is more efficient than the conventional approach, and easier to understand. The feedback from the students has been very encouraging. I share this new approach with the readers of this book, in chapter 11. Basic principles required for a better understanding of the approach to analysis of a rhythm in an EKG have been explained in detail in chapters 9 and 10. Every attempt has been made to make sure that the approach is practical and easy to understand. A series of 25 EKG tracings along with step by step guidance to reach the diagnosis has been provided on pages 287 – 338 for an in-depth understanding of the art of EKG interpretation.

Another important observation concerns the lack of follow up practice of EKG interpretation by the students, due to lack of availability of time to sit down with a cardiologist on a regular basis. A follow up practice is crucial to maintaining the skill, after initial learning of how to read an EKG. This challenge has been met by providing a series of 72 EKG tracings along with interpretation for each tracing, at the back section of the book, whereby, the students can practice and improve their skill at their own convenient time on a regular basis.

Raj K. Anand
MD, FACC, FASLMS

ACKNOWLEDGEMENT

I would like to acknowledge the significance of the contributions made by Dr. Oscar E. Starobin, Professor of Medicine at University of Massachusetts Medical School, that have helped shape my career in cardiovascular medicine. This book would not have been a reality without those contributions. He has been my mentor, and it was his blessings that made it possible for me to receive the fellowship training in cardiovascular medicine at the world's greatest institutions, like Peter Bent Brigham Hospital (now known as Brigham and Women's Hospital) and Massachusetts General Hospital in Boston, Massachusetts. At these institutions I was profoundly influenced by three of the greatest cardiologists of all times — Paul Dudley White, Samuel A. Levine, and David Littman. It was the advice of Dr. Starobin, and my respect and affection for him, that brought me to the University of Massachusetts Medical School in 1972, where I have enjoyed teaching for more than 40 years.

My knowledge in cardiovascular medicine has been enriched through my experiences in teaching. I have decided to pass this knowledge on to the future generations of students in medicine through this book, at the urging of my students. I most sincerely hope that they will benefit from its contents.

Raj K. Anand
MD, FACC, FASLMS

TABLE OF CONTENTS

Chapter 1

Introduction:

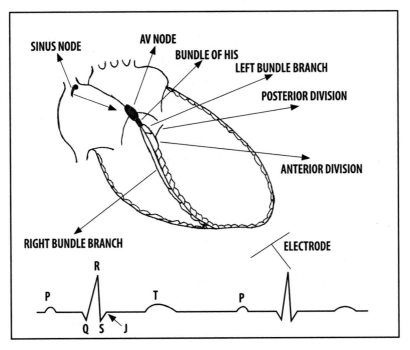

Figure 1

An electrocardiogram is a graphic recording of the electrical activity within the cardiac muscle. EKG (elektrokardiogramm) is a German version of ECG (electrocardiogram) to avoid confusion with EEG. The terminology of P, QRS, and T waves in the EKG tracing was given by Einthoven (in the tradition of Cartesian coordinates) in 1901. Normally an electrical impulse originates at the sinus node, and spreads quickly through the right and the left atrial muscle, on to the AV node. Then, it travels through the AV node and bundle of His, on to the right and the left bundle branches. Right bundle branch distributes the impulse to the lower third of the interventricular septum, the right ventricle, and the inferior surface of the left ventricle through Purkinje fibers. The left bundle branch divides into anterior and posterior divisions, called anterior and posterior fascicles. The anterior fascicle supplies the upper two thirds of the interventricular septum and the anterolateral wall of the left ventricle, and conducts the impulse to these areas through the Purkinje fibers. The posterior fascicle distributes the impulse over the posterior surface of the left ventricle in similar fashion. The spread of electrical impulse through the ventricular muscle leads to depolarization of the myocardial cells, and results in change of polarity of these cells, with sodium ion (+ve charge) moving into the cell and the chloride ion

(-ve charge) moving out of the cell, thus causing contraction of these chambers. This is followed by repolarization, which restores the polarity, followed by a brief period of rest before the cycle begins all over again. The depolarization of the atrial muscle takes 60 – 80 milliseconds and is recorded on the paper as P wave. The horizontal line that follows the P wave is called the PR segment and it represents the time taken by the impulse to travel through the AV node and bundle of His. The time from the start of the P to the end of the PR segment is called the PR interval. It represents the time taken by the impulse to travel from the sinus node to the point where the bundle of His divides into the right and the left bundle branches. Normal PR interval is 0.12 to 0.2 second. The electrical spread from this point onward, to the muscle of the two ventricles is recorded as QRS complex. Normal QRS interval is 0.1 second or less. At the end of the QRS complex, repolarization begins and it is recorded as ST segment and the T wave. The line between the end of the T wave and the beginning of the next P wave is called TP segment, which is the resting period before the next cycle begins. It is considered to be isoelectric. The junction of the S wave and the ST segment is called the "J" point. The T wave is sometimes followed by a prominent wave called the U wave. The interval between the onset of Q wave and the end of the T wave is called the QT interval. One would wonder at this point as to why the depolarization of the AV node is inscribed as a straight line on the EKG tracing, when atrial and ventricular depolarization is inscribed as P and QRS deflections, respectively. It normally takes 80 – 100 milliseconds for the impulse to travel through the ventricular chambers, whereas, it takes 100 – 120 milliseconds to travel through the AV node which is very tiny in comparison to the size of the ventricles. This tremendous slow down shows that the impulse comes to a dead end and somehow struggles through it, thus generating no potential, and therefore a straight line is recorded.

When the electrical spread occurs through atrial and ventricular chambers, the impulse spreads in different directions at the same time. Therefore, at any given time, it is the resultant of all electrical activity, called the instantaneous mean vector (see Figure 2), which determines the direction of various deflections on the EKG paper, like P wave and the QRS complex. If the vector is pointing toward the exploring electrode, an upright deflection is recorded, called a positive deflection; if the vector is pointing away from the exploring electrode, a downward deflection is recorded, called the negative deflection.

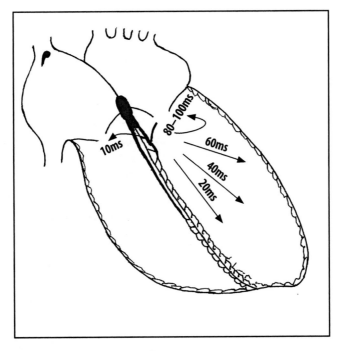

Figure 2

The above diagram (Fig. 2) shows the direction of the electrical mean instantaneous vectors at different times (10, 20, 40, 60, 80, and 100 milliseconds) after the impulse leaves the bundle of His and spreads to depolarize the ventricles. You will note that the 10 msec. vector is directed superiorly and to the right, and activates the interventricular septum. In the horizontal plane it would be directed anteriorly activating the septum from left to the right ventricular side. Since, it points to the right, it gives rise to a Q wave or an initial negative deflection in left sided leads, and a positive initial deflection in right sided leads. The 20, 40, 60, and 80 msec. vectors are directed to the left and posteriorly (left ventricle lies posteriorly and to the left), giving rise to positive deflection by the electrodes placed on the left side of the chest and deep negative deflection by the electrodes placed on the right side of the chest. The terminal or the 100 msec. vector activates the base of the heart and points to the right giving rise to S wave or a terminal negative deflection in left sided leads.

Depolarization of ventricular myocardium starts at the endocardial surface and spreads toward the epicardial surface resulting in ventricular systole. High systolic pressure within the ventricular cavity delays the recovery of the endocardial surface of the myocardium, thus causing the repolarization to start at the epicardial surface and then spread toward the endocardial surface. Thus, depolarization and repolarization occur in opposite directions. The +ve charge is in front during depolarization

(Fig. A), which results in positive deflection on the EKG paper as the process proceeds toward the recording electrode. The – ve charge is in front as repolarization proceeds in opposite direction with the +ve charge facing the recording electrode and gradually moving away from it. This results in initial sharp positive deflection followed by gradual fall in amplitude as the +ve charge moves away from the electrode. That means that when the depolarization and repolarization move in opposite directions, the QRS and the T wave move in the same direction. This explains why the QRS and the T wave are normally concordant. For the same reason, when the depolarization and repolarization move in the same direction (Fig. B), the QRS and the T wave are discordant, as seen with wide QRS complexes (e.g. RBBB, LBBB, IVC delay), where the epicardial depolarization is delayed which allows the endocardial surface of the myocardium to recover before the epicardial surface recovers.

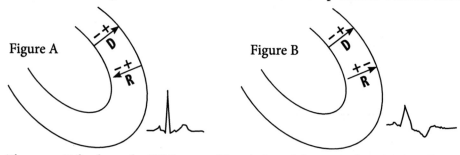

There are 12 leads on the EKG paper (Fig. 3). Six of them are chest leads and are called precordial leads (V1, V2, V3, V4, V5, and V6). The other six are limb leads. Precordial and three of the limb leads (AVR, AVL, and AVF) are unipolar with positive electrode recording the voltage. Lead AVR records voltage at the right shoulder and leads AVL and AVF record the voltage at the left shoulder and the left leg respectively. The remaining three limb leads are bipolar (leads I, II and III). Lead I records the potential difference between left shoulder and the right shoulder, the left shoulder electrode being positive. Lead II records the potential difference between the left leg and the right shoulder, the left leg electrode being positive. Lead III records the potential difference between left leg and the left shoulder, left leg electrode being positive. It should be noted (see Fig. 4) that, while the electrode on the left shoulder serves as positive electrode for lead I, it becomes automatically the negative electrode for lead III.

$$Lead\ I = VL - VR$$
$$Lead\ II = VF - VR$$
$$Lead\ III = VF - VL$$

VL = Voltage at the left shoulder (L).
VR = Voltage at the right shoulder (R).
VF = Voltage at the left leg (LL).

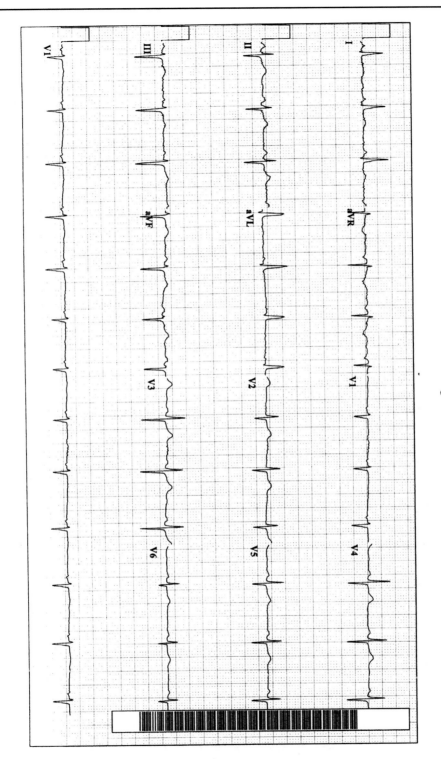

Figure 3

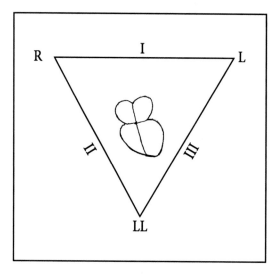

Figure 4

Understanding the EKG paper:

The EKG paper on which the graphic recording is made shows vertical and horizontal lines (see Fig. 2, page 20). Every 5th vertical as well as horizontal line is a thick line. There are 4 thin lines between each successive thick vertical as well as horizontal line. Each consecutive line, vertical or horizontal, is 1.0 mm apart. The electrocardiogram is recorded at the speed of 25 mm per second. That means 25 vertical lines per second. If there are 25 vertical lines in one second, that means each vertical line is 0.04 second apart. Thus, if we want to calculate the PR interval (the distance between the start of the P wave and the end of the PR segment), we simply count the number of lines between these 2 points (starting with zero line) and multiply by 0.04 to get the PR interval. Similarly, we can calculate QRS interval (from the start of the Q wave to the end of S wave) or Q – T interval (from the start of the Q wave to the end of the T wave).

On the left side of an EKG tracing, there is a standardization deflection (see arrow in Fig.1, chapter 7) in the shape of an inverted letter 'U', which represents electronic gain setting in the EKG machine to give 10 mm of deflection for an input of 1.0 mV of potential. If this deflection is 5.0 mm in height, it indicates that the EKG tracing has been recorded at ½ normal standard setting, and therefore, the height of each QRS complex has been reduced to half its standard size.

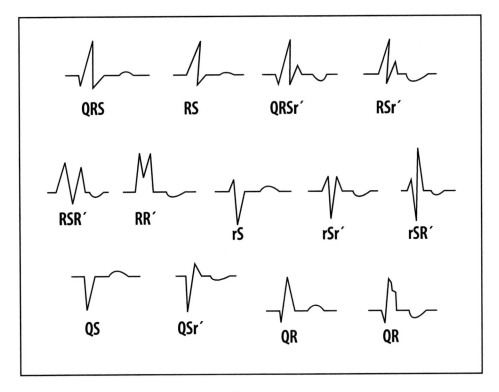

Figure 5

How to read QRS complex morphology (see above):

The first negative deflection is called the Q wave. The first positive deflection after the first negative deflection is called the R wave. If there is no Q wave, and the first deflection is positive, it is called the R wave. If the height of the R wave is less than 5 mm, it is written with the small letter "r" as r wave. The negative deflection after the R wave is called the S wave. The positive deflection after the S wave is called the R prime (R′). If the R prime is small (less than 5 mm), it is written with small letter "r" as r′. When there is entirely negative deflection without R wave, it is referred to as QS complex. For details see Figure 5.

Chapter 2

EKG Leads

A lead is defined as an axis of electrical signals between two electrodes. There are normally ten electrodes in a 12 lead EKG. The 12 EKG leads are divided into 6 limb leads and 6 precordial leads. The limb leads are further divided into 3 standard limb leads and 3 augmented limb leads. The standard limb leads are also called the bipolar limb leads, because they record the difference of electrical potential between two electrodes. The augmented limb leads are sometimes referred to as the unipolar limb leads, because they record the potential at the electrode. The precordial leads are unipolar. The bipolar limb leads have a positive and a negative electrode. Unipolar limb leads and precordial leads have only positive electrode, the negative electrode being a composite of many other electrodes.

The three bipolar limb leads are called lead I, II, and III respectively. Lead I records potential difference between the left and the right shoulders, the left having the positive electrode. Lead II records the potential difference between the left leg and the right shoulder, the left leg having the positive electrode. Lead III records the potential difference between the left leg and the left shoulder, the left leg having the positive electrode. Right leg electrode serves as reference electrode, also called the ground electrode; the ground being infinity which is as close to zero as possible. Addition of various electronic resistors in the ground lead brings its potential to as close to zero as possible in the human body, which is a saline reservoir.

The unipolar limb leads record the potential at the right shoulder, the left shoulder, and the left leg. They are referred to as lead AVR, AVL and AVF, respectively. The letter "A" stands for augmented, and the letter" V" stands for voltage. Due to rather small potential, the unipolar limb leads need to be augmented to achieve bigger deflection on the EKG paper. This is accomplished by averaging the algebraic sum of the remaining two unipolar electrodes and plugging it into a terminal in the EKG machine which serves as the negative electrode for the unipolar limb lead which is being recorded. For example, for lead AVL, it is the algebraic sum of the potential at the right shoulder and the left leg, multiplied by 0.5 to get the average, which is plugged into the negative terminal. This is done automatically and is built inside the EKG machine. This negative terminal is called modification of the Wilson's central terminal. It is based upon the formula that the algebraic sum of the potential at the 3 limb electrodes equals zero i.e. $VL + VR + VF = 0$. The letter "V" refers to voltage. This approach increases the potential by 50 % as explained on the following page.

$$VL + VR + VF = 0$$

$$VL = - (VR + VF)$$

$$VL \times 0.5 = - (VR + VF) \times 0.5$$

$$(VR + VF) \times 0.5 = - (VL \times 0.5)$$

$$AVL = (VL) - \{(VR + VF) \times 0.5)\}$$

$$AVL = (VL) - \{-(VL \times 0.5)\}$$

$$AVL = VL + (VL \times 0.5)$$

$$AVL = VL \times 1.5$$

This is a 50 % increase.

Precordial leads do not need augmentation due to their proximity to the heart. They are unipolar leads with positive electrodes on the chest. The negative electrode is Wilson's central terminal which averages the algebraic sum of leads I, II and III to achieve zero potential. This is based upon Einthoven's Law, which states that lead I + III = II. Thus leads I + III + (- II) = 0. Lead II is reversed for this purpose. This is built into the EKG machine and works automatically.

Leads II, III, and AVF are referred to as inferior leads, because the positive electrode in these leads is located inferiorly. Similarly, leads I, AVL, V5, and V6 are called lateral leads due to lateral location of the positive electrode in these leads. Leads V1, V2, and V3 are referred to as anterior leads for the same reason. Lead V4 is a transitional lead between anterior and lateral leads.

Application of electrodes:

The electrodes are either thin flat metallic conductors with one surface being sticky or they are circular metallic conductor buttons in the center of a patch with sticky back side which adheres to the skin for good contact to transmit electrical signals from the skin to the EKG machine. The electrodes for the limb leads are attached as follows.

Two upper electrodes are attached at the outermost point of the highest site of the two upper limbs, one on each side. Actually the electrode can be attached at any site along the upper extremity up to the wrist, as both limbs are considered to be an extension of the torso in a good conductor body reservoir. All four extremities behave like four wires of a conducting material attached to the torso.

Two lower electrodes are attached at the site just above the pelvis and just lateral to the nipple line, one on each side. The electrode can be attached at any site along the lower extremity up to the ankle.

The black electrode of the limb leads of the EKG machine is attached to the electrode on the left arm. It serves as positive terminal for leads I and AVL, and negative terminal for lead III. The white electrode is attached to the electrode on the right arm. This serves as negative terminal for lead I and II, and positive terminal for lead AVR. The red electrode is attached to the left lower electrode. It serves as positive terminal for leads II, III and AVF. The green electrode is the reference or ground electrode, and attached to the right lower electrode.

Lead I = VL – VR

Lead II = VF – VR

Lead III = VF – VL

The electrodes of Precordial leads are applied on the chest wall as follows:

V1: Fourth intercostal space, next to the right sternal border.

V2: Fourth intercostal space, next to the left sternal border.

V3: Fifth intercostals space, between V2 and V4.

V4: Fifth intercostals space, mid clavicular line.

V5: Fifth intercostals space, anterior axillary line (anterior fold of the arm pit).

V6: Fifth intercostals space, mid axillary line (line in the middle of the arm pit).

The Lewis lead:

This is a bipolar lead, used to detect atrial flutter, when 12 lead EKG does not reveal clear flutter waves. The lead, in this case, is perpendicular to the mean vector of atrial depolarization. The positive electrode is placed in the fourth intercostal space and the negative electrode in the second intercostal space, both next to the right sternal border. The ground electrode is placed in the second intercostal space, next to the left sternal border. One can use the left arm electrode (black) as the positive and the right arm electrode (white) as the negative electrode, and the right leg electrode (green) as ground electrode for this purpose.

Chapter 3

PR Interval

The interval between the start of the P wave and the start of the QRS complex is called PR interval, as shown in the following diagram (Fig. 1). To calculate this interval, count the number of vertical lines on the EKG paper between these two points, starting with zero line, and multiply the number of lines by 0.04 second (which is the interval between two consecutive lines; the paper runs at a speed of 25 mm / second and the distance between two consecutive lines is 1.0 mm) and that would be the PR interval. It should be calculated in all of the three bipolar limb leads, and the longest PR among these leads should be selected as the PR interval. Normal PR interval is 0.12-0.20 second. The PR interval in the EKG tracing (Fig. 2) is 0.18 second.

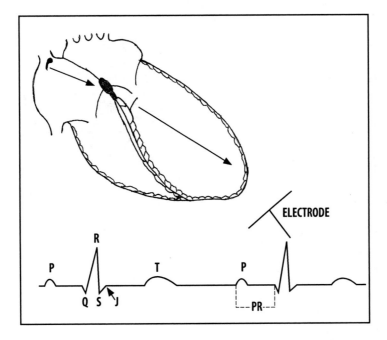

Figure 1

Figure 2

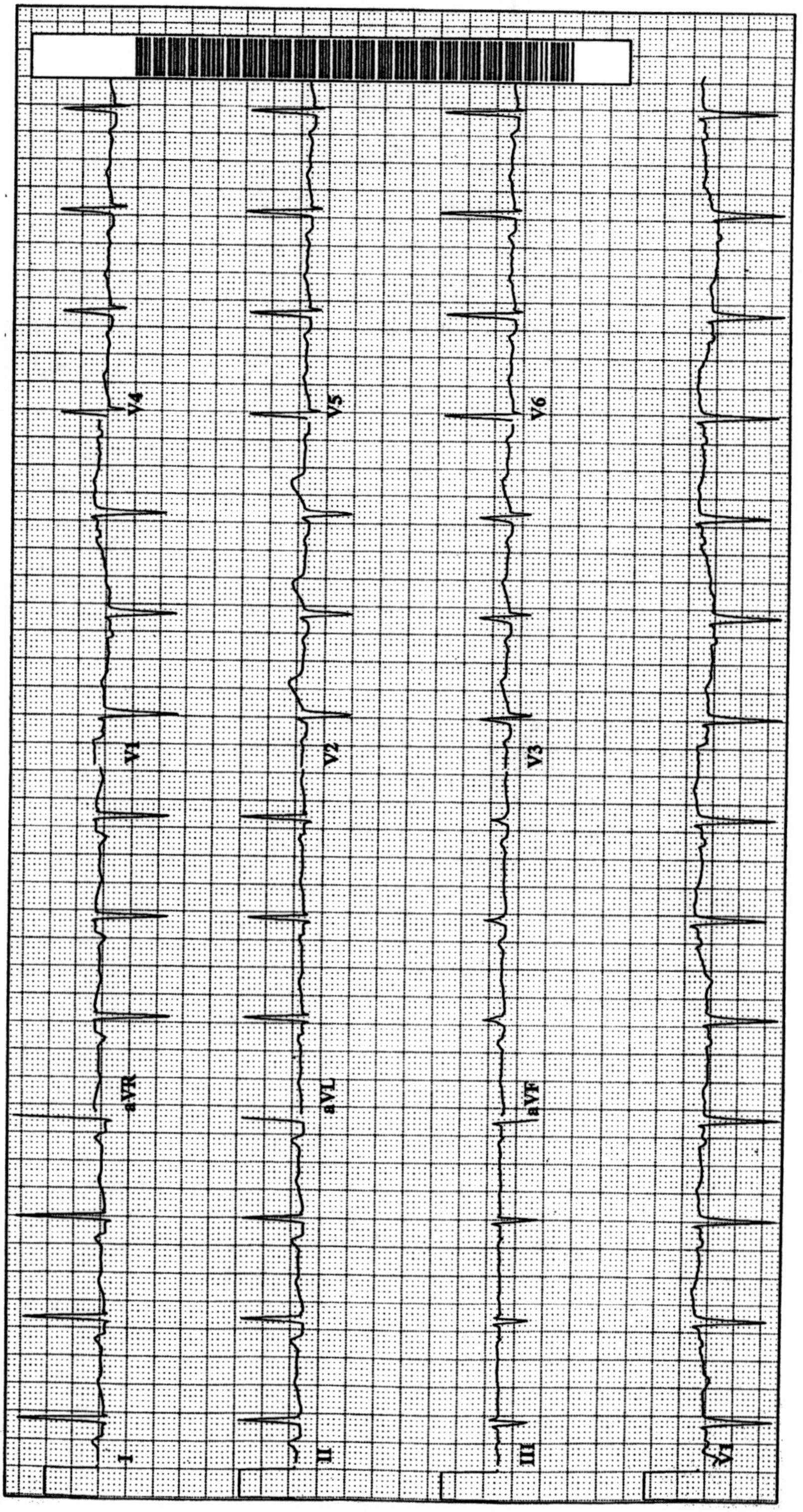

Chapter 4

QRS Interval

QRS interval is the interval between the start of the Q wave (or R wave if there is no Q wave) and the 'J' point of the QRS complex, as shown below in Fig. 1. Count the number of vertical lines between these two points, starting line being the zero line, and multiply by 0.04 to get the QRS interval (each line is 0.04 second apart, as the standard EKG tracing is recorded at a speed of 25 mm/second i.e. 25 lines/second, each vertical line being 1mm apart). Normal QRS interval is 0.10 second or less. Find the QRS interval in all of the three bipolar limb leads, and use the longest of the three as the QRS interval.

A wide QRS interval (0.11 second or greater) is seen with RBBB, LBBB, Intraventricular conduction delay, ventricular rhythm, and electronic ventricular pacing. Premature ventricular contractions (PVCs) also give rise to wide QRS complexes due to slow intraventricular muscular conduction.

The QRS interval in the EKG tracing (Fig. 2) is 0.09 second.

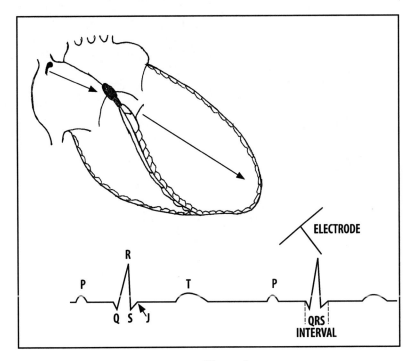

Figure 1

Figure 2

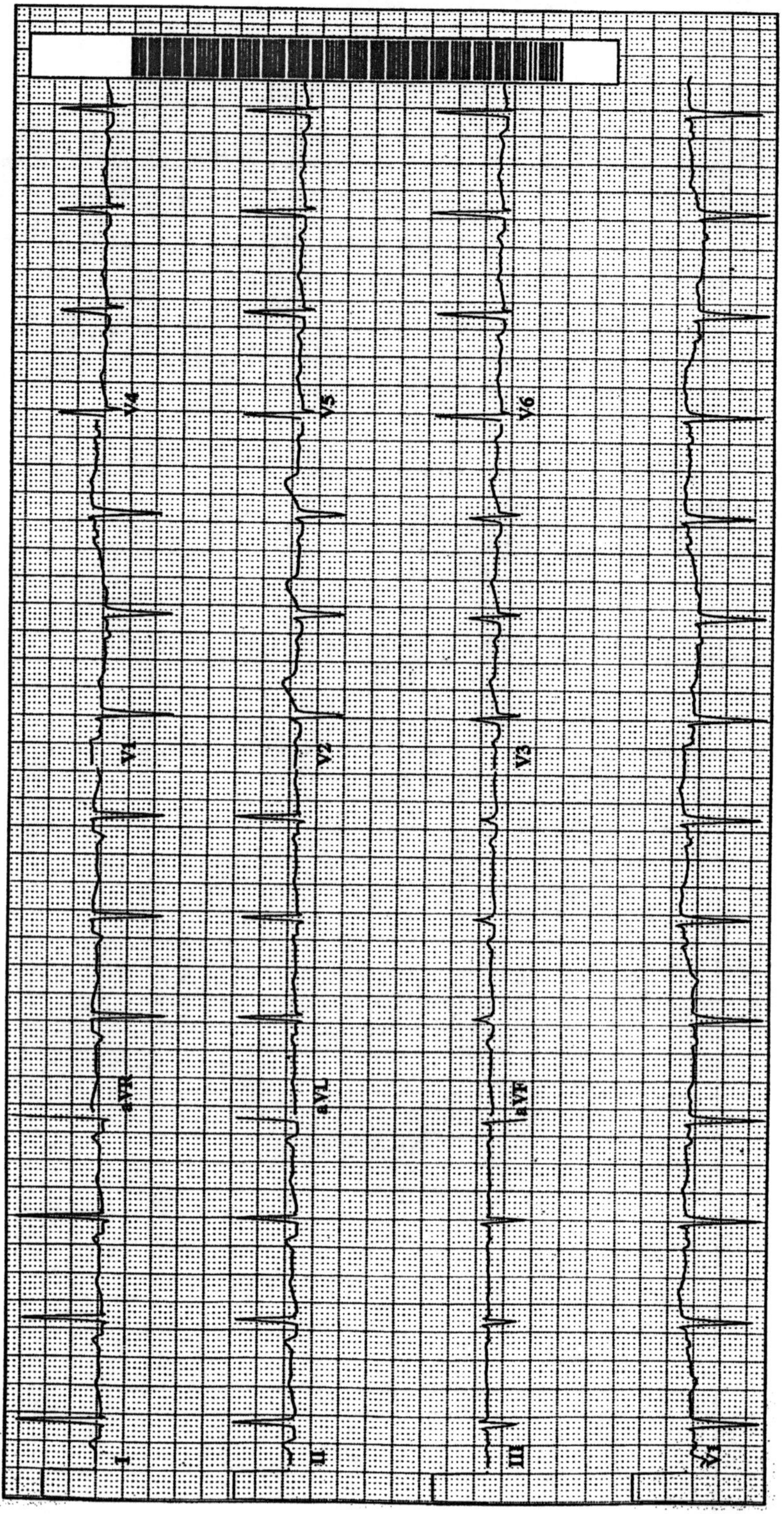

Chapter 5

QT and QTc Intervals

QT interval is the interval between the start of the Q wave (or R wave if there is no Q wave) and the end of the T wave (Fig. 1). Count the number of vertical lines between these two points, starting line being the zero line, and multiply by 0.04 to get the QT interval in seconds. This number has to be corrected for the heart rate to get QTc interval which is more meaningful, because QT interval varies with the heart rate. Divide the QT interval by the square root of the preceding R-R interval to get QTc interval. Normal QTc is 0.44 second or less. QTc interval of 0.48 second or greater is considered to be prolonged and abnormal. Calculate the QTc in all of the three bipolar limb leads, and use the largest number as the QTc interval. In the following EKG tracing (Fig. 2), the QT interval is 0.36 second, and the preceeding R – R interval is 0.72 second. The square root of 0.72 is 0.85; therefore, the QTc is 0.424 second (0.36/0.85 = 0.424).

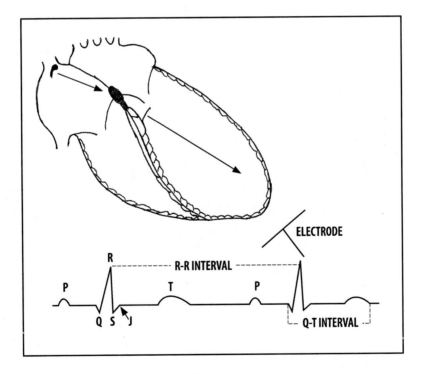

Figure 1

Figure 2

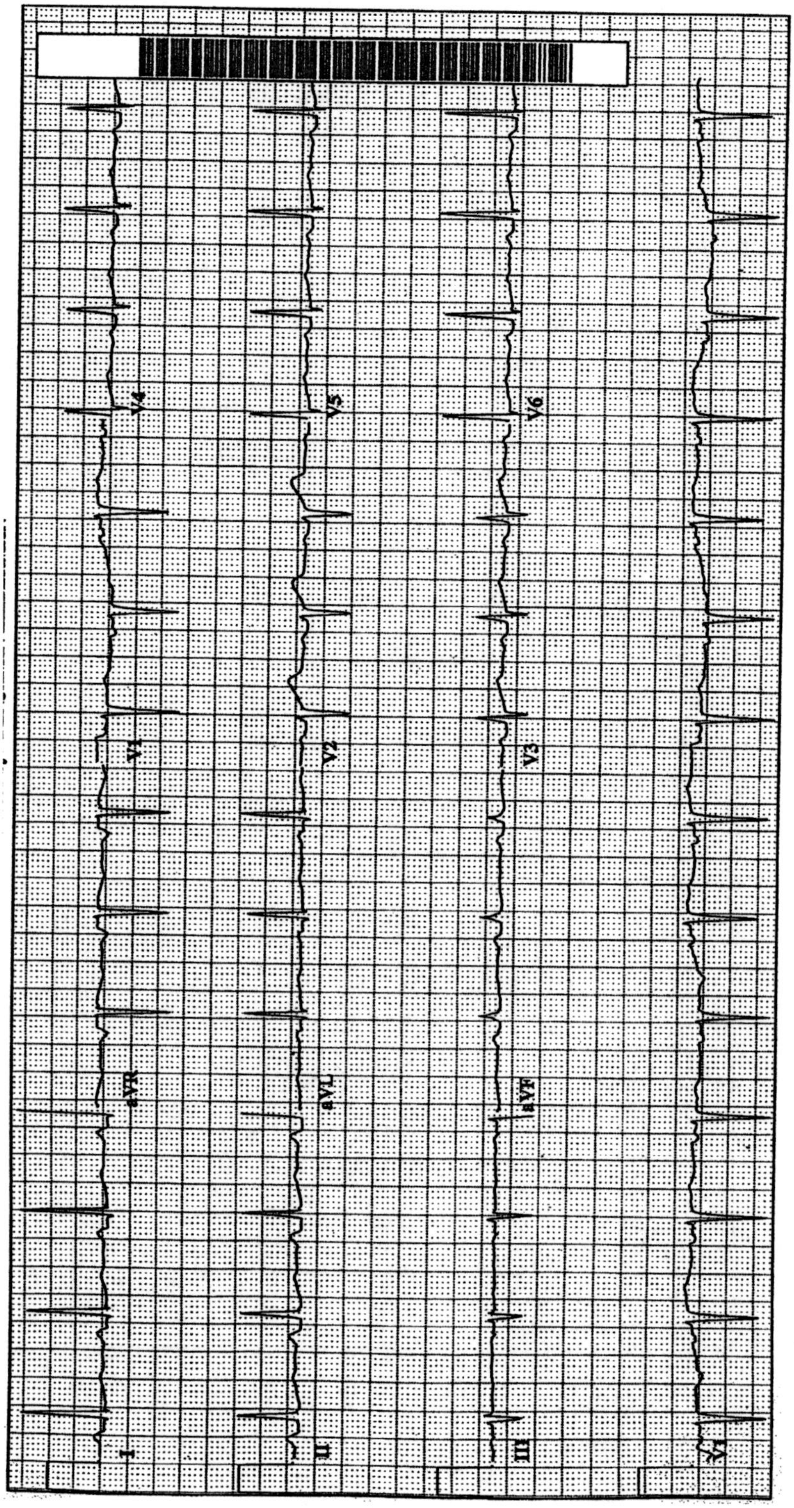

Chapter 6

How to read EKGs

Follow any sequence that you prefer, but stick with it. I recommend the following.

1. Determination of heart rate (beats/min.).

2. Regularity of R – R interval.

3. Cardiac Rhythm.

4. QRS Axis.

5. PR interval.

6. QRS interval.

7. QT / QTc intervals.

8. 12 lead scanning.

Details of PR interval, QRS interval, and QT/QTc intervals have been discussed in chapters 3, 4, and 5 respectively. Other entities mentioned above are detailed individually in the following chapters.

Chapter 7

How to determine the heart rate

There are 3 different ways to calculate the heart rate. When you record an EKG, the paper runs at a speed of 25 mm / sec. Each vertical line on this paper is 1.0 mm apart. That means the paper covers 25 vertical lines / sec. or 1500 lines / minute. If there are 50 QRS complexes recorded in one minute, each complex would be 30 lines apart (1500/50 = 30). This means that if you divide 1500 by the number of lines between 2 consecutive QRS complexes , you will get the heart rate / minute, which in this case would be 1500 / 30 = 50. Since every 5th line on the EKG paper is a thick line, there would be 300 thick lines covered in one minute. Thus if two consecutive QRS complexes are 2 thick lines apart, the heart rate would be 300 / 2 = 150. Keeping this explanation in mind, the following different methods are described.

1. 1500 divided by the number of vertical lines between 2 consecutive QRS complexes excluding the line on which the first QRS complex falls, as it is counted as zero line.

2. 300 divided by the number of thick lines between 2 consecutive QRS complexes excluding the first thick line on which the first QRS complex falls, as it is counted as zero line. Thus if a QRS complex falls on a thick line and the next QRS complex falls on the very next thick line, the heart rate is 300 (300 / 1 = 300). Therefore, the heart rate can be 300, 150, 100, 75, and 60 and so on depending upon the number of thick lines between 2 consecutive QRS complexes. However, this method requires the QRS complexes to fall on the thick lines only, which usually does not happen. Still one can make an approximate guess.

3. Every EKG tracing usually includes a rhythm strip which is recorded over a period of 10 seconds. Counting the total number of QRS – T complexes within the 10 second period and then multiplying this number by 6 will give the heart rate / minute. This method is particularly useful when the heart rate is irregular. Rhythm strip at the bottom of the EKG tracing in Fig.1, starts with a 10 mm standardization deflection on the left. The line on which this deflection ends is a thick line (see arrow). Count this line as zero line. Each successive thick line is 0.2 second apart, as the paper runs at a speed of 25 mm/second. Fifty such lines following the zero line will cover 10 seconds. Note that the start of the bar code on the right side (see arrow) marks the end of 10 second period. Therefore, the number of QRS – T complexes within this period, between standardization deflection on the left and the start of the bar code on the right, is to be multiplied by the number 6 to get

heart rate per minute. In the EKG tracing in Figure 1, there are 9 QRS – T complexes within 10 second period. Therefore, the heart rate is 9 x 6 = 54/min.

Note:

Normal heart rate is 60 – 100 beats per minute. A heart rate below 60/min. is bradycardia, and above 100/min. is tachycardia.

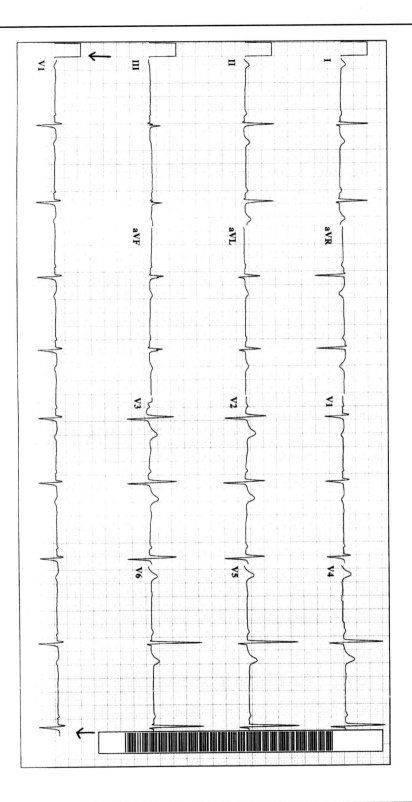

Figure 1

Chapter 8

Regularity of R – R interval

It is important to determine whether the QRS complexes are recorded at regular intervals (R – R interval), or there is a significant irregularity. Sometimes, there is occasional irregularity caused by occasional premature atrial or ventricular complexes. If that is the only irregularity, the basic rhythm in such instances should be considered as regular. Presence of a significantly irregular rhythm points toward the following clinical entities.

1. Atrial fibrillation.

2. Multiple extra systoles in salvos.

3. Changing heart block.

4. Multifocal atrial tachycardia.

5. Wandering atrial pacemaker.

6. Sinus arrhythmia (P – P interval varies).

Further details will be discussed in chapters 9 and 10.

Chapter 9

Cardiac Rhythm

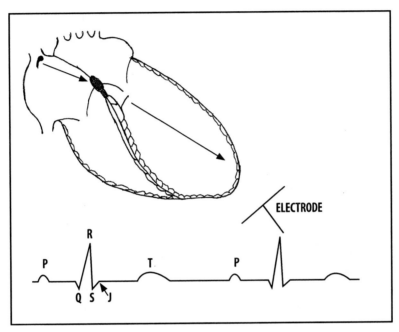

Figure 1

Understanding the fundamentals:

The electrical impulse normally originates at the sinus node and activates both the atrial and the ventricular chambers. It is therefore, called sinus rhythm. Downward conduction of the electrical impulse through the atrial muscle, the AV node, the bundle of His, and the bundle branches is called antegrade conduction. The P wave is referred to as antegrade P wave. It is obvious that the electrocardiogram is made up of three components – P wave, the segment between the P and the QRS (called the PR segment), and the QRS-T complex. P wave represents electrical impulse conduction within the atrial chambers, the PR segment represents AV node and bundle of His conduction, and the QRS complex represents infra nodal conduction within the ventricles. Now let us look at these three components of depolarization phase separately. ST segment and T wave represent ventricular repolarization phase.

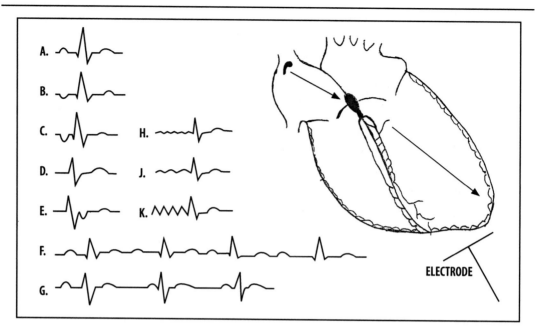

Figure 2

Figure 2.A. shows an EKG tracing with sinus rhythm. Even though, the electrical impulse normally starts at the sinus node, it can originate at any site within the atrial muscle, the AV node, the infra nodal conduction tissue, or the ventricular muscle. Let us now consider a person, in whom the electrical impulse originates at the AV node. The bundle of His is considered to be a part of the AV node. The impulse may originate at the upper end of the AV node, at the mid portion of the AV node, or at the lower end of the bundle of His. When the impulse originates at the upper end of the AV node, it spreads upward to activate the atrial muscle (called retrograde conduction) and an inverted P wave is recorded in inferior leads, as the electrical impulse is moving away from the recording electrode. This is called a retrograde P wave (Fig. 2.C). During the time that the impulse travels upward from the upper end of the AV node, it simultaneously travels downward through the AV node. As the impulse travels in two opposite directions at the same time, there is an overlap and some of the downward conduction through the AV node occurs while the P wave is being inscribed, resulting in shortening of thedistance which the electrical impulse has to travel after the P wave inscription, to reach the lower end of the bundle of His. This leads to shortening of the PR segment that follows the P wave and hence, a short PR interval (distance between start of the P wave and end of the PR segment). Thus an upper nodal rhythm is characterized by an inverted P wave in inferior leads (leads II, III, and AVF) and a short PR interval. When the electrical impulse originates at the mid portion of the AV node, the simultaneous downward and upward spread through the AV node results in inscription of a straight line. Then, as the impulse spreads down the right and the left bundle branches to depolarize the ventricular muscle, it simultaneously spreads upward into the atrial muscle and the

P wave is therefore lost into the QRS complex. Therefore, the EKG tracing shows a row of QRS complexes at regular intervals without any P waves (Fig.2.D).When the impulse originates at the lower end of the bundle of His, it quickly spreads downward to activate the ventricular muscle and the QRS complex is inscribed (Fig.2.E). As this happens, the impulse simultaneously travels upward to reach the upper end of the AV node and then travels upward into the atrial muscle, so that an inverted P wave is inscribed immediately following the QRS complex in the inferior leads (Fig. 2.E). To summarize, an upper nodal rhythm is characterized by an inverted P wave with a short PR interval in the inferior leads; a mid nodal rhythm is characterized by a row of QRS complexes at regular intervals without P waves; and a low nodal rhythm is characterized by a row of QRS complexes with inverted P waves which follow the QRS complexes and therefore located between the end of the QRS complex and the start of the ST segment as shown in Fig. 2.E. Since, the electrical impulse from the AV node activates both the atria and the ventricles, it is referred to as nodal rhythm or junctional rhythm.

Now, let us consider a person in whom the electrical impulse originates from the atrial muscle ,close to the coronary sinus (which lies within the right atrium, close to the AV node), and spreads upward in retrograde manner to activate the atria, and also spreads downward through the AV node, in an antegrade manner, to activate the ventricles. It is called an ectopic atrial rhythm or coronary sinus rhythm. Since the impulse spreads upward to activate the atria in retrograde manner, an inverted P wave (retrograde P) is inscribed in inferior leads (Fig.2.B). During the time the impulse spreads upward, it simultaneously spreads toward the AV node, but the overlap is negligible due to delayed conduction in the AV node. Therefore, the AV conduction time is not affected. Hence, the PR interval remains normal, which is then followed by QRS complex. So, in ectopic atrial rhythm, there will be an inverted P wave in the inferior leads, with normal PR interval and a normal QRS complex (as opposed to upper nodal rhythm, where an inverted P wave is associated with a short PR interval).

The sinus node normally discharges impulses at the rate of 60 – 100 per minute, and it is referred to as normal sinus rhythm. A rate of less than 60/min. is called sinus bradycardia, and above 100 is called sinus tachycardia. Ectopic atrial rhythm above 100/min. is referred to as ectopic atrial tachycardia. AV node discharge rate does not exceed 115/minute. So an inverted P wave before QRS with atrial rate of greater than 115/min. is always an ectopic atrial tachycardia regardless of PR interval (normally PR shortens as the heart rate increases). Similarly, a mid nodal tachycardia above 115/min. is called SVT (supraventricular tachycardia) or AVNRT (AV nodal re-entrant tachycardia). A low nodal tachycardia above 115/min. is referred to as AVRT (AV re-entrant tachycardia).

The electrical impulse can originate at any site within the atrial muscle and may even originate from different sites within the atrial chambers, from one heart beat to the next. When the impulse originates from different foci within the atrial muscle from one heart beat to the next, it is called wandering atrial pacemaker rhythm if the heart rate is normal or slow, and multifocal atrial tachycardia if the heart rate is fast. The shape of the P wave would vary in this situation during different heart beats.

The rate of discharge of the electrical impulse within the atrial muscle may sometimes be so fast that it may lead to contractions of the atrial chambers at a rate of 250 – 350/min. It will give rise to a sawtooth appearance of atrial activation on the EKG tracing, instead of discrete looking P waves. This appearance is called atrial flutter (Fig.2.K). Sometimes the rate of electrical impulse discharge is more than 350/min., and various impulses may be discharged from different foci simultaneously within the atrial muscle. This may lead to chaos, and result in atrial fibrillation. Atrial chambers do not contract in atrial fibrillation, and thus do not empty completely during ventricular diastole. This activity appears on the EKG tracing as a fine (Fig. 2.H) or coarse (Fig. 2.J) serpentine movement, referred to as atrial fibrillation. The morphology of serpentine atrial waves keeps changing due to the chaotic origin of the impulses.

Before reading any further, I would suggest that you pause and familiarize yourself with the morphology of different types of P waves on a real EKG tracing, as well as the appearance of atrial flutter waves and atrial fibrillation. It is a good practice to first look at lead AVF for this purpose, as it is a unipolar lead, and thus a pure inferior lead. Inferior leads (II, III, AVF) differentiate between antegrade and retrograde P waves. An upright P in lead AVF is an antegrade P (impulse coming down from sinus node), whereas an inverted P in lead AVF is a retrograde P (impulse going upwards from AV node or from coronary sinus). Look at figures 4, 5,6,12, 13 and 14 in this chapter for various types of atrial wave morphology in lead AVF. If the morphology is not discrete in lead AVF, it helps to look at the long rhythm strip (lead V1) below the lead AVF, and then trace the P waves up into the lead AVF to find their location and appearance. Figures 4 and 5 show upright P waves in lead AVF suggesting sinus origin to activate the atria (Sinus rhythm). Figure 6 shows inverted P waves in lead AVF suggesting nodal origin of the P wave (nodal rhythm, also called junctional rhythm) or its origin from atrial muscle close to the AV node (coronary sinus rhythm, also called ectopic atrial rhythm). PR interval is short in nodal rhythm, but normal in ectopic atrial rhythm. Figure 12 shows atrial fibrillation – fine serpentine movement in lead AVF and in the rhythm strip. Figure 13 shows coarse atrial fibrillation – coarse serpentine movement in lead AVF and in the rhythm strip. Note the changing morphology of atrial waves in the rhythm strip. Figure 14 shows atrial flutter (sawtooth appearance in lead AVF and in the rhythm strip). Actually, all inferior leads (II, III, AVF) show sawtooth appearance. It is a good practice to look at both, the lead AVF and lead V1 (rhythm strip), because lead V1 is located directly over the right atrium and therefore, gives the clearest view of the shape of the atrial waves, whereas, lead AVF distinguishes between antegrade and retrograde P waves due to its orientation in the frontal plane.

When the electrical impulse activating the ventricles originates at or above the AV node, the rhythm is called supraventricular rhythm. Sinus rhythm, nodal rhythm, ectopic atrial rhythm, atrial flutter, atrial fibrillation, and other rhythms resulting from an electrical impulse originating from the atrial muscle and activating the ventricles – after conduction through the AV node – are broadly classified as supraventricular rhythms. When the ventricles are activated by an impulse originating from a focus within the ventricle, it is classified as ventricular rhythm.

So far, we have discussed variations in the site of origin of the P waves. Now let us consider some of the possible variations in conduction through the AV node. Normally, there is antegrade AV conduction from upper end of the AV node to the lower end of the bundle of His, and the conduction time remains constant from one beat to the next. Thus, the PR interval (time from sinus node to the lower end of bundle of His) also remains constant (0.2 second or less). Sometimes, PR interval is prolonged (greater than 0.2 second), but remains constant from beat to beat. It is referred to as first degree AV block. Sometimes, the time to travel through the AV node may keep changing from beat to beat. The PR interval, in this situation, will also change from beat to beat, resulting in varying PR intervals, but each P will be followed by QRS, because each sinus impulse gets conducted. This condition is called varying AV block. Due to varying PR interval, the R-R interval will also vary and thus become irregular (see Fig. 2.F).

In some individuals, the electrical impulse originates at the sinus node, spreads downward in antegrade manner to the AV node, where it gets blocked, and cannot travel any further. If it is only an occasional impulse which gets blocked, it is called second degree AV block. But if all such impulses are blocked, it is called complete AV block (Fig.2.G). Atrial contractions will occur in a patient with a complete AV block, and P waves will be inscribed on the EKG. But, there has to be another focus, which would discharge electrical impulses to activate the ventricles. Such a focus may lie in the AV node below the site of the block, or in the ventricular muscle. If the focus lies in the AV node, the impulse generated from this focus will travel down the normal infra nodal conduction pathway to activate the ventricles. This will be called sinus rhythm with complete AV block and nodal escape rhythm. Due to two foci, one activating the atria and the other activating the ventricles, the atria will beat at their own rate, and the ventricles will beat at their own rate, quite independent of each other. Thus, there will be no relationship between P waves and the QRS complexes, and therefore, the PR will not remain constant. It will vary from beat to beat just like in varying AV block. The shape of the P wave in inferior lead will be upright, and the QRS complexes will remain normal in duration due to normal conduction below the AV node. The findings will remain the same if the second focus were to be within the ventricular muscle instead of the AV node, except that the QRS duration will increase due to relatively slower intramyocadial conduction, resulting in wide QRS complexes (greater than 0.1 sec.). R-R interval is usually regular in complete AV block, as atria and ventricles are activated independently from two different foci; each beating at its own rate. This is in sharp contrast to the varying AV block (see Figs.2.F and 8A), where R-R interval always remains irregular. This is an important point to differentiate between these two conditions. Exceptions to this rule are rare, but do exist, such as in case of sinus rhythm with complete AV block and nodal arrhythmia where the second focus does not discharge impulses at regular intervals. In case of varying AV block, each P wave is conducted through the AV node, although with varying PR interval. Therefore, each P must be followed by a QRS and each QRS must be preceded by a P Wave in varying AV block (see Fig. 8A). If that is not the case, i.e. each P wave is not followed by a QRS complex or each QRS complex is not preceded by a P wave, it is not a varying AV block but a complete AV block with second focus (activating the ventricles) not discharging impulses at regular intervals (see Fig. 8B). This would help differentiate between these two conditions, when R–R intervals are irregular. Please see Fig. 8B in this chapter and read the note underneath the EKG tracing to get a better understanding. Another posssibility to be considered is Mobitz 1 AV block. A detailed description of heart blocks will follow in the next chapter. Normal AV conduction, varying AV block, and how to differentiate varying AV block from complete AV block have been discussed above in this chapter.

The conclusions from above discussion are as follows:

• Shape of the P wave in lead AVF helps differentiate between antegrade and retrograde P wave.

• A constant PR indicates antegrade AV node conduction. Normally PR is constant.

• A varying PR indicates:

> Varying AV block (R-R is irregular; each P is followed by a
> QRS, and each QRS is preceded by a P wave).

> OR

> Complete AV block (R-R is usually regular).

At this time, let me explain the meaning of aberrant conduction before we discuss the third component of the electrocardiogram, the QRS complex.

Aberrant Conduction:

This terminology refers to the conduction of the electrical impulse below the AV node. The conduction is normally very fast, because the conduction tissue is a specialized myocardial tissue with this special property. It is for this reason, that the normal QRS complexes are narrow in duration (0.1 sec. or less), as compared to the QRS complexes which result from the conduction of the impulse through the ventricular muscle, which is relatively slower, resulting in wide QRS complexes (0.11 sec. or greater in duration). If there is blockage in the right or the left bundle branch (resulting in detour of the conduction), or the conduction through the Purkinje fibers is delayed, it is referred to as aberrant conduction of the impulse originating from a supraventricular focus. When the impulse gets blocked at the right bundle branch, the impulse travelling along the left bundle branch pierces through the interventricular septum from the left side and activates the right ventricle in addition to activating the left ventricle. This results in a wide QRS complex. Same would happen when there is blockage in the left bundle branch, except that in this situation, the impulse travelling along the right bundle branch will enter the interventricular septum and activate the left ventricle in addition to activating the right ventricle. If the conduction through Purkinje fibers is slower than normal, QRS duration will increase, resulting in wide QRS complexes. This abnormal conduction due to right bundle branch block (RBBB) or left bundle branch block (LBBB), or a slower conduction through Purkinje fibers resulting in wide QRS complexes is called aberrant conduction of the impulse originating from a supraventricular focus, and the rhythm is referred to as a supraventricular rhythm with aberrant conduction or simply supraventricular rhythm with aberrancy.

Now, let us turn to the third component of the impulse conduction, the Infra nodal conduction. The QRS complex is inscribed during the time when electrical impulse is travelling below the lower end of the AV node, along the right and the left bundle branches and Purkinje fibers. This conduction normally takes up to 0.1 second. Therefore, normal QRS interval is 0.1 sec. or less, and the normal QRS complex is referred to as a narrow QRS complex. A narrow QRS complex, therefore, suggests a normal infranodal conduction of the impulse from a supra-ventricular focus, called the supraventricular rhythm. A wide QRS (>0.1 sec.) is seen when there is aberrant conduction of a supraventricular impulse or when it is a ventricular rhythm. Thus a wide QRS indicates a supraventriculr rhythm with aberrant conduction (also referred to as supraventricular rhythm with aberrancy), or a ventricular rhythm (which is associated with complete AV block or AV dissociation).

Conclusion:

• Narrow QRS complexes indicate a supraventricular rhythm with normal infra-nodal conduction.

• Wide QRS complexes indicate a supraventricular rhythm with aberrancy, or a ventricular rhythm associated with complete AV block or AV dissociation.

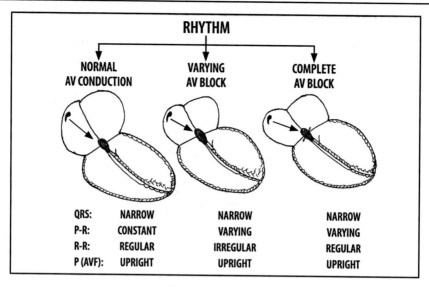

Figure 3A

Approach to the diagnosis of cardiac rhythm:

The above illustration (Fig. 3A) shows hearts of three members of a family. Sinus node activates the atria in all the three hearts. The heart on the left has normal AV node conduction. The heart in the middle has varying AV node conduction time from beat to beat, called varying AV block. The heart on the right has complete AV block with second focus in the AV node below the block which activates the ventricles. Infra nodal conduction is normal in all the three hearts. EKG findings in each case are listed below each heart. You will note that QRS complex is narrow in all the three cases due to normal infra nodal conduction. PR interval is constant in the heart on the left due to normal antegrade AV conduction, but there is varying PR in other two hearts because of varying AV block in the heart in the middle and complete AV block in the heart on the right with atria and the ventricles beating independent of each other in response to stimuli from two different foci (causing loss of relationship between P and QRS). Among these two hearts, the one in the middle with varying AV block has irregular R – R interval due to changing AV conduction time from beat to beat, and each P wave should be followed by a QRS complex and each QRS complex must be preceded by a P wave with PR segment, whereas the heart on the right with complete AV block has regular R – R interval as the ventricles beat at a regular rate in response to stimuli from AV node at regular intervals. Thus, by looking at the PR (constant or varying) and the R–R (regular or irregular), we can differentiate between all the three hearts.

The illustration below (Fig. 3B) shows hearts of three members of another family. Like the previous family, sinus node activates the atria in all the three hearts. Also like the previous family, the heart on the left has normal AV conduction, the heart in the middle has varying AV block, and the heart on the right has complete AV block. However, unlike the previous family, this family has abnormal infra nodal conduction due to RBBB in the heart on the left and the heart in the middle, resulting in aberrant infra nodal conduction; the heart on the right with complete AV block has second focus in the left ventricle activating the ventricles, thus causing abnormal infra nodal conduction. EKG findings are listed below each heart. You will note that the only difference in findings between the two families is the QRS morphology. Previous family reveals narrow QRS complexes in all the three hearts, whereas the family below shows wide QRS complexes in the heart of all its members. Again, by looking at the PR (constant or varying) and the R – R (regular or irregular), we can differentiate between all the three hearts of the family below. Thus, by looking at QRS complexes (narrow or wide), we can separate the two families, and then by looking at PR (constant or varying) and the R – R (regular or irregular), we can separate all the six individuals. The shape of the P wave in lead AVF in each case will tell us about origin of atrial activation.

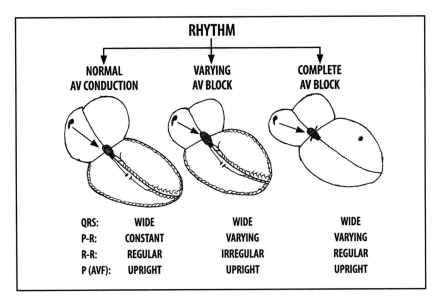

Figure 3B

We can conclude from the above observation, that the following four steps are necessary to determine the cardiac rhythm in a given EKG tracing in addition to the heart rate.

1. The shape of the QRS complexes: Narrow (up to 0.1 sec.) or wide (greater than 0.1 sec.).

2. The rate and the shape of the P waves in inferior leads (lead AVF is preferred, as it is unipolar and thus, pure inferior lead) and lead V1: The rate will indicate the atrial rate. Atrial and ventricular rates are usually the same, but they may be different, e.g. in complete AV block.

3. PR interval: Constant or varying.

4. R – R interval: Regular or irregular.

Above discussion also teaches us the following:

1. Narrow QRS complexes indicate a supraventricular rhythm with normal infranodal conduction. Wide QRS complexes indicate a supraventricular rhythm with aberrancy or a ventricular rhythm associated with complete AV block or AV dissociation.

2. When the rhythm is supraventricular with narrow QRS complexes, the shape of the P wave in lead AVF and V1 will indicate the site of origin of the impulse activating the atria; a constant PR will indicate antegrade AV node conduction; a varying PR interval will indicate either varying AV block, or complete AV block with nodal rhythm. Regular R – R interval will indicate complete AV block with nodal rhythm, whereas irregular R – R interval will suggest varying AV block. In case of varying AV block, each P must be followed by QRS, and each QRS must be preceded by a P wave with PR segment, otherwise, it is a complete AV block with nodal rhythm or Mobitz I AV block – as described on page 109.

3. When QRS complexes are wide, the rhythm is supraventricular with aberrancy or ventricular. The shape of the P wave in lead AVF and V1 will indicate the site of origin of the impulse activating the atria; a constant PR will indicate antegrade AV node conduction with aberrancy; a varying PR will indicate either varying AV block with aberrancy, or a complete AV block with ventricular rhythm. Regular R – R interval will indicate complete AV block with ventricular rhythm, whereas irregular R – R will suggest varying AV block with aberrant conduction. To qualify for the diagnosis of varying AV block with aberrant conduction, each P must be followed by QRS, and each QRS must be preceded by a P wave with PR segment, otherwise, it is a complete AV block with ventricular rhythm or Mobitz I AV block with aberrancy.

In summary, we first look at QRS complexes (narrow or wide) to see what is happening in the infra nodal area (the ventricles), then at the rate and shape of P wave in lead AVF and V1 to determine the atrial rhythm, and then at P R (constant or varying) and R – R (regular or irregular) in the rhythm strip to evaluate AV node conduction. Rhythm strip is preferred due to the presence of multiple QRS complexes. Once we know what is happening in the ventricles, the atria, and the AV node, we can reach the diagnosis of cardiac rhythm. The following chart highlights this approach.

Rhythm

– Heart Rate
– Regularity (R–R)
+
1. Shape of the QRS complexes:
Narrow vs. Wide (>0.1 sec)
2. Rate and Shape of P waves in lead AVF and V1
3. P-QRS relationship:

Constant PR – Antegrade AV conduction
(with aberrancy if wide QRS)

Varying PR – Varying AV Block: R-R is irregular; P ⇌ QRS
(with aberrancy if wide QRS) ↖ PR
OR
Complete AV Block: R-R is regular
with Nodal rhythm (narrow QRS)
OR
Ventricular rhythm (wide QRS)

Chart 1

It has been pointed out that a varying PR with regular R – R intervals indicates a complete AV block. This block is usually pathologic in nature and the ventricles are activated by a focus in the AV node or in the ventricular muscle. The ventricular rate, therefore, is slower than the atrial rate due to the inherent physiologic properties of the cardiac tissue. However, if an individual develops an accelerated nodal or ventricular rhythm in the absence of a pathologic AV block, and the ventricular rate is higher than the atrial rate, the supraventricular impulse may find the AV node refractory each time an atrial impulse arrives at the AV node, and may be blocked from further antegrade conduction. This kind of physiologic AV block resulting in independent beating of the atrial and the ventricular chambers is called AV dissociation. Thus, while the atrial rate is higher than the ventricular rate in complete AV block, reverse is true in AV dissociation. This differentiates between these two conditions when faced with an EKG tracing showing a varying PR with regular R – R intervals. Sometimes, the atrial and the ventricular rates, though different, but may be almost identical, and it may present a dilemma whether it is a complete AV block or AV dissociation (also called isorhythmic AV dissociation due to almost identical atrial and ventricular rates). Under these circumstances, it is prudent to call it "Isorhythmic AV dissociation, ? complete AV block" when ventricular rate is less than 50/minute; when it is greater than 50/minute, it is isorhythmic AV dissociation.

The following page shows an algorithm to demonstrate a schematic approach to the EKG diagnosis of a rhythm.

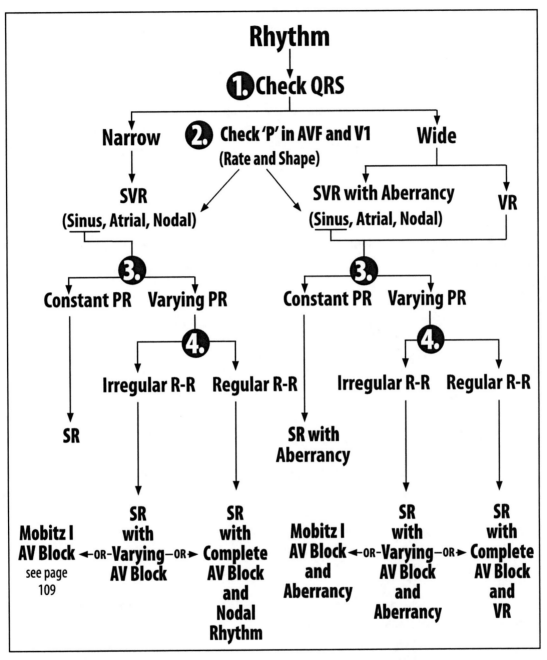

Rhythm

1. Check QRS

Narrow — 2. Check 'P' in AVF and V1 (Rate and Shape) — Wide

SVR (Sinus, Atrial, Nodal)

SVR with Aberrancy (Sinus, Atrial, Nodal) — **VR**

3. Constant PR — Varying PR

3. Constant PR — Varying PR

4. Irregular R-R — Regular R-R

4. Irregular R-R — Regular R-R

SR

SR with Aberrancy

Mobitz I AV Block see page 109 ◄–OR–**Varying**–OR► **SR with Complete AV Block and Nodal Rhythm**

SR with Varying AV Block

Mobitz I AV Block and Aberrancy ◄–OR–**Varying**–OR► **SR with Complete AV Block and VR**

SR with Varying AV Block and Aberrancy

SVR = Supraventricular Rhythm
VR = Ventricular Rhythm
Complete AV Block (? AV Dissociation)
SR = Sinus Rhythm

See page 115

Algorithm Key

1: Infra-Nodal Conduction
2: Atrial Rhythm
3 & 4: AV Node Conduction

It would be appropriate at this time to briefly revisit the aberrant conduction. Right bundle branch block (RBBB), left bundle branch block (LBBB), and intraventricular conduction delay (IVC delay) are the three causes of aberrant conduction. The RBBB is characterized by the presence of RSR-prime (written as RSR′)or rSr-prime (rSr′) in lead V1. A QRS interval of 0.09 to 0.11 second indicates incomplete RBBB; a QRS interval of 0.12 sec. or greater indicates complete RBBB. The morphology of QRS complexes in lead V1 in RBBB is referred to as that of two rabbit ears (see Fig. 9). LBBB is characterized by wide and bizarre looking QRS complexes (0.12 sec. or more in duration) in leads I and V6 (see Fig. 10); looking like a sore thumb or a tomb stone. If there is no evidence of RBBB or LBBB, the aberrancy is considered to be due to IVC delay (see Fig. 11).

Now, as we know the causes of aberrancy, it would be more appropriate to write down the EKG diagnosis in case of sinus rhythm with aberrancy as sinus rhythm with RBBB, or sinus rhythm with LBBB, or sinus rhythm with IVC delay, thus replacing the word "aberrancy" with its cause.

Aberrant Conduction
(Aberrancy)

» RBBB

» LBBB

» IVC Delay (Intraventricular Conduction Delay)

Chart 2

Atrial Fibrillation:

Electrical impulses originate from atrial muscle at a rate of more than 350/min. in atrial fibrillation, and vary in potential. Impulses of stronger potential are conducted through the AV node, whereas the weaker impulses with low potential get blocked, thus creating a varying AV block, which results in irregular R – R interval. Therefore, an irregular R – R interval is expected in atrial fibrillation. The appearance of atrial activation in EKG tracing is like a serpentine movement with varying morphology, instead of discrete P waves. The presence of wide QRS complexes with irregular R – R in atrial fibrillation, indicates atrial fibrillation with aberrancy. A regular R – R interval would indicate atrial fibrillation with complete AV block and nodal or ventricular escape rhythm. QRS complexes would be narrow in case of nodal rhythm, and wide in case of ventricular rhythm. Thus, looking at the QRS complexes (narrow vs. wide) and the shape of serpentine atrial waves with varying morphology in lead AVF and the rhythm strip, in addition to R – R being irregular, will give the diagnosis. Since, there are no P waves in atrial fibrillation, the question of looking at the PR interval (constant or varying) does not arise. Please note that the steps to follow to reach the diagnosis are similar as when P waves are present, i.e. QRS morphology (narrow vs. wide), and shape of atrial activity in leads AVF and V1. The step to check whether PR is constant is replaced by checking the regularity of R – R interval, which is irregular in atrial fibrillation.

Atrial Fibrillation

R-R Interval:

» **IRREGULAR: Expected to be irregular (with aberrancy if wide QRS)**

» **REGULAR: Complete AV Block:
with Nodal Escape Rhythm (Narrow QRS)
OR
Ventricular Escape Rhythm (Wide QRS)**

Chart 3

Atrial Flutter:

Electrical impulses in atrial flutter originate from the atrial muscle, and remain uniform in their electrical potential. Due to very fast atrial rate (250 to 350 per minute), all of the impulses cannot get conducted through the AV node, resulting in a ratio between atrial waves (flutter waves) and the ventricular waves (QRS complexes), e.g. 2:1, 3:1, 4:1 etc. Thus, one would see 2, 3 or 4 flutter waves, before each QRS complex. The appearance of flutter waves is like teeth of a saw; hence it is called a sawtooth appearance. Morphology of the QRS complexes (narrow or wide), the sawtooth shape of the flutter waves in leads AVF and V1, and regularity of R-R will give the diagnosis. Irregular R – R interval would indicate atrial flutter with varying AV block, whereas a regular R – R interval would suggest atrial flutter with 2:1, 3:1, or 4:1 AV conduction.

Flutter waves to QRS complex ratio will vary in varying AV block. Atrial flutter with complete AV block will also result in a regular R – R interval, but the interval between the flutter wave which immediately precedes the QRS complex and the following QRS complex will vary in complete AV block (atria and ventricles are activated from two different foci and beat independently of each other), whereas it will remain constant in case of fixed 2:1, 3:1, or 4:1 AV conduction. In the case of atrial flutter with complete AV block and nodal escape rhythm, the QRS complexes would be narrow, whereas in case of atrial flutter with complete AV block and ventricular escape rhythm, the QRS complexes would be wide.

The atrial rate in atrial flutter is usually 250 – 350 BPM. However, sometimes the atrial rate may be below 250 BPM. It may then present a challenge to differentiate from paroxysmal atrial tachycardia (PAT) where the atrial rate is 150 – 250 BPM. The P waves are always upright in inferior leads in PAT with a straight line between the consecutive P waves (see Figs. 16A and B), whereas P waves are inverted in these leads in atrial flutter with slow atrial rate of <250 BPM (see Fig. 16C). A slow atrial flutter has also to be differentiated from ectopic atrial tachycardia with inverted P waves in lead AVF. Saw-tooth appearance in lead V1 indicates atrial flutter, and its absence suggests atrial tachycardia (see Fig. 17B).

Atrial Flutter

R-R Interval:

» **IRREGULAR: Varying AV Block**
(with aberrancy if wide QRS)

» **REGULAR: Flutter waves: QRS ratio - fixed**
(with aberrancy if wide QRS)
OR
Complete AV block
(with Nodal or Ventricular Escape Rhythm)

Chart 4

What if there are only QRS complexes and no atrial waves?

When there are no atrial waves and the R – R is irregular, it is always atrial fibrillation. If QRS complexes are wide, it would be atrial fibrillation with aberrancy in the presence of irregular R – R interval. If the R – R interval is regular and there are no P waves, it is nodal rhythm, nodal tachycardia, or SVT (supraventricular tachycardia) – depending upon the heart rate – when QRS complexes are narrow; and it is idioventricular rhythm or wide QRS tachycardia when the QRS complexes are wide. Heart rate will be slow in idioventricular rhythm and fast in wide QRS tachycardia. Wide QRS tachycardia is always assumed to be ventricular in origin until proven otherwise. Nodal tachycardia with heart rate > 115 BPM is referred to as SVT or AVNRT (AV nodal re-entrant tachycardia).

What if only QRS complexes?
» R-R irregular:
   Atrial fibrillation
   (with aberrancy if wide QRS)
» R-R regular:
   Nodal rhythm or SVT (narrow QRS)
   Vent. Rhythm or Wide QRS tachycardia

Chart 5

Following are some examples of various cardiac rhythms. I would suggest to go through each example judiciously for a good understanding. Always remember to follow the 5 steps mentioned below, in the same sequence as they are written, when you try to find the rhythm. Consider them as 5 step by step commandments for diagnosis of a rhythm.

1. Heart rate.

2. Regularity: R – R is regular or irregular.

3. QRS: Narrow or wide.

4. P wave in lead AVF and V1: Rate and morphology.

5. PR interval: constant or varying.

Figure 4

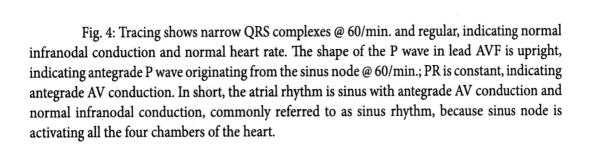

Fig. 4: Tracing shows narrow QRS complexes @ 60/min. and regular, indicating normal infranodal conduction and normal heart rate. The shape of the P wave in lead AVF is upright, indicating antegrade P wave originating from the sinus node @ 60/min.; PR is constant, indicating antegrade AV conduction. In short, the atrial rhythm is sinus with antegrade AV conduction and normal infranodal conduction, commonly referred to as sinus rhythm, because sinus node is activating all the four chambers of the heart.

Figure 5

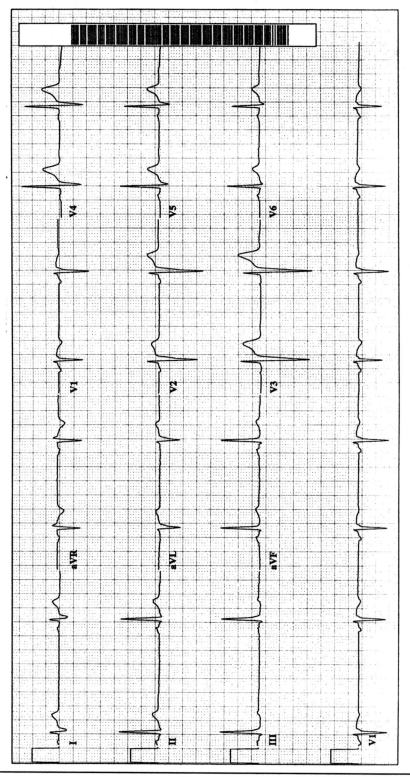

Fig. 5: Tracing shows heart rate of 48/min., indicating bradycardia. The R–R interval is irregular. QRS complexes are narrow, suggesting normal infranodal conduction. The P wave is upright in lead AVF (antegrade P) @ 48/min., indicative of sinus bradycardia activating the atrial chambers. PR is constant, suggesting antegrade AV conduction of sinus impulse. Therefore, it is sinus bradycardia with antegrade AV conduction and and normal infranodal conduction, commonly referred to as sinus bradycardia. R-R is irregular because P–P is irregular due to sinus arrhythmia (sinus node is not discharging electrical impulses at regular intervals). Therefore, the diagnosis is sinus bradycardia with sinus arrhythmia.

Figure 6

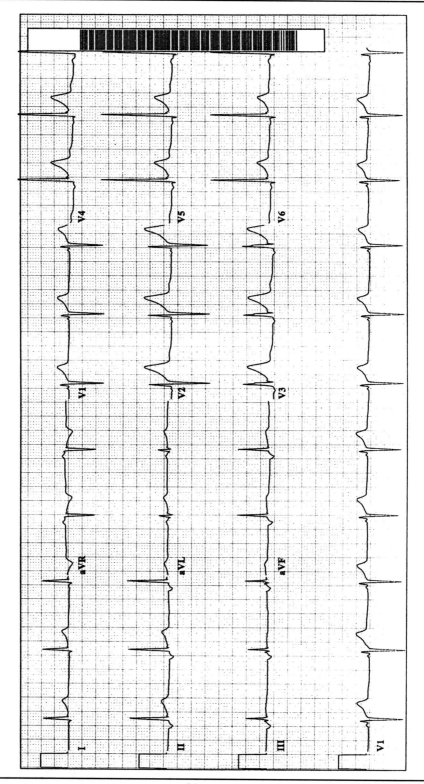

Fig. 6: Tracing shows heart rate of 63/min. and regular. QRS complexes are narrow, suggesting normal infranodal conduction. The P wave is inverted in AVF indicating a retrograde P wave activating the atria. Short PR interval is consistent with nodal origin of the P wave. PR is constant, indicating antegrade AV conduction. Hence, it is nodal rhythm with antegrade AV conduction and normal infranodal conduction, called nodal rhythm. Note: If PR interval was normal (0.12-0.2 sec.), it would indicate the origin of the impulse from the atrial muscle close to the coronary sinus and the rhythm would have been called coronary sinus rhythm or ectopic atrial rhythm instead of nodal rhythm.

Figure 7

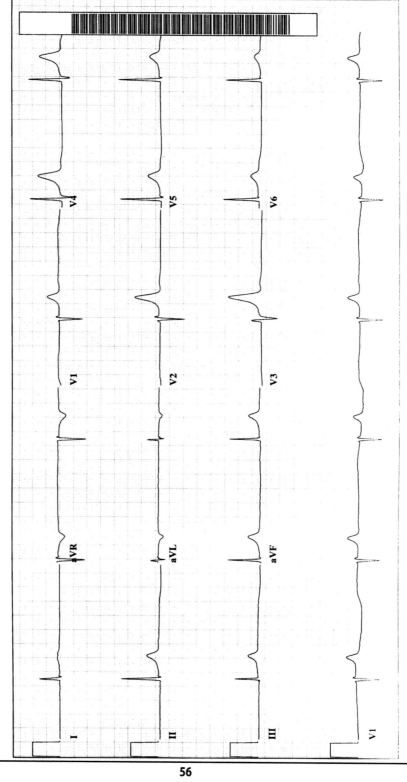

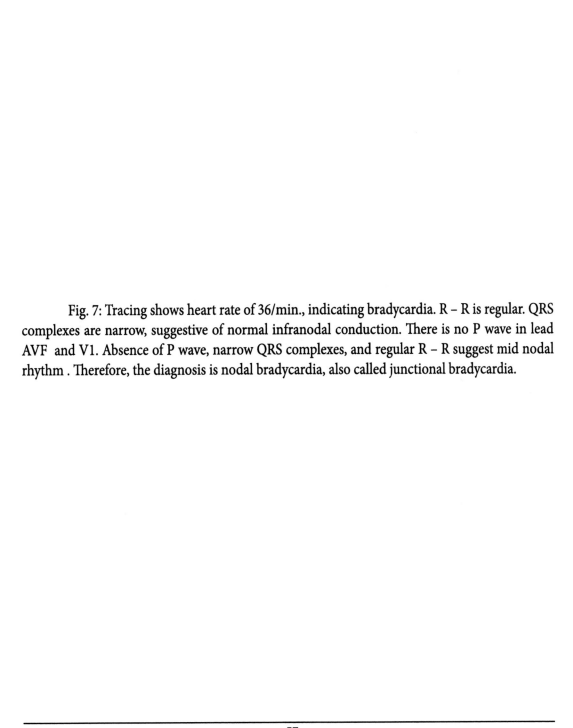

Fig. 7: Tracing shows heart rate of 36/min., indicating bradycardia. R – R is regular. QRS complexes are narrow, suggestive of normal infranodal conduction. There is no P wave in lead AVF and V1. Absence of P wave, narrow QRS complexes, and regular R – R suggest mid nodal rhythm . Therefore, the diagnosis is nodal bradycardia, also called junctional bradycardia.

Figure 8A

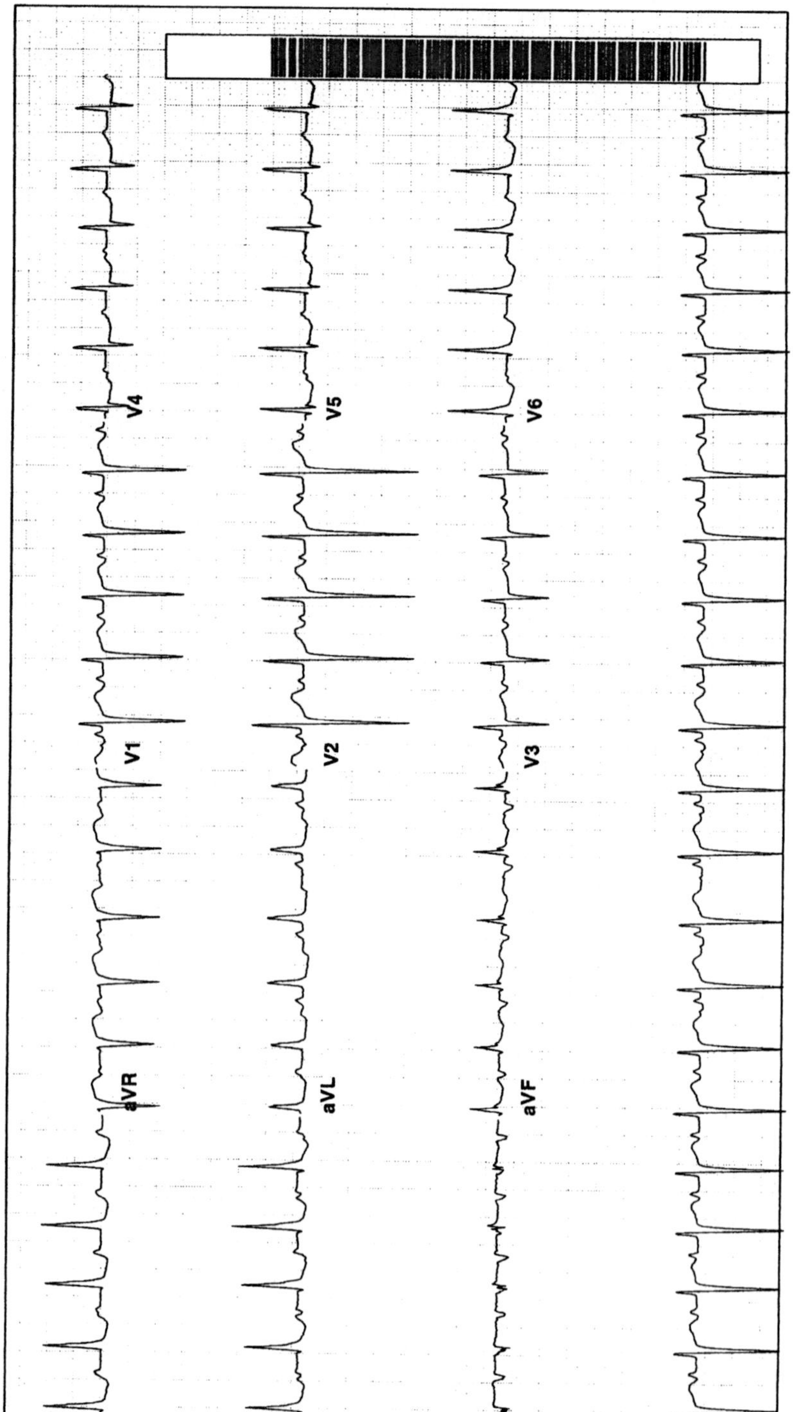

Fig. 8A: The tracing shows heart rate of 132/min. and irregular. QRS complexes are narrow, suggesting normal infranodal conduction. The P wave in lead AVF is inverted (retrograde P), and the atrial rate is 132/minute; findings consistent with ectopic atrial tachycardia. Thus the atrial rhythm is ectopic atrial tachycardia. PR interval is varying and   R – R interval is irregular. The diagnosis is ectopic atrial tachycardia with varying AV block. Please note that each P wave is followed by a QRS complex, and each QRS complex is preceded by a P wave with PR segment (a requirement for the diagnosis of varying AV block). Also, please read page 212 to differentiate from nodal (junctional) tachycardia.

Figure 8B

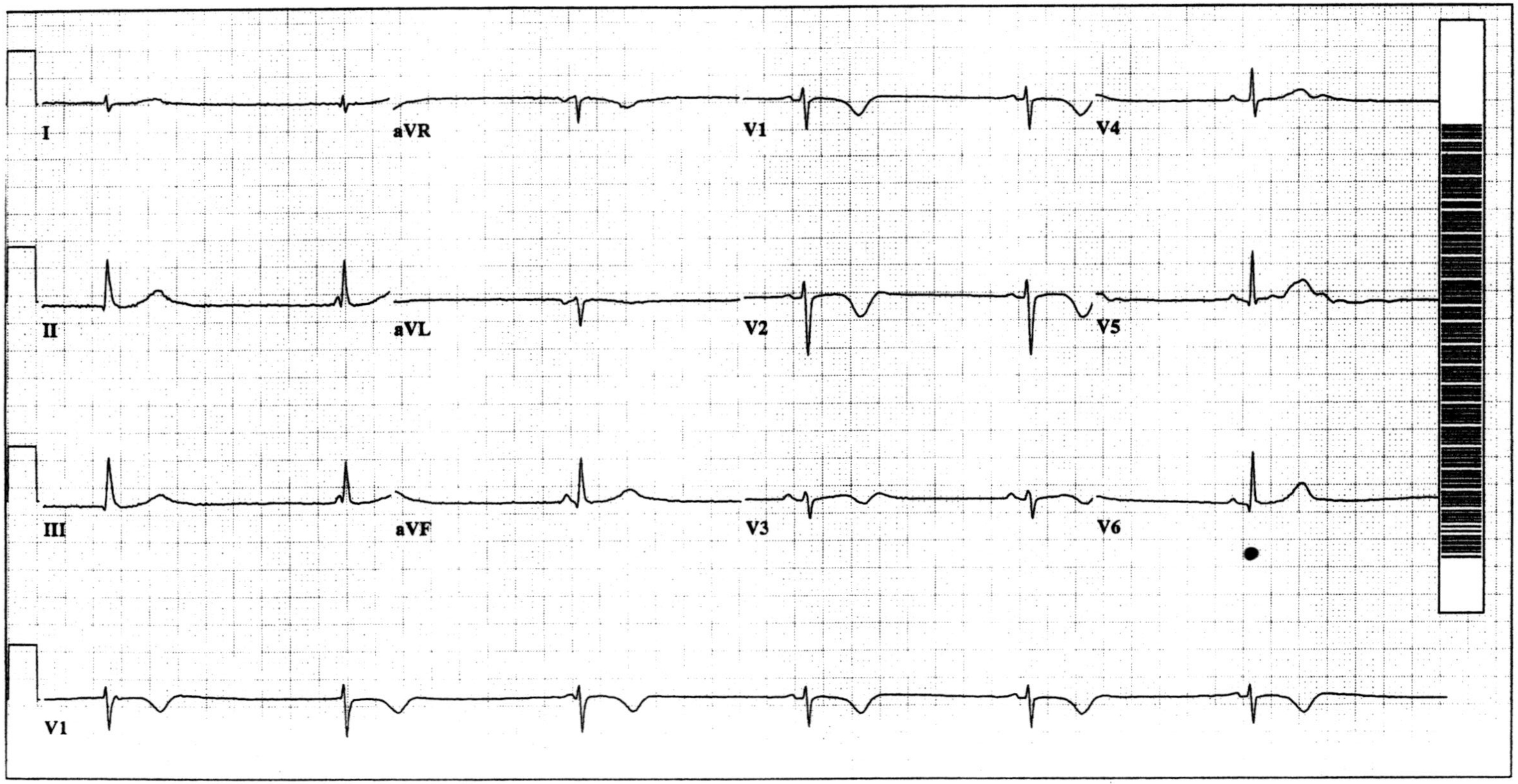

Fig. 8B: Tracing shows heart rate of 36/min., indicating bradycardia. R-R is irregular. QRS complexes are narrow, suggestive of normal infranodal conduction. P wave is upright in lead AVF @ 39/min., indicating sinus bradycardia activating the atrial chambers. PR is varying, indicating varying AV block or complete AV block. Since, R-R is irregular, it favors the diagnosis of varying AV block. However, even though each P wave is followed by a QRS complex, the first and the second QRS complexes in the rhythm strip from the left side are not preceded by a P wave. Hence, it is not a varying AV block. It is therefore, a complete AV block (isorhythmic AV dissociation as atrial and ventricular rates are almost identical). AV node is not firing the impulse at regular intervals, making the R-R intervals irregular. The diagnosis in this case would be sinus bradycardia with isorhythmic AV dissociation, and nodal arrhythmia. If the R – R were to be regular in this case, the diagnosis would have been sinus bradycardia with isorhythmic AV dissociation, and nodal rhythm. Since, the ventricular rate is less than 50/minute, the correct diagnosis in this case is sinus bradycardia with isorhythmic AV dissociation, ?complete AV block, and nodal arrhythmia. Please see pages 44 and 115 for the description of AV dissociation.

Note:

Since, there is only one P wave in lead AVF, the atrial rate was obtained from the rhythm strip at the bottom (1500/39 = 39).

Figure 9

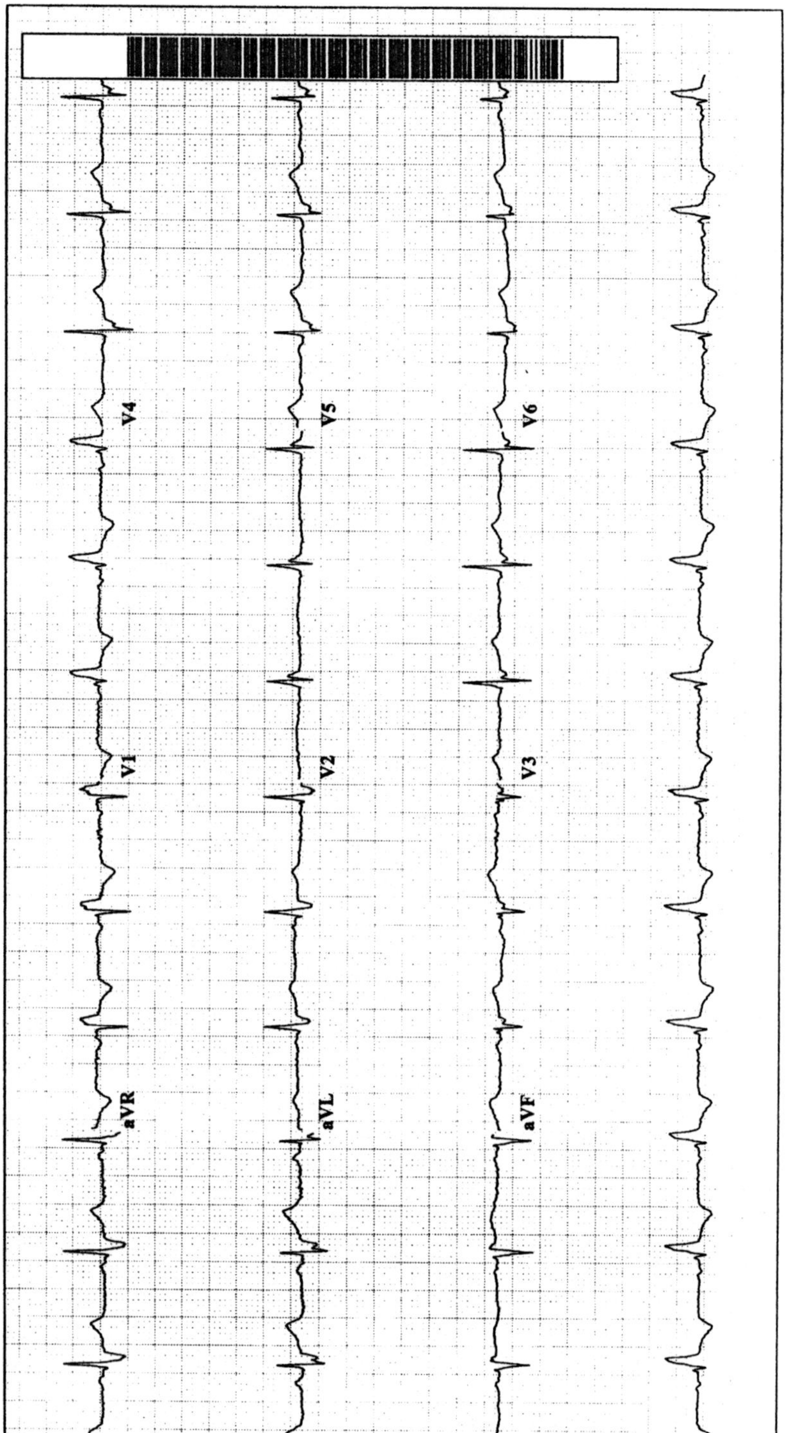

Fig. 9: Tracing shows heart rate of 72/min. and regular. QRS complexes are wide, indicating aberrant infranodal conduction or a ventricular rhythm. P waves are upright in lead AVF suggesting sinus rhythm activating atrial chambers; PR is constant, indicating antegrade AV conduction. Therefore, it is antegrade AV conduction with aberrancy, and not a ventricular rhythm (PR varies in ventricular rhythm as atria and ventricles beat independent of each other). These findings suggest sinus rhythm with aberrancy. The morphology of QRS in lead V1 is consistent with RBBB which explains the cause of aberrant conduction. Therefore, the diagnosis is sinus rhythm with RBBB.

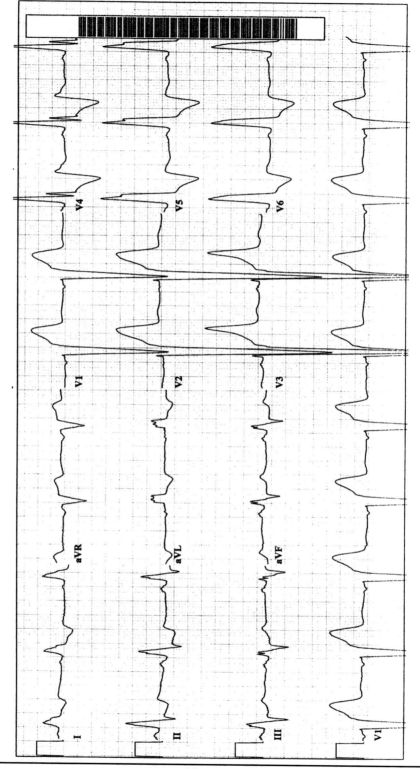

Figure 10

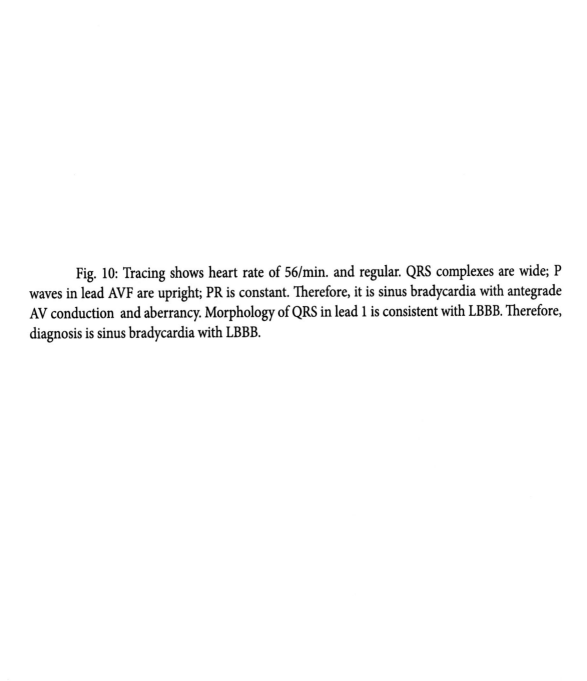

Fig. 10: Tracing shows heart rate of 56/min. and regular. QRS complexes are wide; P waves in lead AVF are upright; PR is constant. Therefore, it is sinus bradycardia with antegrade AV conduction and aberrancy. Morphology of QRS in lead 1 is consistent with LBBB. Therefore, diagnosis is sinus bradycardia with LBBB.

Figure 11

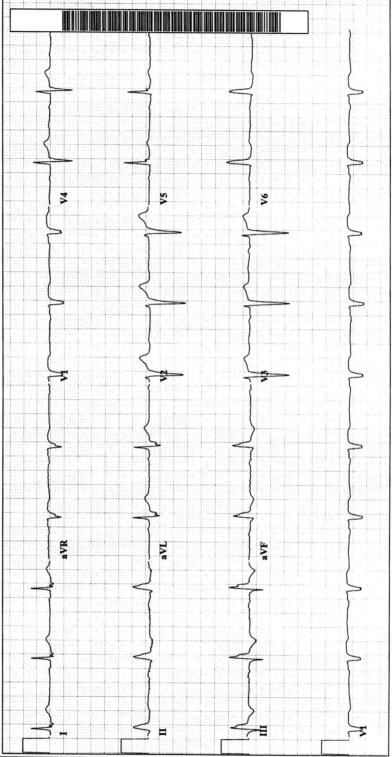

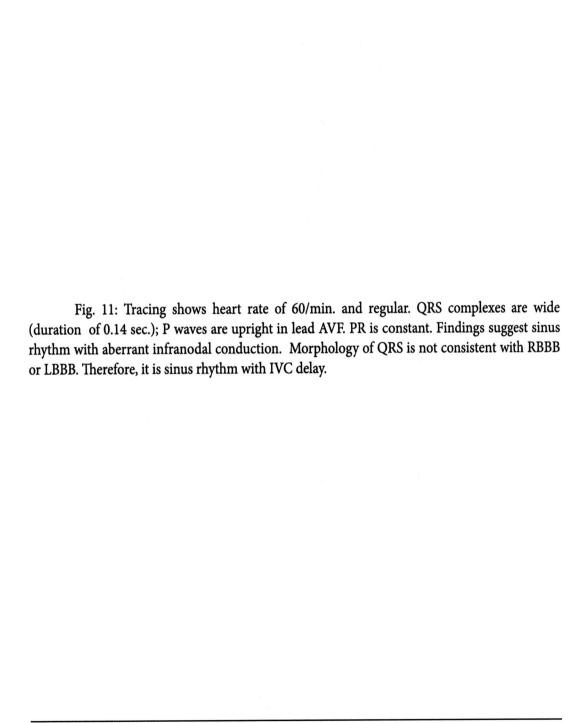

Fig. 11: Tracing shows heart rate of 60/min. and regular. QRS complexes are wide (duration of 0.14 sec.); P waves are upright in lead AVF. PR is constant. Findings suggest sinus rhythm with aberrant infranodal conduction. Morphology of QRS is not consistent with RBBB or LBBB. Therefore, it is sinus rhythm with IVC delay.

Figure 12

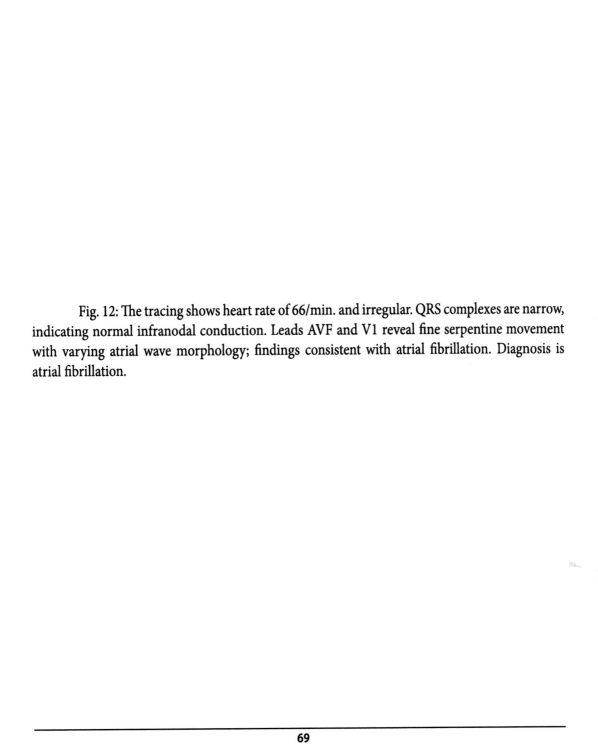

Fig. 12: The tracing shows heart rate of 66/min. and irregular. QRS complexes are narrow, indicating normal infranodal conduction. Leads AVF and V1 reveal fine serpentine movement with varying atrial wave morphology; findings consistent with atrial fibrillation. Diagnosis is atrial fibrillation.

Figure 13

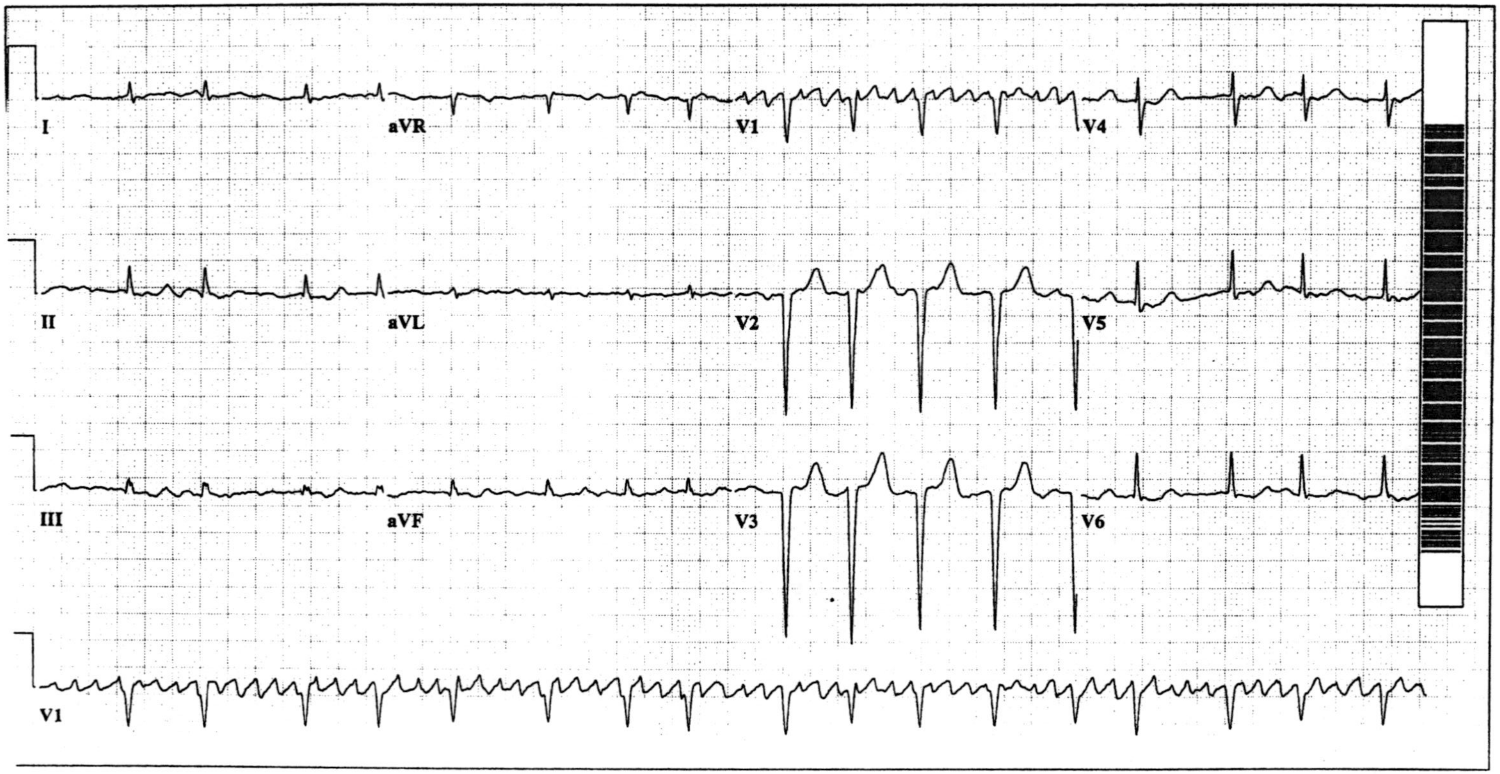

Fig. 13: The tracing shows heart rate of 102/min. and irregular. QRS complexes are narrow. Leads AVF and V1 reveal serpentine movement with varying morphology; findings consistent with atrial fibrillation. The rate of atrial waves is 375–500/min. The serpentine morphology in lead V1 is coarse in comparison to the morphology in Fig. 12, where it is a fine movement. The diagnosis is coarse atrial fibrillation with rapid heart rate. Some of the atrial activation waves in rhythm strip (lead V1) have sharp sawtooth appearance, while others are more rounded. This varying morphology makes it atrial fibrillation and differentiates it from atrial flutter where the morphology of atrial waves does not vary. The rate of atrial waves is also against the diagnosis of atrial flutter.

NOTE:

If a rhythm strip shows coarse atrial fibrillation with intermittent brief periods of atrial flutter (atrial rate of 250–350/min.), it is called atrial flutter - fibrillation.

Figure 14

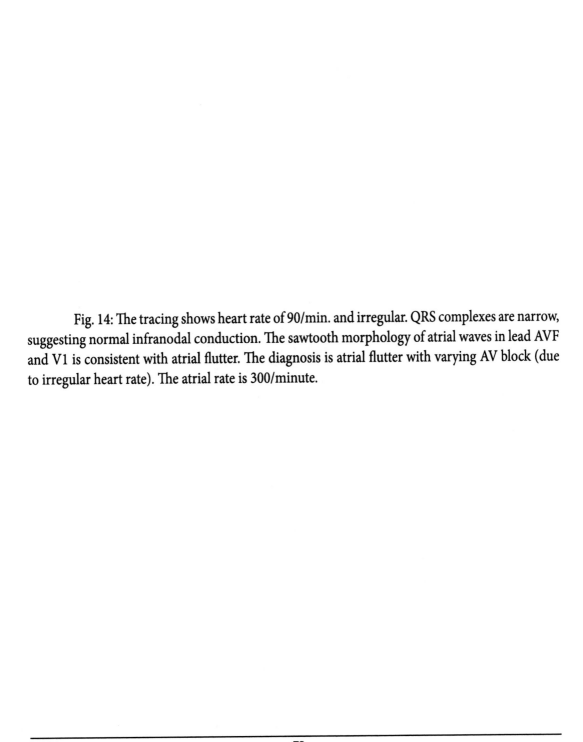

Fig. 14: The tracing shows heart rate of 90/min. and irregular. QRS complexes are narrow, suggesting normal infranodal conduction. The sawtooth morphology of atrial waves in lead AVF and V1 is consistent with atrial flutter. The diagnosis is atrial flutter with varying AV block (due to irregular heart rate). The atrial rate is 300/minute.

Figure 15

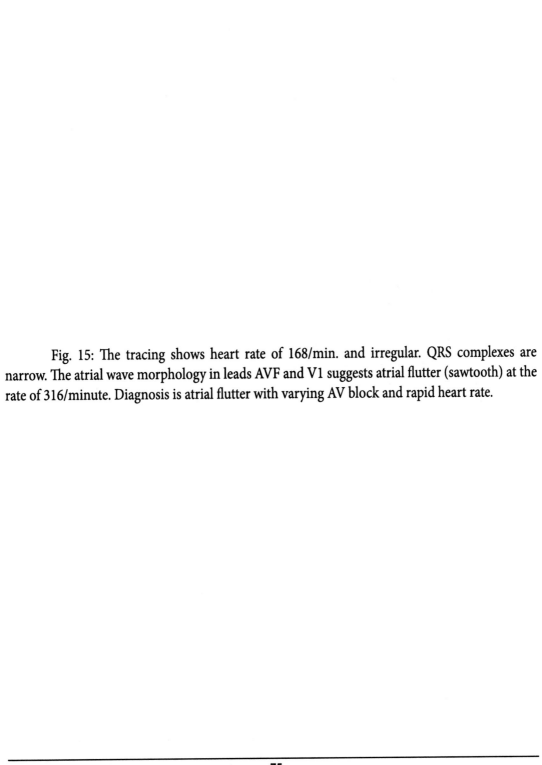

Fig. 15: The tracing shows heart rate of 168/min. and irregular. QRS complexes are narrow. The atrial wave morphology in leads AVF and V1 suggests atrial flutter (sawtooth) at the rate of 316/minute. Diagnosis is atrial flutter with varying AV block and rapid heart rate.

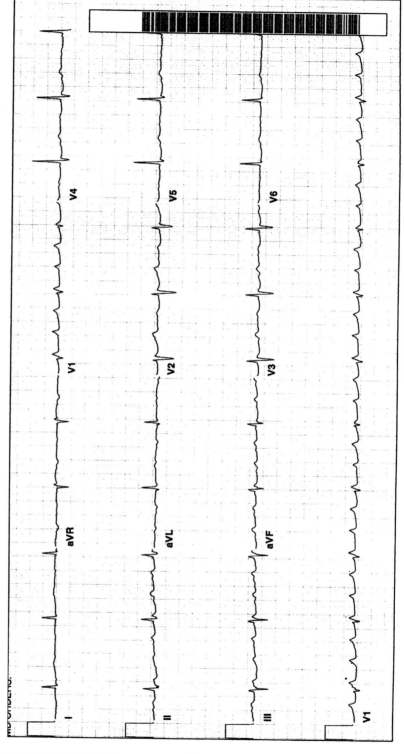

Figure 16A

Fig. 16A: The tracing shows heart rate of 63/min. and regular. QRS complexes are narrow, suggesting normal infranodal conduction. P waves are abnormal looking in the rhythm strip (lead V1) at the bottom of the EKG, and give the first impression of being atrial flutter. But, in lead AVF and other inferior leads, the P waves are upright with a round top and the line between each consecutive P wave is straight. That makes it PAT (paroxysmal atrial tachycardia) with atrial rate of 188/minute. Therefore, the diagnosis is PAT with 3:1 AV conduction. In atrial flutter, the P waves (called flutter waves) are sawtooth in appearance in lead V1but either inverted or sawtooth in lead AVF – never upright with a round top like a sinus P wave in AVF. The atrial rate is usually 150 to 250 per minute in PAT. For more details on PAT, see pages 48, 78 and 79. The impulse in PAT arises from the atrial muscle close to the sinus node with antegrade atrial conduction while depolarizing the tissue around the sinus node simultaneously.

Figure 16B

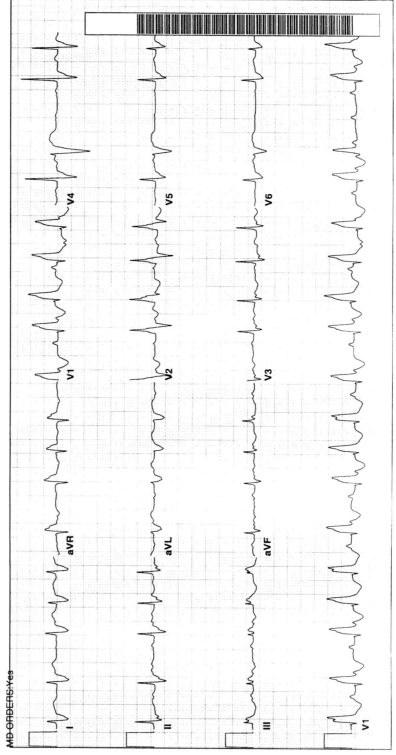

Fig. 16B: The tracing shows heart rate of 106/min. and irregular. QRS complexes are wide. The rhythm strip shows atrial rate of 167/min. with abnormal looking P wave morphology and a straight line between consecutive P waves (near the end of the rhythm strip). P wave in inferior leads is upright. These findings suggest paroxysmal atrial tachycardia, also referred to as PAT (P wave is inverted in slow atrial flutter in inferior leads). R – R is irregular and some P waves are not followed by QRS complex. This suggests second degree AV block which appears to be varying between 2:1, 3:1 and Mobitz 1 AV block, i.e. it is varying within second degree AV block. Therefore, the diagnosis is PAT with varying second degree AV block. Wide QRS is due to RBBB. A detailed description of heart block follows in the next chapter.

Atrial Tachycardia
(PAT and Ectopic)

R-R Interval:

» **IRREGULAR: Varying AV Block, 1:1 AV Conduction**
OR
Varying Second Degree AV Block
OR
Mobitz Type 1 AV Block
(with aberrancy if wide QRS complexes)
» **REGULAR: Fixed AV Conduction, 2:1, 3:1, or 4:1…**
(With aberrancy if wide QRS complexes)
OR
Complete AV Block
(With Nodal or Ventricular Escape Rhythm)

Chart 6

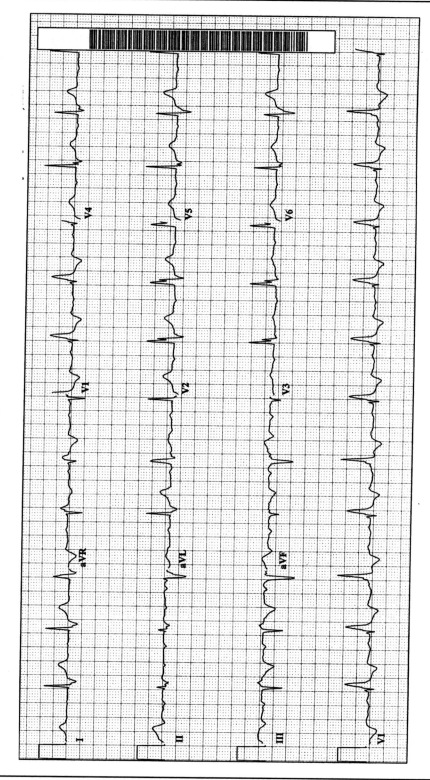

Figure 16C

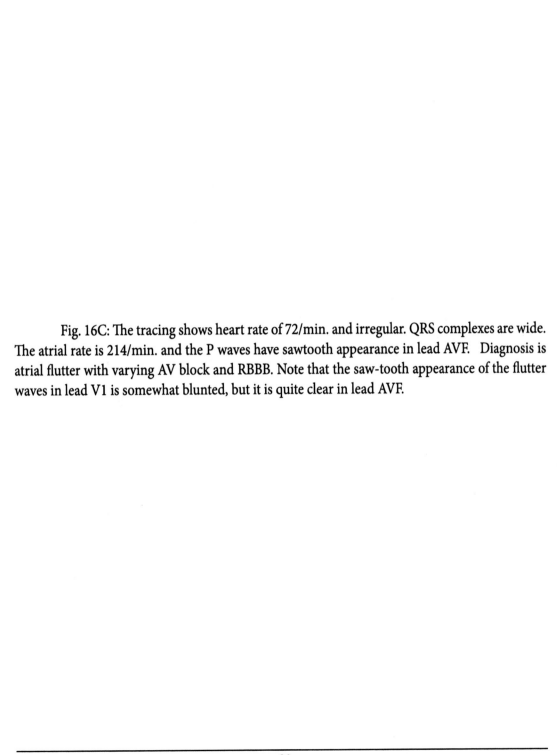

Fig. 16C: The tracing shows heart rate of 72/min. and irregular. QRS complexes are wide. The atrial rate is 214/min. and the P waves have sawtooth appearance in lead AVF. Diagnosis is atrial flutter with varying AV block and RBBB. Note that the saw-tooth appearance of the flutter waves in lead V1 is somewhat blunted, but it is quite clear in lead AVF.

Figure 17A

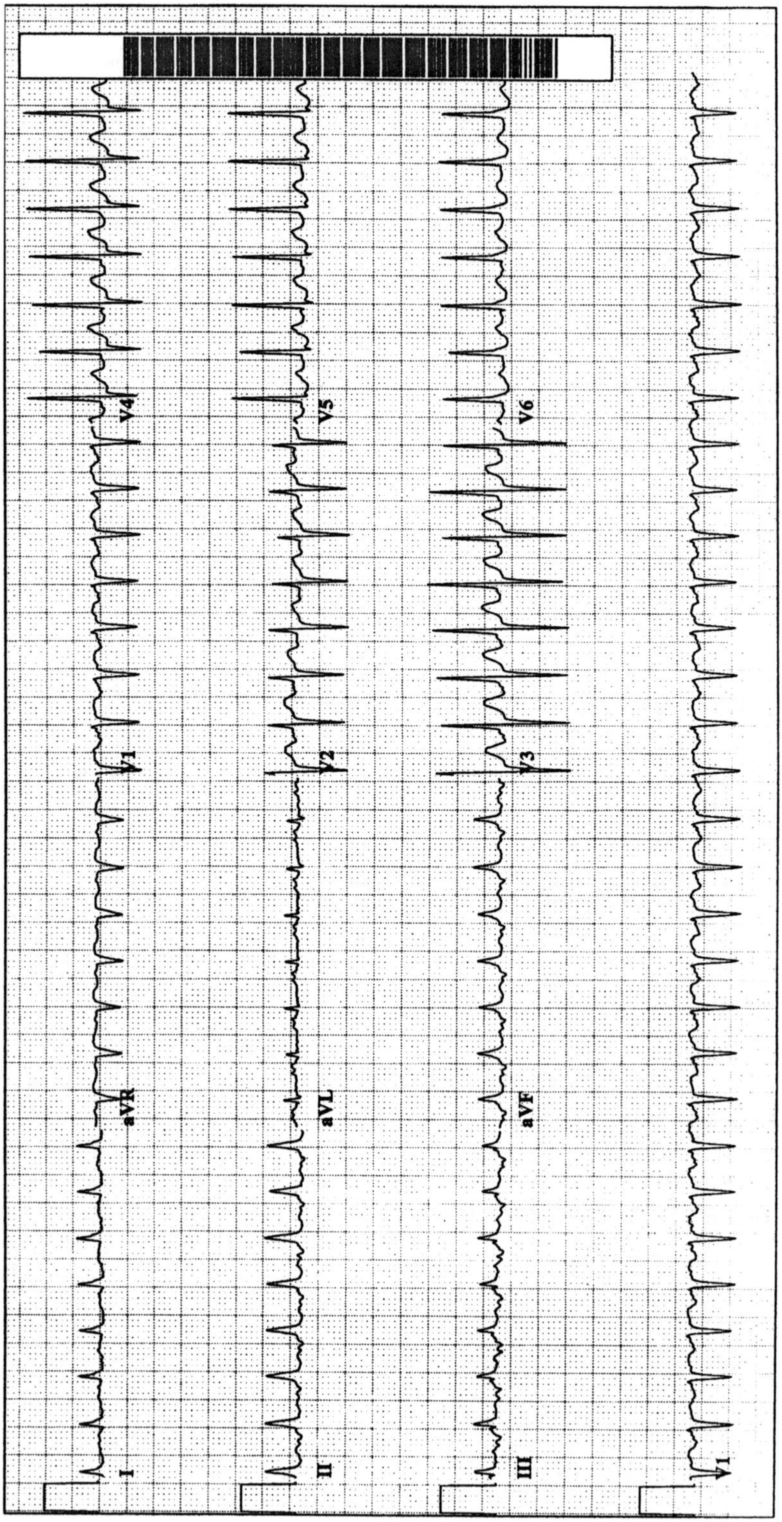

Fig. 17A: The tracing shows heart rate of 180/min. and regular. QRS complexes are narrow, suggesting normal infranodal conduction. The shape of the P wave in lead AVF shows a retrograde P wave @ 180/min., with short PR interval; findings suggesting atrial rhythm to be an ectopic atrial tachycardia. PR is constant, suggesting antegrade AV conduction of all P waves. Therefore, it is ectopic atrial tachycardia with antegrade AV conduction and normal infranodal conduction. Thus, the diagnosis is ectopic atrial tachycardia. It is not a nodal tachycardia because the atrial rate is greater than 115 BPM.

Figure 17B

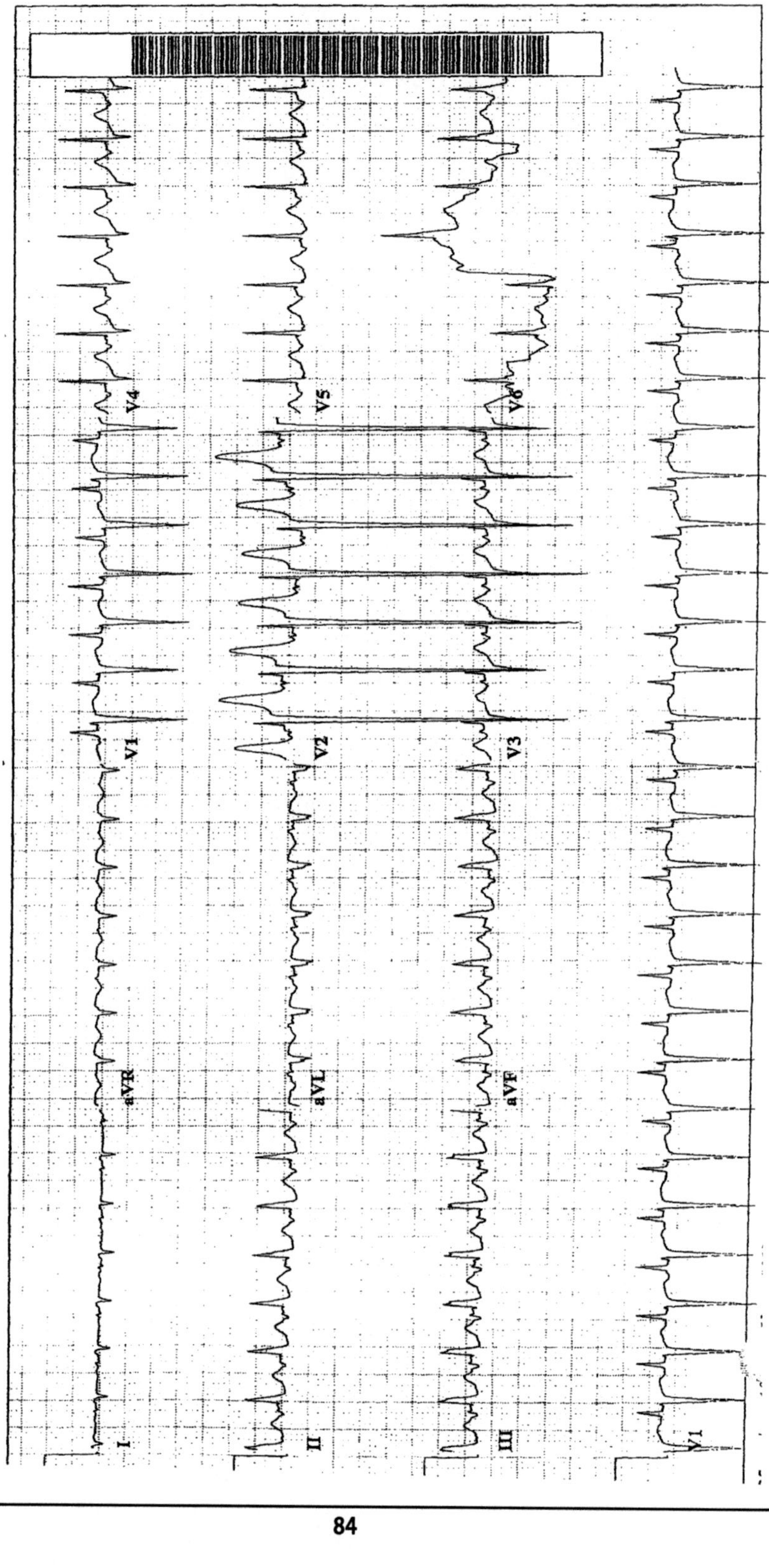

Fig. 17B: The tracing shows heart rate of 171/min. and regular. QRS complexes are narrow, suggesting normal infranodal conduction. The shape of the P wave in lead AVF shows a retrograde P wave @ 171/min., with short PR interval, suggesting atrial rhythm to be ectopic atrial tachycardia. PR is constant, suggesting antegrade AV conduction of all P waves. Therefore, it is ectopic atrial tachycardia (also called atrial tachycardia) with antegrade AV conduction and normal infranodal conduction. Thus, the diagnosis is ectopic atrial tachycardia, which means that it is the ectopic focus within the atrium which is activating all the four cardiac chambers at a fast rate. Note the abnormal shape of the P waves in lead V1, which supports the diagnosis of atrial tachycardia. P waves in lead AVF in atrial tachycardia may be inverted, biphasic or upright and abnormal in appearance, depending upon the site of origin of the impulse in the atrial muscle, but the absence of saw-tooth appearance in lead V1 differentiates it from atrial flutter.

Figure 18

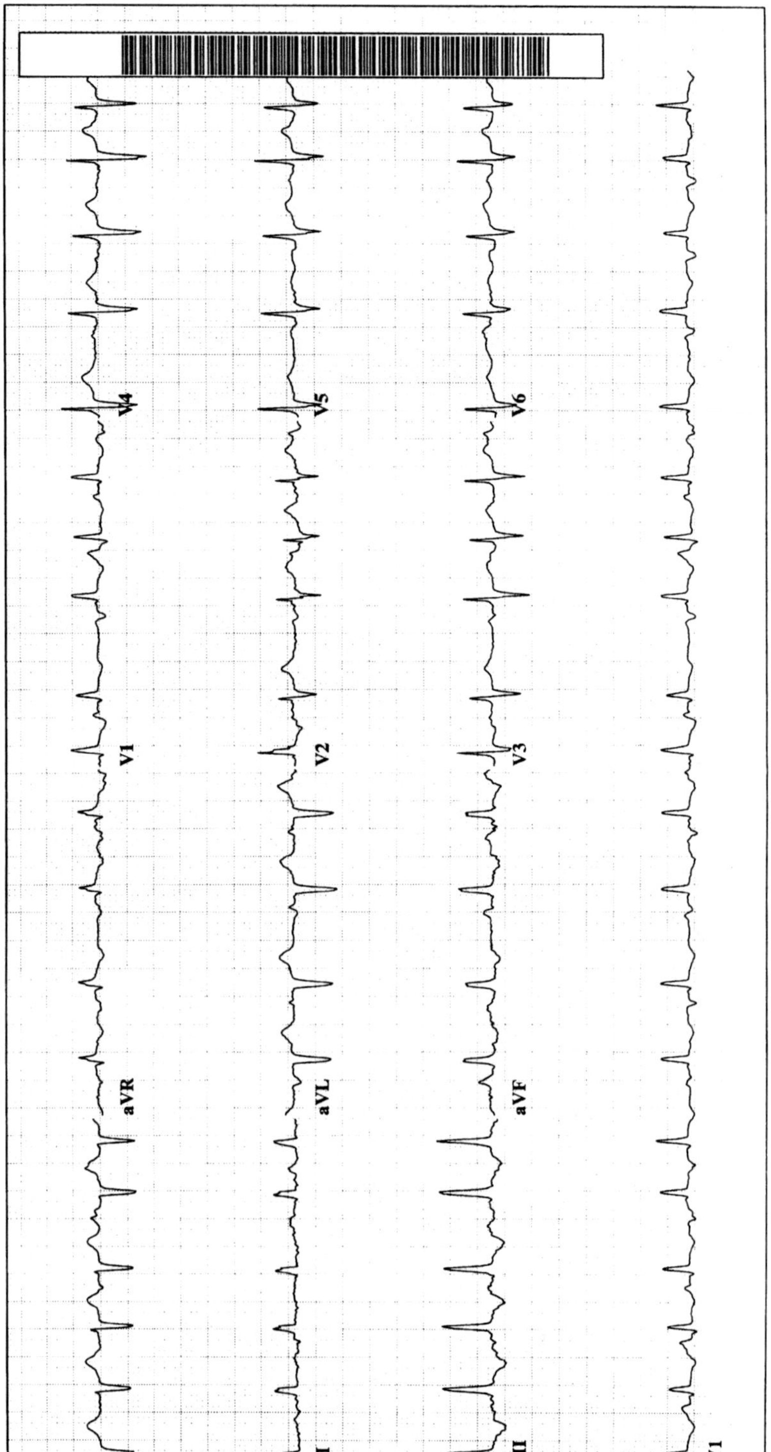

Fig. 18: The tracing shows heart rate of 120/min. and irregular. QRS complexes are narrow, suggesting normal infranodal conduction. The shape of the P waves in leads AVF and V1 is varying, suggesting multiple foci of origin of the electrical impulse activating the atria. The rate of the P waves is 120/minute. Thus, the rate and the shape of P waves in leads AVF and V1 suggests atrial rhythm to be multifocal atrial tachycardia. PR interval is varying and the R – R is irregular; findings consistent with varying AV block. Thus, the diagnosis is multifocal atrial tachycardia with varying AV block.

Figure 19

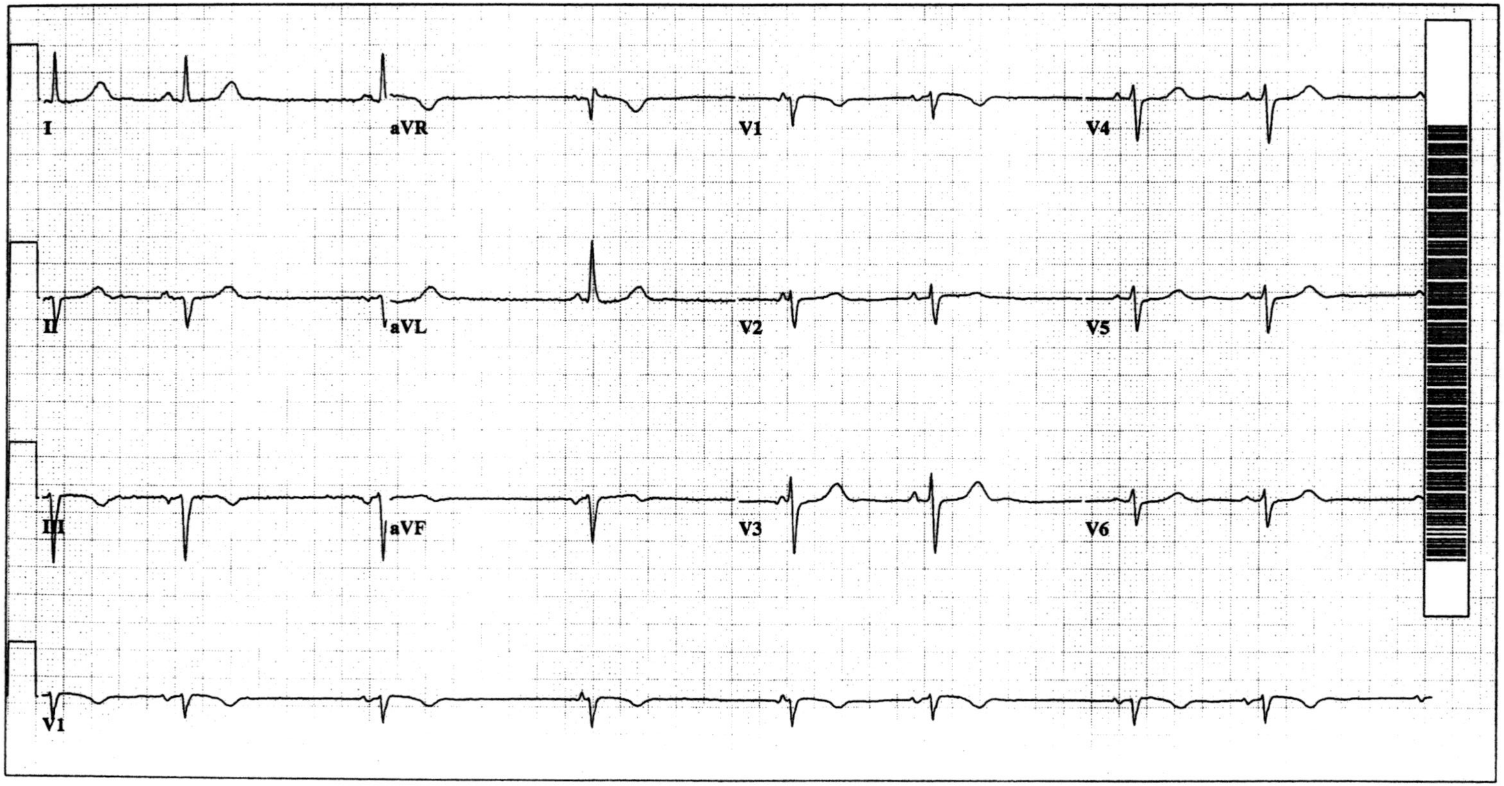

Fig. 19: The tracing shows heart rate of 48/min. and irregular. QRS complexes are narrow, suggesting normal infranodal conduction. The rate and the shape of the P waves in lead V1 are varying, suggesting two foci of origin of these P waves at different rates, called wandering atrial pacemaker. The diagnosis is sinus bradycardia with sinus arrhythmia and pacemaker wandering between sinus and the AV node. PR is varying due to varying site of origin of the impulse. The complexes with short PR are AV nodal in origin. This tracing can also be interpreted as sinus bradycardia with sinus arrhythmia and nodal escape complexes (see page 100 for description of nodal escape phenomenon).

Figure 20

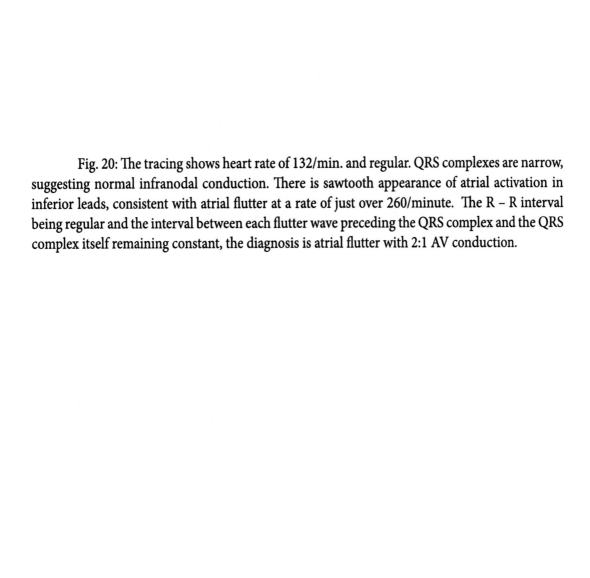

Fig. 20: The tracing shows heart rate of 132/min. and regular. QRS complexes are narrow, suggesting normal infranodal conduction. There is sawtooth appearance of atrial activation in inferior leads, consistent with atrial flutter at a rate of just over 260/minute. The R – R interval being regular and the interval between each flutter wave preceding the QRS complex and the QRS complex itself remaining constant, the diagnosis is atrial flutter with 2:1 AV conduction.

Figure 21

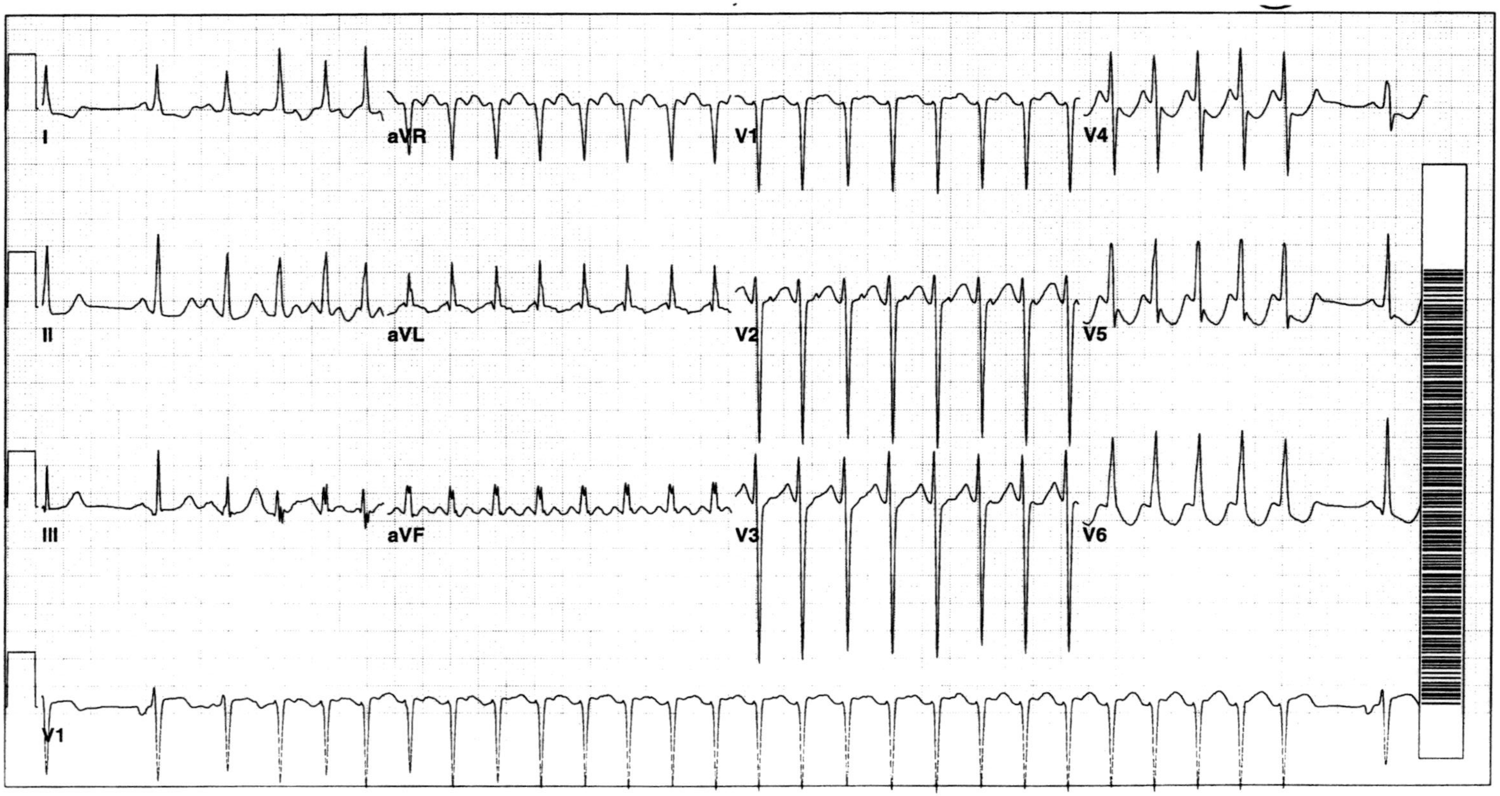

Fig. 21: The tracing shows heart rate of 162/minute. With the exception of the first two beats of the rhythm strip starting from the left and the last beat on the right, the R – R interval is regular with a fast heart rate, and the QRS complexes are narrow, suggesting some kind of a supraventricular tachy-arrhythmia with normal infranodal conduction. Since no P waves are visible, that makes it SVT. The P – QRS complexes before the start of the SVT and after the end of the SVT are normal sinus rhythm complexes. Hence, the diagnosis is sinus rhythm with a prolonged burst of SVT. It is commonly known as paroxysmal supraventricular tachycardia.

Diagnosis of various cardiac rhythms associated with normal AV conduction, prolonged AV conduction, and varying AV conduction (varying AV block) have been discussed in this chapter. Differentiation of varying AV block from complete AV block has also been discussed. Thus, the discussion has covered those conditions where each P wave is followed by a QRS complex (even though each QRS complex, sometimes, may not be preceded by a P wave). Next chapter (chapter 10) will deal with conditions where some P waves are followed by a QRS complex and some P waves are not followed by a QRS complex – second and third degree heart blocks.

Premature atrial and ventricular contractions:

No description of cardiac arrhythmias is complete without the discussion about premature atrial contractions (PACs) and premature ventricular contractions (PVCs), also called atrial and ventricular extra-systoles, respectively. As the name implies, these beats occur prematurely. In the presence of sinus rhythm, a focus in the atrial or ventricular muscle may discharge an electrical impulse before the next sinus impulse is due to be discharged, and depolarize the atrial and ventricular chambers, thus rendering the muscle of these chambers refractory to the next impulse from the sinus node. Sometimes, even the sinus node may be depolarized by the premature impulse, as it is getting ready to discharge the next impulse, and may have to recycle itself for discharge of the next impulse. If the sinus node is not depolarized, it discharges its impulse on schedule, but the impulse just cannot propagate as it finds the atrial muscle refractory. In such a scenario, the cycle of the sinus node impulse discharge is not affected, and the next impulse is discharged on schedule, making the interval between the QRS preceding the premature QRS complex and the QRS complex following the premature QRS complex twice as long as the R – R interval between two normal consecutive QRS complexes. The pause that follows the premature QRS complex is called a compensatory pause, because it compensates for the prematurity of the premature complex. This phenomenon occurs only with PVCs, as the likelihood of premature sinus node depolarization is remote due to the distance which a PVC impulse has to travel in retrograde fashion before it can depolarize the sinus node. That is why a P wave is sometimes seen in the terminal part of the QRS complex of a PVC indicating that a part of the atrial chambers was depolarized by the impulse from the sinus node. PVCs are not always associated with a compensatory pause, because it depends upon whether the sinus node gets depolarized by the PVC or not. Premature atrial contractions (PACs) are usually not associated with a compensatory pause due to their proximity to the sinus node, which usually gets depolarized in the process, by the PAC.

Sometimes, the ventricular ectopic focus may discharge an impulse as the sinus node impulse exits the AV node and starts activation of the ventricles. In that case, the ventricles would be depolarized partly by the ventricular impulse and partly by the sinus impulse. The resulting P-QRS complex will be called a fusion complex. A wide premature QRS complex in this situation will be accompanied by a P wave before it without appreciable change in PR interval.

How to differentiate between PAC and PVC:

A narrow QRS complex in a premature beat indicates premature atrial contraction (PAC). If there is a premature P wave before such PAC, it indicates atrial origin of the PAC, whereas an absence of such a P wave suggests nodal origin of the PAC, also called nodal premature contraction (NPC). A wide QRS complex in a premature beat could be a PAC with aberrant conduction or a PVC. A premature P wave (P comes before its time in the P–P cycle) before the premature QRS complex indicates that it is a PAC, regardless of whether the QRS complex of the premature beat is narrow or wide (greater than 0.1 second). A wide premature QRS complex is usually a PVC, unless there is a premature P before it. A P wave embedded in the terminal portion of the premature wide QRS complex means it is a PVC. If a wide premature QRS complex has the morphology of RBBB pattern, try hard to see if there is a premature P wave before it, which, if present, indicates that it is a PAC with aberrancy, otherwise it is a PVC. Premature atrial or ventricular complexes can occur occasionally or frequently, or as couplets or triplets, or in salvos. When an alternate QRS complex is a premature complex, it is referred to as atrial or ventricular bigeminy.

Some examples follow (see Figures 22, 23, 24).

Parasystole:

Sometimes, an independent ectopic focus may exist within the atrial or ventricular muscle which is capable of discharging an electrical impulse of its own, in total disregard to the sinus node, resulting in a competition between these two foci. This ectopic focus is usually protected by a block around it, so that it cannot be depolarized by the sinus node impulse. However, this block may sometimes be partial, making the ectopic focus vulnerable to depolarization by the sinus impulse. Since the ectopic focus is usually protected, the ectopic R – R interval (also called ectopic coupling interval) is a multiple of a common denominator. For example, if you find four ectopic QRS complexes with coupling intervals of 0.6 second, 0.9 second, 1.8 second, and 3.0 seconds respectively, the common denominator is 0.3 second. Narrow QRS indicates an atrial parasystole, whereas a wide QRS suggests a ventricular parasystole. Presence of fusion complexes should raise the suspicion of its being a ventricular parasystole rather than a PVC. Usually a long rhythm strip is required for the diagnosis of a parasystole.

NOTE:

Those students who are just beginning to learn the interpretation of EKGs would find it worthwhile at this point to go back to chapter 8 and spend a few moments reading about regularity of R – R intervals for a better understanding of the importance of finding whether R – R is regular or irregular in the diagnosis of arrhythmias.

Fig. 22 (right): EKG tracing shows fifth QRS complex from the left (see rhythm strip at the bottom) is a premature complex followed by a pause. The QRS complex is narrow, and preceded by an inverted P wave in lead III. This P wave is also premature on the P –P cycle. This is a PAC.

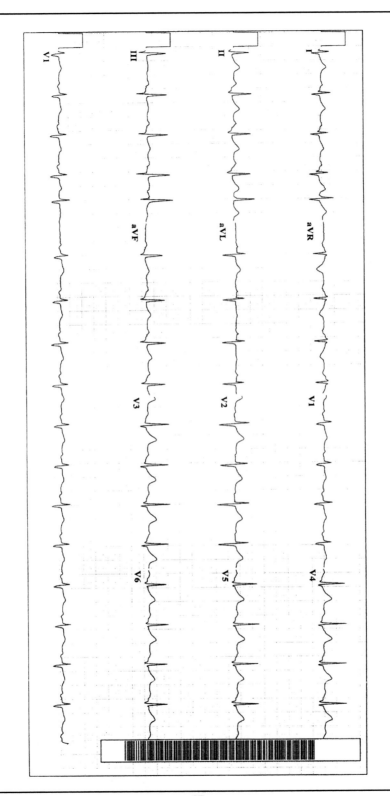

Figure 22

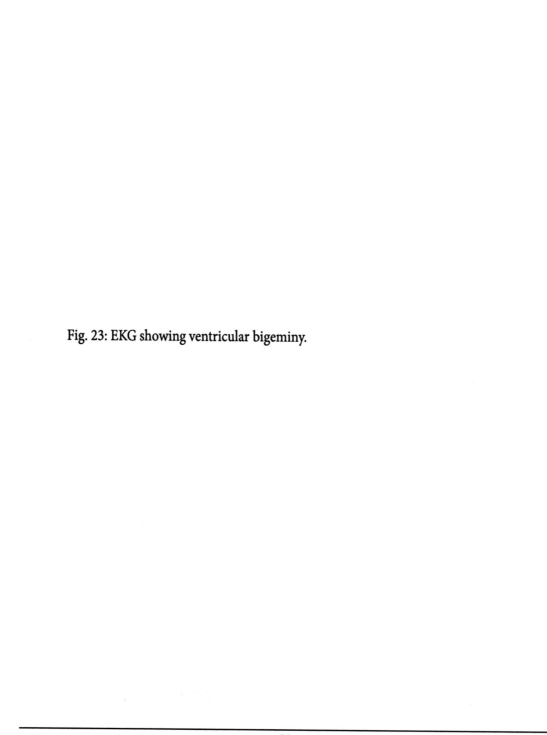

Fig. 23: EKG showing ventricular bigeminy.

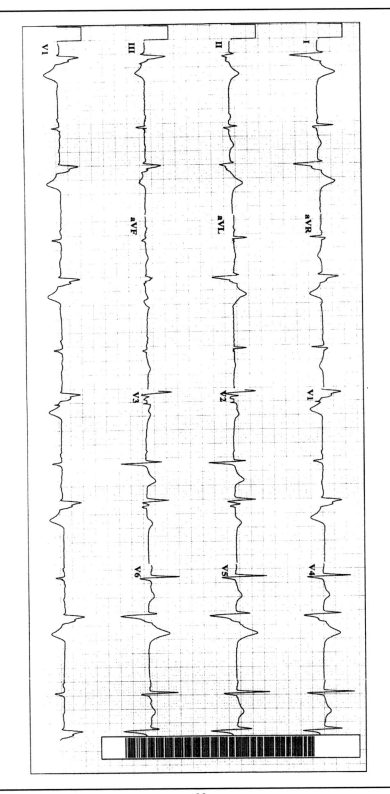

Figure 23

Nodal and Ventricular escape phenomenon:

Sinus node normally activates the atria and the ventricles. It achieves this dominance through suppression of automaticity of other potential foci. In case of failure or significant delay on the part of the sinus node to discharge an impulse, it may provide an opportunity for the AV node or the potential ventricular focus to escape the continuous suppression by the sinus node, and discharge its own impulse to activate the ventricular chambers. Atrial chambers may be activated by this focus in retrograde manner or by the sinus node or both. The QRS complex which results from such escape phenomenon is called nodal or ventricular escape complex, according to the site of origin of the impulse. If several such complexes occur in succession, it is called nodal or ventricular escape rhythm, respectively. This phenomenon is also seen in complete AV block, where nodal or ventricular escape rhythm must come into action for survival. Figure 25 illustrates severe sinus bradycardia with nodal escape complexes (see arrows).

Fig. 24: EKG tracing with 7th and 12th QRS complexes from the left (see rhythm strip) looking wider and different from the rest. There is a premature P wave before each of these two complexes which appears abnormal in morphology. Therefore, these are PACs with aberrant conduction. All other premature QRS complexes are narrow. They are also preceded by abnormal looking respective P waves. These are PACS occurring in salvos. The 2nd, 11th and 13 through 16th complexes are normal sinus driven QRS complexes. The P wave on top of the T wave of the first QRS complex on the left is a non-conducted PAC (without QRS). This P wave came prematurely and did not get conducted through the AV node due to refractoriness.

Fig. 25: The tracing (see page 102) illustrates severe sinus bradycardia with nodal escape complexes (see arrows).

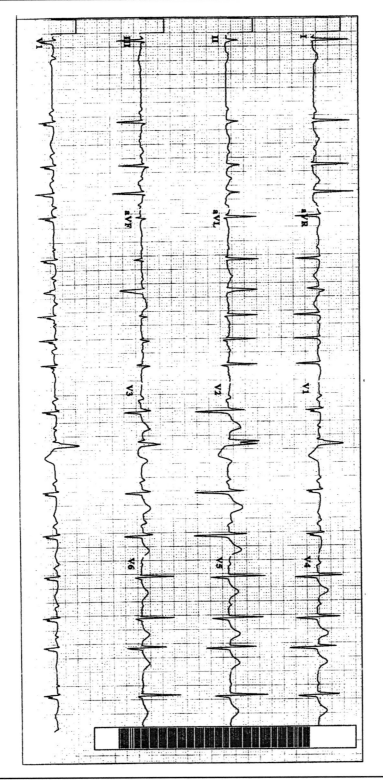

Figure 24

Figure 25

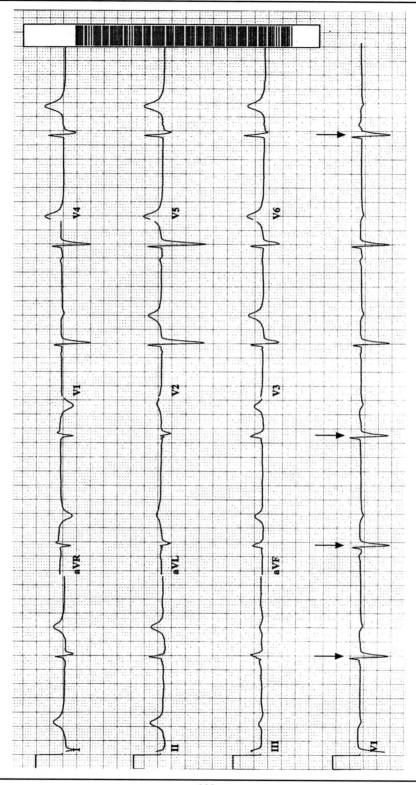

Chapter 10

Heart Blocks

Heart block is defined as blockage at any level of the conduction tissue. It includes blockage at the sinus node (also called sinoatrial node or SA node), AV node, or below the AV node (called infra nodal or infrahisial i.e. below the bundle of His). Infra nodal blocks include right bundle branch block, left bundle branch block, left anterior hemiblock, left posterior hemiblock, and intra ventricular conduction delay. SA block and AVnodal block are discussed in detail in this chapter. A detailed description of infra nodal blocks will follow in chapter 14. Hemiblocks are discussed in chapters 14 and 11.

SA Block:

Sinus node discharge is suppressed during atrial fibrillation and atrial flutter. In case of sinus exit block, the sinus node discharges the impulse, but the impulse cannot depolarize the atria due to blockage around the sinus node, or due to the atrial muscle having been rendered refractory by a PAC or PVC (with retrograde atrial conduction). This is referred to as SA exit block. There are 3 types of SA exit blocks as follows.

1. Wenckeback (type 1) sinus exit block: P - P interval shortens until a P drops. The pause between the P before and the P after the dropped P is not twice the P – P interval.

2. Type II sinus exit block: There is occasional drop of a P wave, and the pause between the P before and the P after the dropped P is twice the P – P interval. There is no shortening of P – P interval.

3. Complete sino-atrial block: There is a complete exit block at the sinus node, and therefore, a junctional or idioventricular escape rhythm takes over.

Note: The term sinus arrest is used when there is no discharge of sinus node impulse and the EKG tracing shows a straight line until another focus, usually a ventricular focus, takes over. The term sick sinus syndrome (also called brady-tachy syndrome) refers to a tendency for periodic tachy and brady arrhythmias.

AV Block:

AV blocks are classified as first degree, second degree, third degree, and varying AV block. Third degree AV block is also called a complete AV block. In first degree AV block, each P wave gets conducted through the AV node, but takes longer than normal time, and the conduction time remains constant for each impulse. Therefore, PR is prolonged and remains constant from beat to beat. In varying AV block, each P wave gets conducted through the AV node, but the conduction time varies from beat to beat. Therefore, the PR does not remain constant. However, in both of these situations – first degree AV block as well as varying AV block – each P wave is followed by a QRS complex, and each QRS complex is preceded by a P wave and PR segment, because all of the P waves are conducted. In second degree AV block, some P waves get conducted through the AV node, and some are blocked. Therefore, some P waves are followed by a QRS complex and some P waves are not followed by a QRS complex (called P with dropped QRS). An occasional P with dropped QRS will also qualify for a second degree AV block. In third degree AV block, none of the P waves gets conducted through the AV node. Therefore, a second focus, located within the AV node below the site of the blockage or within the ventricle, activates the ventricles, resulting in beating of the ventricles at a rate which is different from the atrial rate. Atria and the ventricles beat independent of each other. That leads to a loss of relationship between P and the QRS complexes. The PR, therefore, does not remain constant, just as in varying AV block. However, R – R interval is usually regular in complete AV block (as the ventricles beat independently at a regular rate) but always irregular in varying AV block. Further details are discussed below.

The AV node conduction is classified as follows:

1. Normal AV conduction: Each P wave is followed by a QRS complex; PR interval is normal (0.12 – 0.2 sec.) and remains constant from beat to beat.

2. First degree AV block: Each P wave is followed by a QRS complex; PR interval is prolonged (more than 0.2 sec.) and remains constant from beat to beat.

3. Varying AV block: Each P wave is followed by a QRS complex and PR interval varies. R – R interval is irregular due to varying PR interval. Each QRS complex must also be preceded by a P wave and PR segment for the diagnosis of varying AV block (see Fig. 7A), otherwise it is Mobitz I AV block or a complete AV block (see Fig. 7B and read footnote for a better understanding). In atrial flutter with irregular R – R interval, the changing ratio between flutter waves and the QRS complexes is also due to varying AV block. Similar phenomenon is seen in PAT (paroxysmal atrial tachycardia) with varying AV block (see Fig.16B, chapter 9).

4. Second degree AV block: There is occasional to frequent drop of QRS complex after the P wave (P wave without QRS complex).

5. Complete AV block: It is also called complete heart block or third degree AV block. None of the P waves is conducted through the AV node. The ventricles are activated by the impulse from a second focus, and thus atria and the ventricles beat independently of each other at different rates. Therefore, there is no relationship between P and the QRS; PR interval varies from beat to beat; R – R usually remains regular due to independent ventricular activation from a second focus. If R – R is irregular due to the irregular discharge of impulse by the second focus activating the ventricles, there would be some P waves without the QRS complex or some QRS complexes which are not preceded by a P wave or PR segment. This would differentiate it from varying AV block where each QRS complex must be preceded by a P wave and PR segment, and each P wave must be followed by a QRS complex (see Fig. 7B for a better understanding).

When PR interval is 0.21 second or greater, it is considered as prolonged, and referred to as first degree AV block. Each P wave is followed by a QRS complex with prolonged PR interval. However, the PR interval remains constant for each P-QRS complex. Should the PR remain prolonged and vary from one P-QRS complex to the next, it is called varying first degree AV block.

Looking at the rhythm strip, if you find that some P waves are followed by QRS complex and some P waves are not followed by QRS complex, and the P waves which are not followed by QRS complex are not premature P waves (non-conducted PACs), it is always a second or third degree heart block. To distinguish between these two, one should always follow the following sequence.

If R-R intervals are regular and the PR intervals are varying, it is a third degree heart block (see Fig. 1 on following page), otherwise it is a second degree heart block.

Figure 1

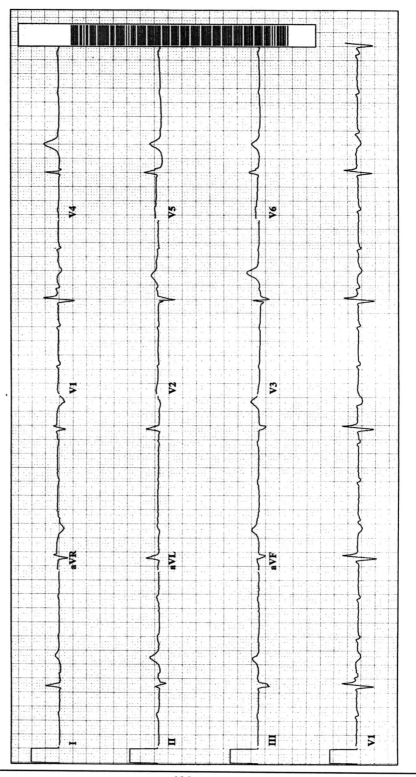

Fig. 1: The tracing shows that some P waves are followed by QRS and some are not, in the rhythm strip at the bottom of the EKG tracing. The P waves which are not followed by QRS complex are not premature P waves. This indicates AV block. R – R interval is regular and the PR interval is not regular. That makes it third degree AV block. The ventricles are being activated by a focus in the AV node (QRS complexes are narrow), below the site of the AV block. Therefore, the diagnosis is sinus tachycardia (atrial rate is 107/minute) with complete AV block, and nodal (or junctional) rhythm (also referred to as nodal escape rhythm). See page 100 for detailed description of "escape phenomenon".

NOTE:

P – P interval in complete AV block remains constant. However, sometimes the P wave that follows the QRS complex may appear slightly before time due to vascular perfusion of sinus node from ventricular systole, resulting in relatively early recovery of the sinus node. This is called ventriculo-phasic sinus arrhythmia. The morphology of such a sinus P wave will be similar to the morphology of other sinus P waves on the rhythm strip, whereas, the morphology of a non-conducted premature atrial contraction (PAC) will differ from the morphology of other sinus P waves. This will help differentiate between these two kinds of P waves.

Figure 2

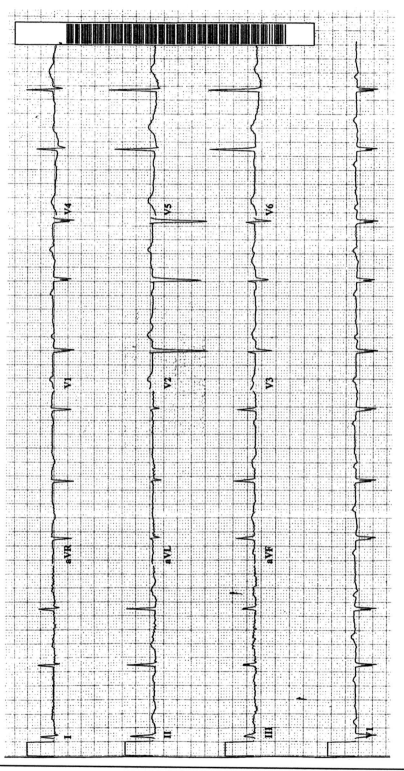

Second degree heart block is divided into 3 categories:

1. Mobitz type I (also known as Wenckebach block).

2. Mobitz type II.

3. High grade 2nd degree AV block.

Mobitz type I (Fig. 2):

In this type of block, successive PR intervals get longer and longer until there is a P wave which is not followed by QRS complex. This completes the cycle and next cycle starts in a similar fashion. These cycles continue to repeat in this pattern. It is noteworthy that each cycle from its start to finish has one more P wave than the number of QRS complexes in the cycle. Thus, the ratio between the number of P waves and the QRS complexes in each cycle is 3:2, 4:3, 5:4 or 6:5 and so on.

Fig. 2: The tracing shows that some P waves are followed by QRS, and some P waves are not, and those P waves which are not followed by QRS complex are not premature P waves. This indicates 2nd or 3rd degree AV block. To qualify for 3rd degree AV block, R–R should be regular and PR should not be regular. Here, the R–R is irregular. Therefore, it is not third degree AV block. Therefore, it is a second degree AV block. The successive PR intervals get longer and longer until the P wave is not followed by QRS complex; the cycle begins all over again. In each cycle, the P to QRS ratio is 3:2, i.e. one P wave more than the number of QRS complexes. That makes it Mobitz type 1 AV block.

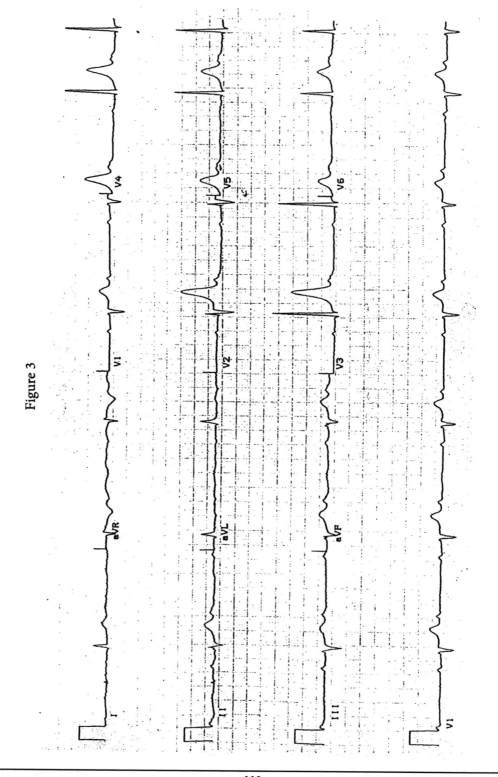

Figure 3

Mobitz type II (Fig. 3):

While Mobitz type 1AV block is located in the AV node, type II is usually located in the infra nodal conduction tissue, and associated with relatively less favorable prognosis. Unlike Mobitz type I, the PR interval usually stays constant, associated with an occasional drop of QRS complex following the P wave. If there is frequent drop of the QRS complex, the P to QRS ratio always shows one more P wave than the number of QRS complexes, e.g. 2:1, 3:2, 4:3 or 5:4 and so on. Should the PR interval vary, it does not follow a set pattern seen in Mobitz type 1 AV block. A good rule to follow is that, in case of an AV block, if third degree AV block has been excluded, and it is neither Mobitz type 1, nor a high grade second degree AV block (see page 113), it is Mobitz type II.

Fig. 3: The tracing shows that some P waves are followed by QRS complex and some P waves are not followed by QRS complex. The P waves which are not followed by QRS complex are not premature P waves. This indicates 2nd or 3rd degree AV block. This is not a third degree AV block, because, in third degree AV block, the R – R interval is regular and PR interval is not; in this tracing, both the R – R interval and the PR interval are essentially regular (the only exception is the last PR on the right side). Therefore, it is a second degree AV block. P to QRS ratio is 2:1, and PR interval remains essentially constant. That makes it Mobitz type II AV block. The P – QRST complex on extreme right in the rhythm strip shows first degree AV block. Thus, the diagnosis in this patient is heart block changing between second degree (Mobitz type II) and first degree.

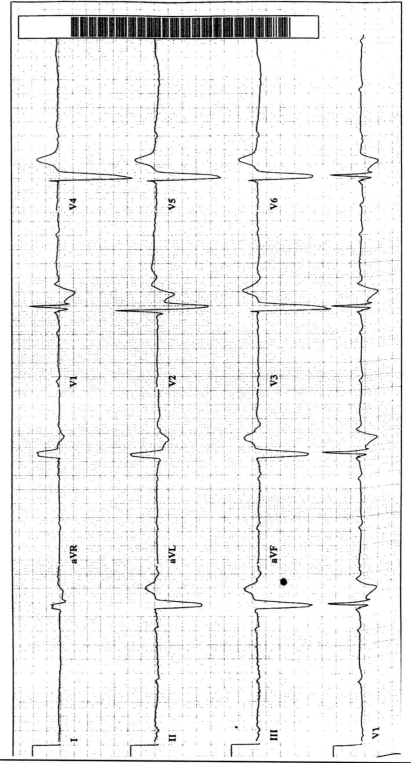

Figure 4

High grade 2nd degree AV block (Fig. 4):

In high grade 2nd degree AV block, there are too many successive P waves without the corresponding QRS complexes, and the P to QRS ratio may be 3:1, 4:1, or more. It is considered most serious of the 3 types of 2nd degree AV block due to the possibility of an impending complete AV block. Note that in Mobitz type II AV block when one P drops the QRS, the next P wave is followed by a QRS, whereas in high grade 2nd degree AV block, 2 or more consecutive P waves drop the QRS complex.

Fig. 4: EKG tracing shows 3:1 P to QRS ratio. It is not a third degree AV block, because PR is regular (in third degree AV block, R – R is regular and PR is not regular). This is high grade 2nd degree AV block.

NOTE:

Sometimes, the second degree AV block may vary between Mobitz-I and Mobitz-II block, or between Mobitz-II and high grade 2nd degree block in the same EKG strip. This is referred to as 2nd degree AV block varying between Mobitz type I and type II, or between Mobitz type II and high grade, as the case may be; or simply as varying 2nd degree AV block.

Controversies:

In a typical case of Mobitz I, as the PR interval gets longer and longer, the R-R interval gets shorter and shorter until there is a P wave without the QRS and the cycle keeps repeating itself (see Fig. 5 below and read foot note for details).

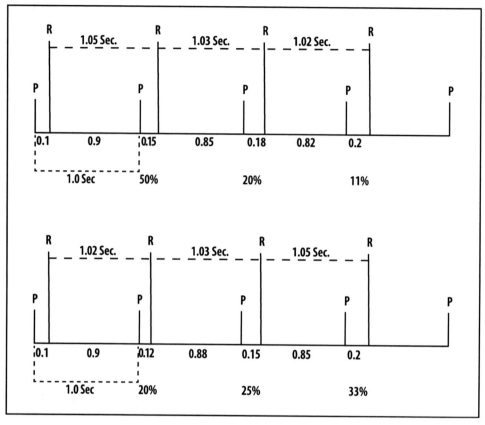

Figure 5

Fig. 5: The diagram shows two illustrations, one at the top and one at the bottom. Both illustrations assume a patient with atrial rate of 60 BPM. Thus, the P – P interval in each patient is 1.0 second. The successive PR intervals in the top patient are 0.1, 0.15, 0.18, and 0.2 second respectively. The successive PR intervals in the bottom patient are 0.1, 0.12, 0.15, and 0.2 second respectively. You can see that PR interval increases in successive beats in both patients, but R – R interval progressively decreases in the top patient while it increases in the bottom patient. The top patient qualifies for Mobitz type 1 AV block. It is controversial whether the bottom patient should be labeled as Mobitz type 1 (Wenckebach AV block). This may be regarded as a variant of Mobitz type I, but some individuals may disagree with that interpretation. However, it makes no difference as far as the medical treatment of the patient is concerned. The explanation for the difference in these two cases is that even though there is a progressive increase in the absolute value of subsequent PR intervals in each case, the percent increase progressively decreases in the typical case of Mobitz type I (50%, 20%, 11%), and it increases in the atypical case (20%, 25%, 33%).

It may be noted that Wenckebach reported Mobitz type 1 AV block in 1899 and called it Wenckebach phenomenon. What is known as Mobitz type II second degree AV block was first described as heart block in 1906 by Wenckebach (Dutch born Austrian), and by John Hay, an English physician, in 1905, independently. Wenckebach reported observing occasional P waves without the following QRS complex and called it heart block. Woldemar Mobitz , a Russian born German surgeon (born on May 31, 1889), later separated the second degree heart block into Mobitz type I (Wenckebach phenomenon) and Mobitz type II, as he considered it to be two different manifestations of 2nd degree heart block.

A Practical Approach To The Diagnosis Of Heart Block:

Whenever there are some P waves followed by QRS and some P waves not followed by QRS, and the P waves which are not followed by QRS are not premature P waves (premature P wave indicates premature atrial complex--PAC), it is always a 2nd or 3rd degree heart block. Always ask yourself first, whether it is a third degree AV block, because it is easier to include or exclude this diagnosis. That way, the problem gets simplified. If R-R intervals are regular and the PR intervals are varying, it is a 3rd degree heart block; otherwise, it is 2nd degree heart block. It is that simple. Then, If it is a 2nd degree heart block, look for criteria of Mobitz type 1 and criteria of a high grade second degree AV block. If these are excluded, call it Mobitz type II AV block.

A-V Dissociation:

In a complete heart block, there is an organic block at the AV node resulting in dissociation of atrial and ventricular contractions. Thus, atria beat at their own rate and the ventricles beat at their own rate, independently of each other. Since, the focus activating the ventricles lies within the AV node or in the ventricles, it discharges impulses at a slower rate than the sinus node. Therefore, the ventricular rate is slower than the atrial rate in complete heart block. Sometimes, there is no organic block at the AV node, but the AV node or the ventricle starts discharging electrical impulses at a rate faster than the sinus node, resulting in ventricular rate faster than the atrial rate. Under such circumstances, impulses from the sinus node may find the AV node refractory upon their arrival, and thus may be blocked from antegrade conduction. This creates a physiologic block at the AV node even though there is no organic block. This condition is called AV dissociation. The difference between complete AV block and the AV dissociation is that the ventricular rate in AV dissociation is higher than the atrial rate, whereas the reverse is true in complete AV block. PR interval varies in both cases, as atria and the ventricles are activated from two different foci at different rates in each case. Sometimes, the atrial and the ventricular rates, though different, but are very close to each other in AV dissociation. That is called isorhythmic AV dissociation (see Fig. 6). During AV dissociation, sometimes the P wave may occasionally get conducted through the AV node and activate the ventricles (Dressler beat). When that happens, it is called interference dissociation. When ventricular rate is less than 50/min. and atrial and ventricular rate are almost identical, it is very difficult to differentiate between isorhythmic AV dissociation and complete AV block. Hence, the diagnosis should be "Isorhythmic AV dissociation, ? complete AV block". (See Figure 7B)

NOTE:

Whenever you think of complete AV block, always keep the possibility of AV dissociation in mind as the differential diagnosis.

Fig. 6: EKG tracing shows varying PR interval. R – R is regular. Differential diagnosis is complete AV block vs. AV dissociation. Ventricular and atrial rates are almost identical. Ventricular rate is 60/min. Diagnosis is isorhythmic AV dissociation. Complete diagnosis is sinus rhythm with isorhythmic AV dissociation and underlying ventricular rhythm.

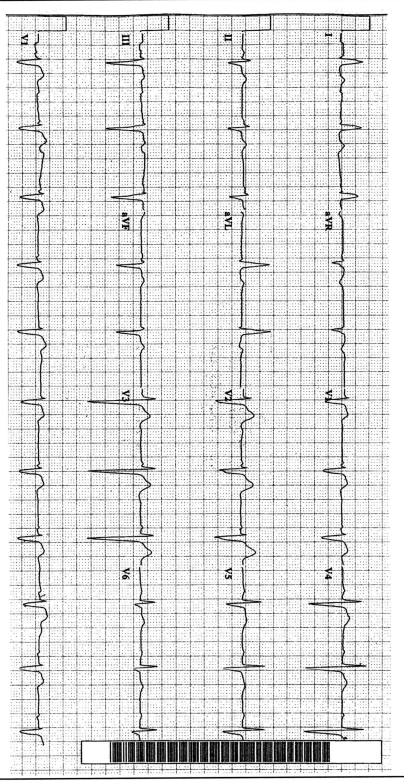

Figure 6

Fig. 7A: The tracing shows a heart rate of 132/min. and irregular. QRS complexes are narrow, suggesting a supraventricular rhythm with normal infra nodal conduction. The P wave in lead AVF is inverted (retrograde P), and the atrial rate is 132/min. PR interval is varying. The diagnosis is ectopic atrial tachycardia with varying AV block. Please note that each P wave is followed by a QRS complex, and each QRS complex is preceded by a P wave and PR segment (a requirement for the diagnosis of varying AV block).

Figure 7A

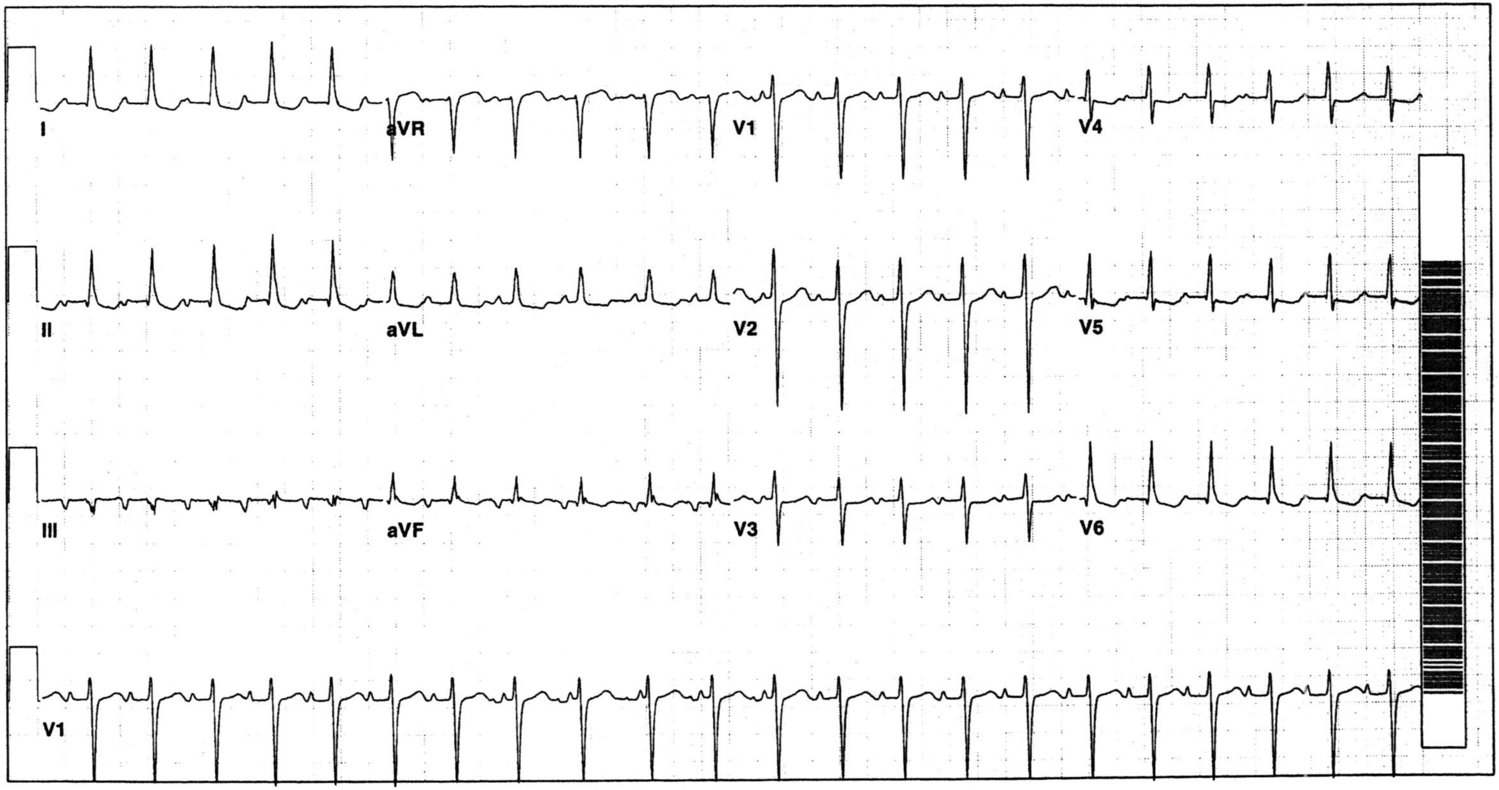

Fig. 7B: Tracing shows heart rate of 36/min., indicating bradycardia. R-R is irregular. QRS complexes are narrow, suggestive of supraventricular rhythm (focus activating the ventricles is located at or above the AV node). P wave is upright in lead AVF @ 39/min., indicating sinus bradycardia. PR is varying, indicating varying AV block or complete AV block. Since, R-R is irregular, it favors the diagnosis of varying AV block. However, first and second QRS complexes in the rhythm strip from the left side are not precede by a P wave. Hence, it is not a varying AV block. It is a complete AV block (?AV dissociation), where AV node is not firing the impulse at regular intervals. Since the atrial and the ventricular rates are almost identical, it is isorhythmic AV dissociation. However, the ventricular rate is less than 50/minute. Therefore, the diagnosis is isorhythmic AV dissociation, ? complete AV block. The complete diagnosis in this case therefore, is sinus bradycardia with isorhythmic AV dissociation, ? complete AV block, and slow nodal arrythmia. If R–R interval were to be regular in this case, the diagnosis would have been sinus bradycardia with isorhythmic AV dissociation, ? complete AV block, and slow nodal rhythm.

Note:

Since, there is only one P wave in lead AVF, the atrial rate was obtained from the rhythm strip at the bottom (1500/39 = 39).

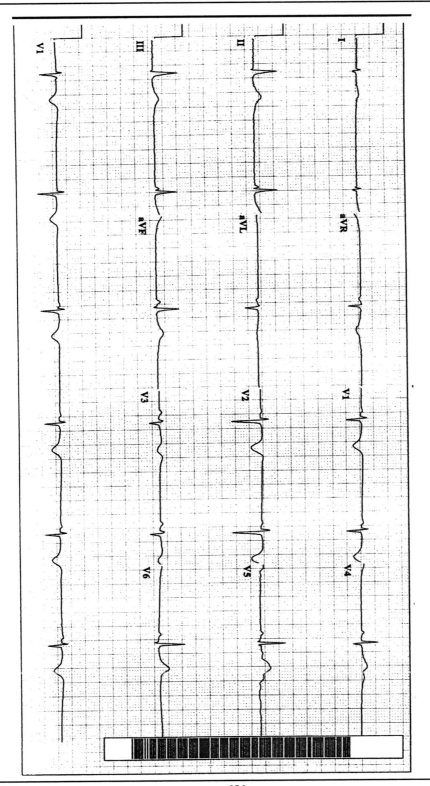

Figure 7B

Chapter 11

QRS axis

QRS axis is the net result of all electrical depolarization of the ventricular muscle. It uses the Law of parallelogram (see Fig. 1 below), which states that if two forces are pulling at the same point from two different directions, the resultant force pulls midway between them along the diagonal of a parallelogram, the two forces forming the two sides of the parallelogram. This resultant diagonal force, in the case of heart, is called the mean QRS vector or QRS axis, as seen in the frontal plane.

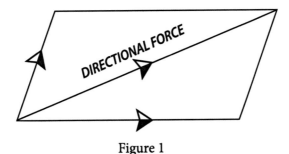

Figure 1

The location of QRS axis is described by measuring the angle between the mean QRS vector and the horizontal line drawn at the level of the heart, called the reference line (Fig. 2). The angle above the reference line is indicated with minus (-) sign and the angle below the reference line is indicated with plus (+) sign, e.g. the QRS axis in Fig. 2 is +45 degrees. A QRS axis of – 30 degrees indicates that the QRS axis lies at 30 degrees above the reference line, and +30 degrees indicates the QRS axis at 30 degrees below the reference line in the frontal plane. Normal QRS axis is located in the area between less than –30 degrees and +90 degrees (Fig. 3).

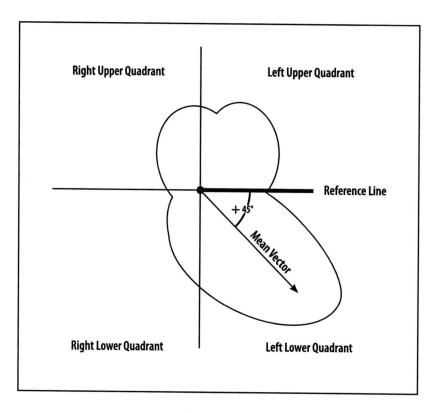

Figure 2

Figure 2: The diagram above shows a QRS axis of +45°.

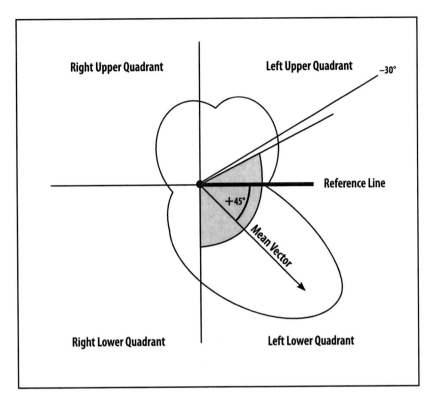

Figure 3

Figure 3: The diagram above shows a QRS axis of +45°.

Remember that the plus and minus signs used above are only to describe whether QRS axis is located in the positive or negative field of lead AVF. When the vector points downward, it gives a positive deflection in lead AVF and when the vector points upward, it gives a negative deflection in lead AVF. Hence, an angle below the reference line is located in the +ve field of lead AVF and indicated with the plus sign, and similarly, an angle above the reference line is located in the –ve field of lead AVF and indicated with the minus sign. Plus and minus signs have no mathematical value. An angle of – 60 degrees is greater than –30 degrees angle. The successive angles above the reference line moving counterclockwise are referred to as –30, –60, –90, –120, –150 and –180 degrees respectively. Similarly, the successive angles below the reference line moving clockwise would be referred to as +30, +60, +90, +120, +150 and +180 degrees respectively.

Why is it important to determine QRS axis?

In the previous illustration (Fig. 3), there are 4 quadrants. The QRS axis of most of the normal human beings is located in the left lower quadrant and called normal axis. If the QRS axis falls in any of the other 3 quadrants, it is usually considered abnormal and may indicate investigation for a heart disease, though some of the normal adults with no heart disease may have their QRS axis fall in the lower part of the upper left quadrant. Thus QRS axis is a screening marker in the diagnosis of heart disease. It may be important to point out at this time, that simply finding out the quadrant in which the mean QRS vector (called QRS axis) is located is not enough, as it gives very little information beyond being normal or abnormal, and may even give erroneous information, as the QRS axis of some of the normal hearts may lie in the lower part of the left upper quadrant. Therefore, it is important to determine the precise location of the QRS axis in terms of how many degrees above or below the reference line. If QRS mean vector is parallel to the reference line, it is called a QRS axis of zero degree.

How to determine QRS axis:

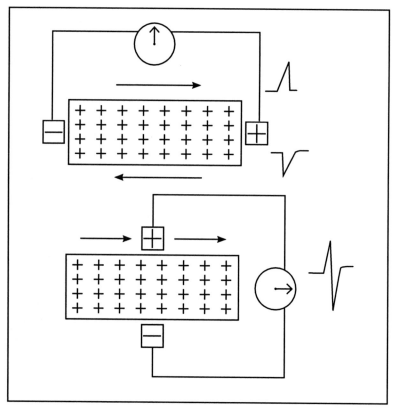

Figure 4

Let us first understand some basic rules about the relationship between mean QRS vector and the QRS morphology recorded on the EKG paper. As shown in the upper experiment in Fig. 4, there is a strip of live myocardial tissue with positive electrode on the right and the negative electrode on the left. A galvanometer is placed in the middle of these electrodes. If an electrical impulse spreads through the muscle from left to right, the positive electrode will record a positive deflection; if the direction of the impulse is reversed and it spreads from right to left, the positive electrode will record a negative deflection. Now, if the position of the electrodes is changed, as shown in the lower experiment, and the positive electrode is placed against the middle of the muscle strip, and the negative electrode opposite to the positive electrode, the electrode lead would now be perpendicular to the direction of spread of the electrical impulse (the vector). The positive electrode, in this case, would initially record a positive deflection as the impulse spreads from left to right and approaches the electrode, followed by a negative deflection as the impulse moves away from the electrode resulting in a biphasic, isoelectric deflection. Therefore, one can conclude that the QRS complexes in an EKG tracing would be isoelectric in the lead which is perpendicular to the mean vector. In other words, the mean vector would be perpendicular to the lead which shows isoelectric QRS complexes. This is the principle used to determine the QRS axis. Fig. 5 shows leads I, II and III. If the QRS complexes are isoelectric in any one of these leads, that means the mean QRS vector is located perpendicular to it, and the angle between this vector and the reference line is the angle of QRS axis.

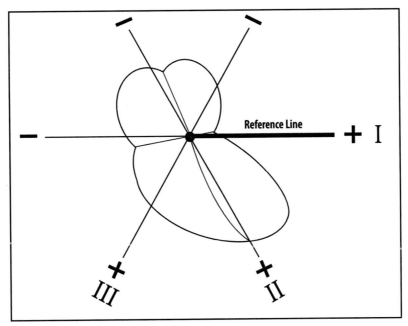

Figure 5

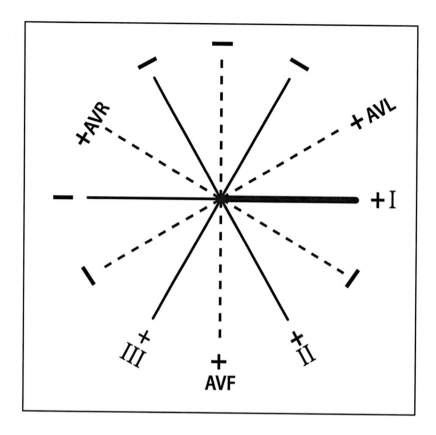

Figure 6

As shown in the hexa-axial diagram, Fig. 6, lead AVL is perpendicular to lead II, lead AVR is perpendicular to lead III, and lead AVF is perpendicular to lead I, and vice versa i.e. lead II is perpendicular to lead AVL, lead III is perpendicular to lead AVR, and lead I is perpendicular to lead AVF. Since the information is too crowded in Fig. 6, it is spread out in Fig. 7, where the diagram on the left shows mutually perpendicular relationship between leads II and AVL, and similarly the diagram on the right shows similar relationship between leads III and AVR. Both diagrams show similar relationship between leads I and AVF.

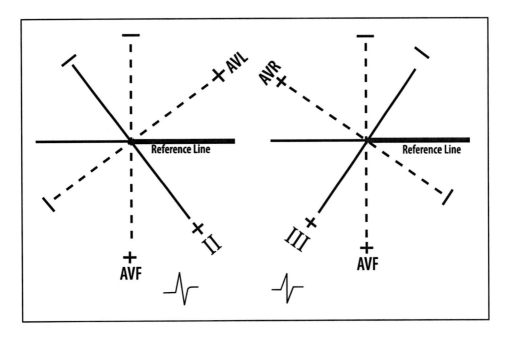

Figure 7

The determination of QRS axis is done by finding the limb lead showing isoelectric QRS complexes; the lead perpendicular to it would indicate the direction of the mean QRS vector. The angle between this perpendicular lead and the reference line is the angle of QRS axis. It is this angle which provides more useful information for clinical purposes in the diagnosis of heart disease. For example, in Fig. 7, if the QRS complexes in lead II are isoelectric, the QRS axis being perpendicular to this lead would lie along lead AVL. The angle that lead AVL makes with the reference line is the angle at which the QRS axis is located in relation to the reference line. Lead AVL makes two angles with the reference line, a 30 degree angle which is above the reference line and a 150 degree angle which is below the reference line. For the purpose of description, any angle above the reference line is designated with minus (-) sign and any angle below the reference line is designated with plus (+) sign. Therefore, in this case, the QRS axis is located at either –30 degrees or + 150 degrees from the reference line. A QRS mean vector at –30 degrees is pointed superiorly and to the left and thus located in the negative field of lead AVF, whereas a mean vector at +150 degrees is pointed inferiorly and to the right, and thus located in the positive field of lead AVF. If QRS complexes in lead AVF show more positive deflection, the QRS axis would be +150 degrees in this case, whereas if QRS complexes in lead AVF are more negative, the QRS axis would be –30 degrees. Therefore, by finding a limb lead with isoelectric QRS complexes or closest to being isoelectric, then finding the lead perpendicular to it and then looking at the lead AVF we can determine the location of the QRS axis in relation to the reference line.

In the diagram in Figure 7, if lead III is isoelectric, the lead perpendicular to it is lead AVR. The QRS axis lies along lead AVR. The angle between lead AVR and the reference line is the angle of QRS axis. However, you will note that there are two angles that lead AVR makes with the reference line (lead I); one lies below the reference line (+30 degrees) and the other lies above this line (–150 degrees). So the QRS axis is either +30 degrees or –150 degrees. If the QRS complexes in lead AVF are more negative, use the negative number, i.e. –150 degrees, andif QRS complexes are more positive in lead AVF, use the positive number, i.e. +30 degrees. Thus, to determine the QRS axis, you first find a limb lead which is isoelectric, then find the lead perpendicular to this lead and the angle between the latter and the reference line, either above or below the reference line, is the angle of QRS axis. If lead AVF is more positive, use the angle with the +ve sign, and if lead AVF is more negative, use the angle with –ve sign. It is that simple. Following this exercise further (see Fig. 7.), one would see that isoelectric QRS complexes in lead AVR would mean a QRS axis of –60 or +120 degrees. Isoelectric QRS complexes in lead AVL would mean a QRS axis of +60 or –120 degrees. Similarly, isoelectric QRS complexes in lead AVF would mean a QRS axis of zero degree, and isoelectric QRS complexes in lead I would mean QRS axis of +90 or – 90 degrees. For further clarification, see Fig. 8. Since the sum of the two numbers of each set (ignore the plus and the minus sign) equals 180, you do not have to memorize all the numbers. If you remember only one number for each limb lead, the other number has to be 180 minus this number along with the opposite sign. Therefore, you have to only remember the numbers as –30, +30, –60, +60, and + or – 90, as shown in Fig. 9. You must make a permanent mental picture of this illustration for future use, when you need to determine the QRS axis.

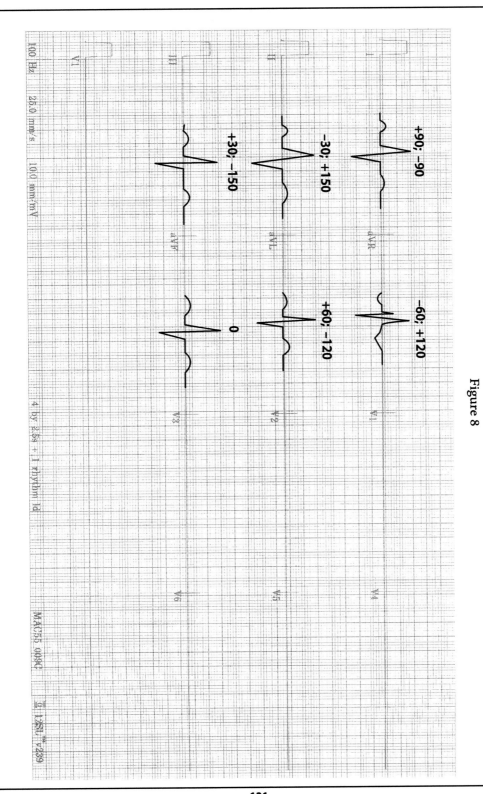

Figure 8

131

Figure 9

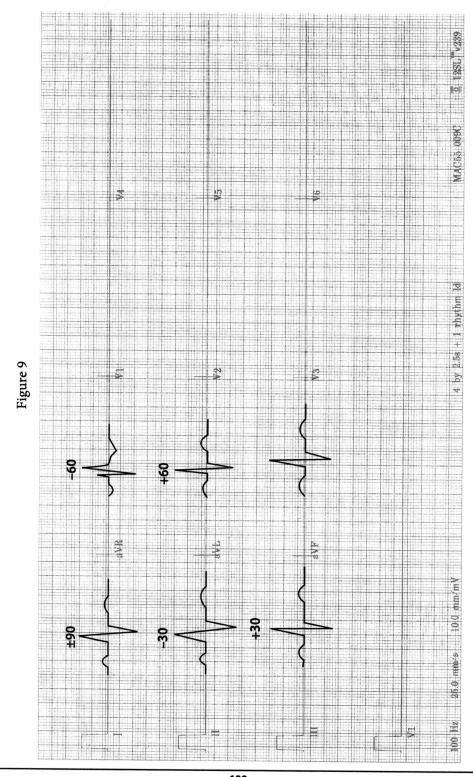

More often than not, you would find that QRS complexes are not quite isoelectric. They are either more positive or more negative. That means that the actual QRS axis in this situation is slightly different from what you might have concluded. Under these circumstances, after you find one of the limb leads which is closest to being isoelectric, first calculate the QRS axis as if it were isoelectric. Then, increase or decrease the number of degrees. If the lead used as closest to being isoelectric is lead I, II or AVL and it shows more negative deflection (area under the negative deflection greater than the area under the positive deflection), increase the number and do the same if the lead used as closest to being isoelectric is lead III or AVR and it shows more positive deflection. Do the reverse, if situation is reverse, i.e. decrease the number in case of leads I, II, and AVL if the lead shows more positive deflection, and in case of lead III and AVR if there is more negative QRS deflection. Do this regardless of whether there is a plus or minus sign in front of the number of degrees. To make it easier to remember, leads I, II and AVL are arranged in the shape of the letter "L" on the EKG paper. In these leads, the more negative the QRS complexes in the lead used, the higher the number, whereas in leads III and AVR, the more positive the QRS complexes, the higher the number. Reverse would be true in opposite situation, as explained above. This approach has been formulated by me. Therefore, it would not be inappropriate to refer to it as the "Anand approach" for the purpose of comparison with the conventional approach, which is discussed in the following pages of this chapter. The Anand approach is an attempt to make the approach more efficient and easier to understand.

NOTE:

The Anand rule states that "the more negative the QRS complexes in lead I, II, or AVL, or more positive in lead III or AVR, the higher the number, regardless of the plus or minus sign; opposite is true if situation is reverse."

The next question is by how much to increase or decrease the number. The answer is as follows. Suppose, lead AVF is more negative, and lead II is closest to being isoelectric but it is more negative than positive. This means that the QRS axis is greater than – 30 degrees. Now ask yourself whether the negative area in lead II is no greater than 1 ½ time the positive area, more than 1 ½ time but no more than twice, more than twice but no more than 2 ½ times, or greater than 2 ½ times the positive area. Increase the number by 5 if it is up to 1 ½ time, by 10 if up to twice, by 15 if up to 2 ½ times, and by 20 if it is greater than 2 ½ times the positive area. Similarly, decrease the number if lead II were to be more positive than negative. Decrease by 5 if positive area is up to 1 ½ time the negative area, by 10 if up to twice, by 15 if up to 2 ½ times, and by 20 if greater than 2 ½ times. Now suppose that lead AVF is more positive and lead I is closest to being isoelectric but it is more negative than positive. In this case the QRS axis is greater than + 90 degrees. Increase the number by 5, 10, 15 or 20 depending upon whether the negative area in lead I is up to 1 ½ time, up to twice, up to 2 ½ times, or more than 2 ½ times the positive area, respectively. Similarly, in case of lead AVL, increase the number if it is more negative and decrease if it is more positive, regardless of + or – sign in front of the number. In case of leads III and AVR, increase if it is more positive and decrease if more negative. When in doubt whether to increase or decrease by 5 or 10, use the average and thus increase or decrease by 7, and so on.

Summary:

An isoelectric lead AVF indicates zero or indeterminate QRS axis. Otherwise, look at other 5 limb leads and find an isoelectric or closest to isoelectric lead, then apply the corresponding memorized number along with the plus or minus sign (–30, +30. –60, +60, + or –90) according to lead AVF, and then use the Anand rule. Anand rule states that "the more negative the QRS complexes in lead I, II or AVL, or more positive in lead III or AVR, the higher the number, regardless of the plus or the minus sign; opposite is true if situation is reverse".

Note:

Sometimes, none of the limb leads is isoelectric or close to being isoelectric, as shown in Fig. 17B. Sometimes it may be difficult to choose between 2 limb leads for the one being closest to isoelectric. Under these circumstances, first look at lead AVF to see if it is predominantly negative or positive. If it is negative, you know that the QRS axis is with the minus number. The smallest memorized negative number is –30 degrees. So go to lead II and ask yourself whether the axis is less or more than   –30 degrees. If it is less, apply the Anand rule and find out the axis; if it is more than –30 degrees, go to lead AVR and ask yourself whether the axis is more or less than –60 degrees. If it is less than –60 degrees, it is between –30 and – 60 degrees; i.e., –45 degrees. If it is more than –60 degrees, go to lead I and ask yourself if it is more or less than –90 degrees. If it is less than –90 degrees, it is between –60 and –90 degrees; i.e., –75 degrees. If it is more, go to lead AVL to see if it is between –90 and –120 degrees or more than –120 degrees. This way, you should be able to find out the location of the QRS axis. Similarly, if lead AVF is positive, go to lead III to find out if the axis is less or more than +30 degrees. If it is more, go to lead AVL, and then onto lead I if it is more than +60 degrees. Continue on in this manner until you find the QRS axis.

Following are some examples for practice and clear understanding.

Fig. 10: The tracing shows lead II as isoelectric; lead AVF is negative. Therefore, the number is –30 degrees. The QRS axis is –30 degrees.

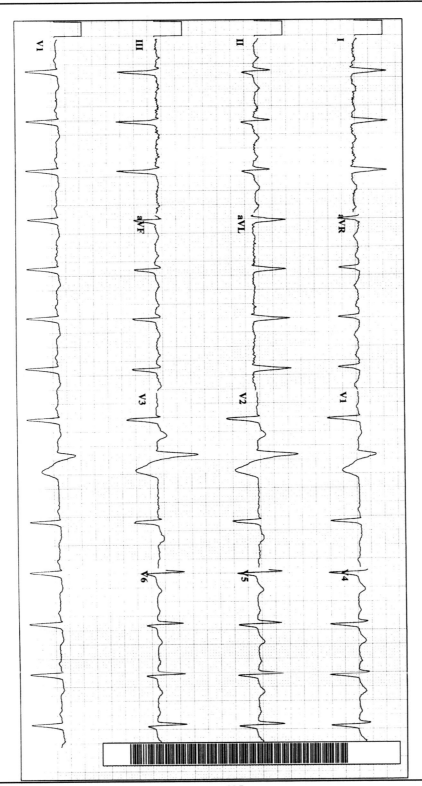

Figure 10

Fig. 11: Tracing shows lead II as closest to being isoelectric among the limb leads; lead AVF is negative. Therefore, the number is –30 degrees. But lead II is more negative than positive. Hence, according to Anand rule, you increase the number (ignore the minus sign), which means that the number should be more than 30. Since the negative area is almost twice the positive area, add 10 and that makes the QRS axis of –40 degrees. If the negative area were to be up to 1½ times the positive area, you would add 5 and that would make the QRS axis of –35 degrees.

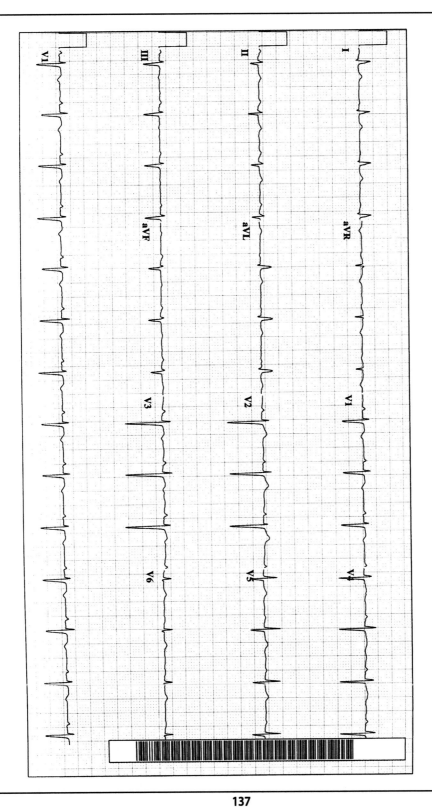

Figure 11

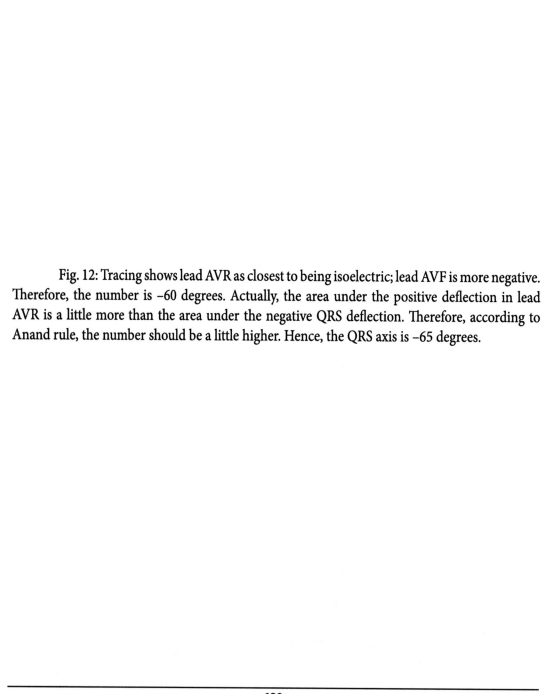

Fig. 12: Tracing shows lead AVR as closest to being isoelectric; lead AVF is more negative. Therefore, the number is –60 degrees. Actually, the area under the positive deflection in lead AVR is a little more than the area under the negative QRS deflection. Therefore, according to Anand rule, the number should be a little higher. Hence, the QRS axis is –65 degrees.

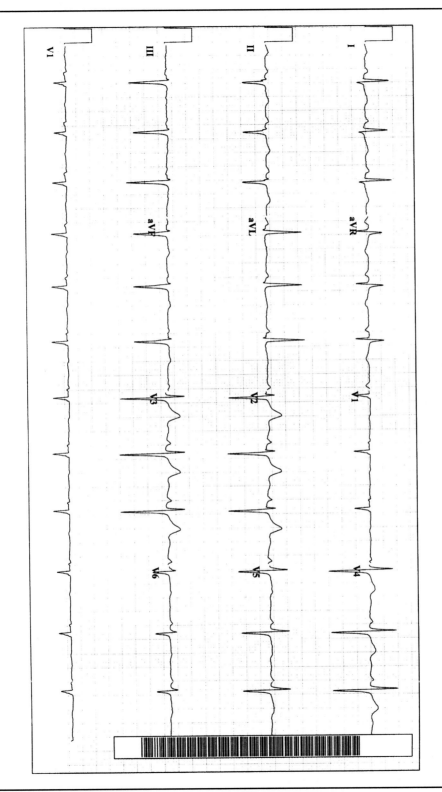

Figure 12

Fig. 13: Tracing shows lead AVL as closest to being isoelectric; lead AVF is positive. Therefore, the number is +60. Since, lead AVL is actually more negative, the actual number, according to Anand rule, should be higher. The area under the negative deflection appears to be close to twice the area under the positive deflection in lead AVL. Therefore, the actual number should be +70 degrees. Hence, the QRS axis is +70 degrees.

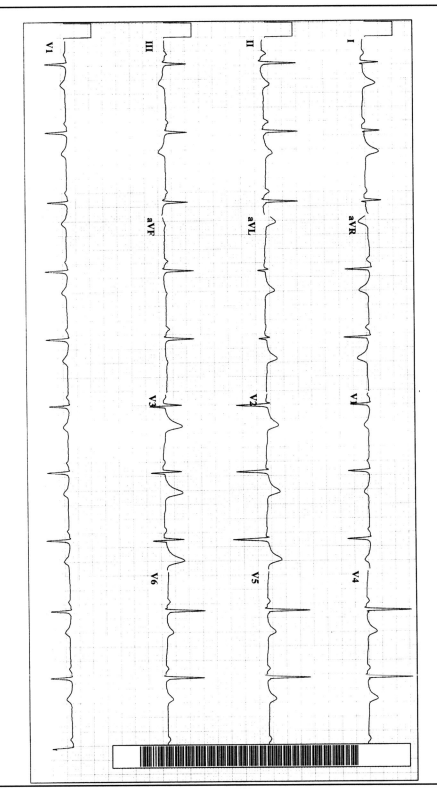

Figure 13

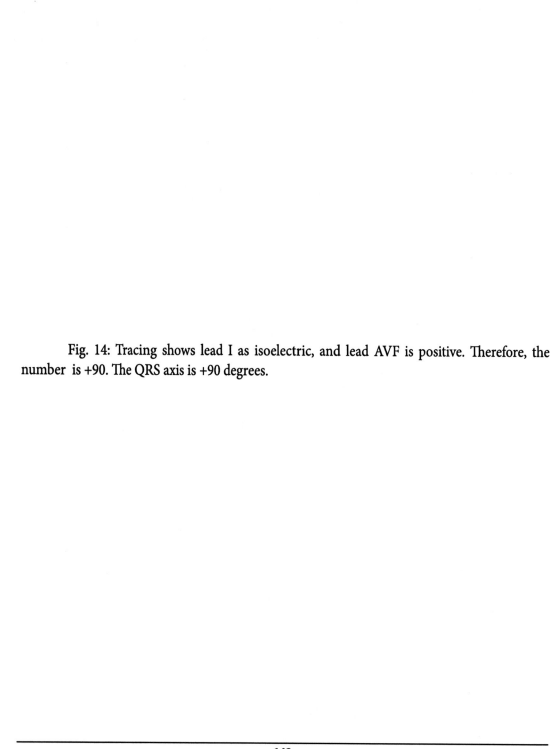

Fig. 14: Tracing shows lead I as isoelectric, and lead AVF is positive. Therefore, the number is +90. The QRS axis is +90 degrees.

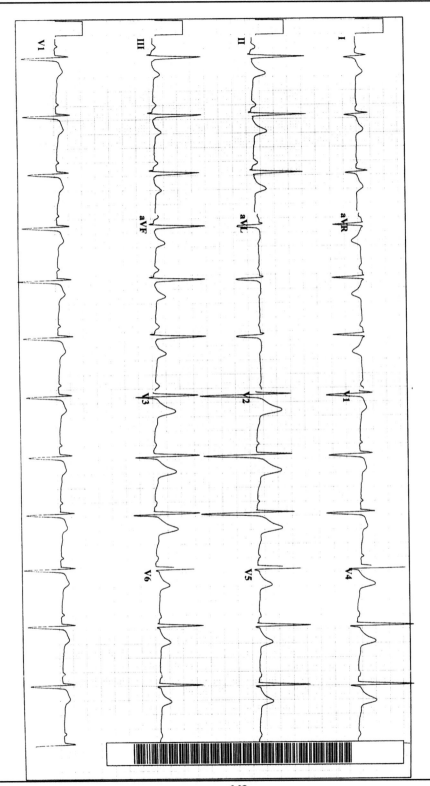

Figure 14

Fig. 15: Tracing shows lead AVR as closest to being isoelectric among the limb leads, and the lead AVF is positive. Therefore, the number should be +120 (memorized number is –60, but lead AVF is positive; therefore, 180 – 60 = 120 i.e. +120). But lead AVR is predominantly negative (almost 2 ½ times the positive deflection area).Therefore, according to Anand rule, the number should be decreased by 15. Thus, the number is +105. Hence, the QRS axis is approximately +105 degrees. If it appears to someone that the area under the negative deflection is greater than 2 1/2 times that under the positive deflection, then decrease by 20, and the QRS axis would be +100 degrees. A variation of 5 degrees between different observers is quite acceptable.

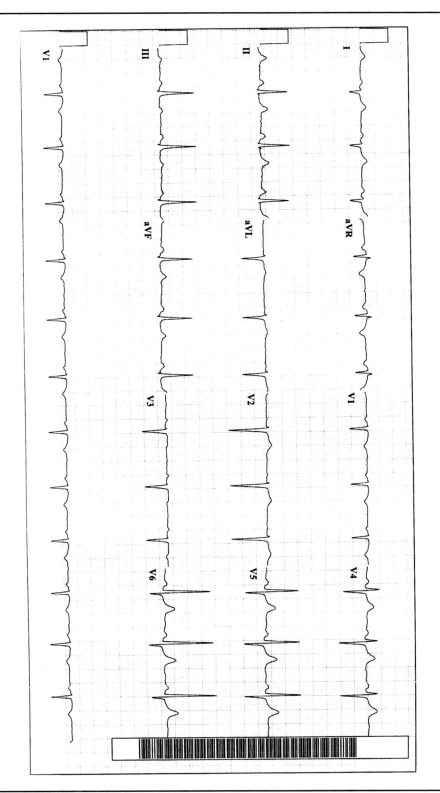

Figure 15

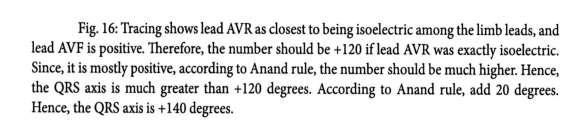

Fig. 16: Tracing shows lead AVR as closest to being isoelectric among the limb leads, and lead AVF is positive. Therefore, the number should be +120 if lead AVR was exactly isoelectric. Since, it is mostly positive, according to Anand rule, the number should be much higher. Hence, the QRS axis is much greater than +120 degrees. According to Anand rule, add 20 degrees. Hence, the QRS axis is +140 degrees.

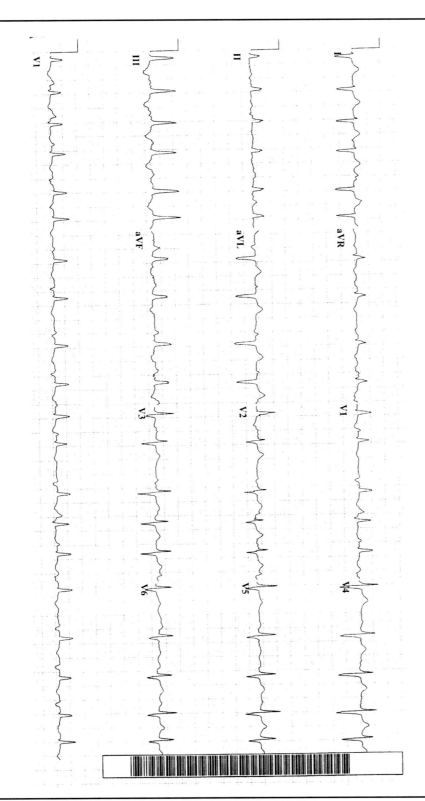

Figure 16

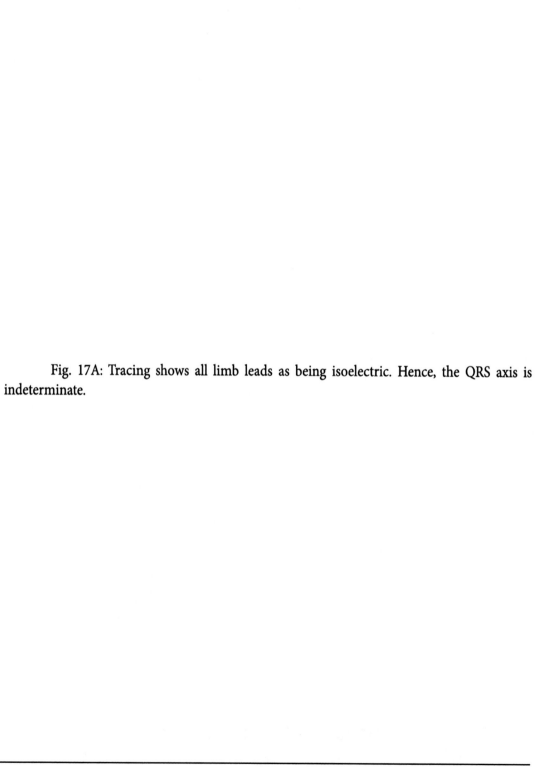

Fig. 17A: Tracing shows all limb leads as being isoelectric. Hence, the QRS axis is indeterminate.

Figure 17A

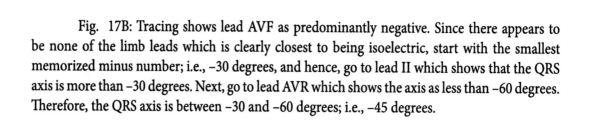

Fig. 17B: Tracing shows lead AVF as predominantly negative. Since there appears to be none of the limb leads which is clearly closest to being isoelectric, start with the smallest memorized minus number; i.e., –30 degrees, and hence, go to lead II which shows that the QRS axis is more than –30 degrees. Next, go to lead AVR which shows the axis as less than –60 degrees. Therefore, the QRS axis is between –30 and –60 degrees; i.e., –45 degrees.

Figure 17B

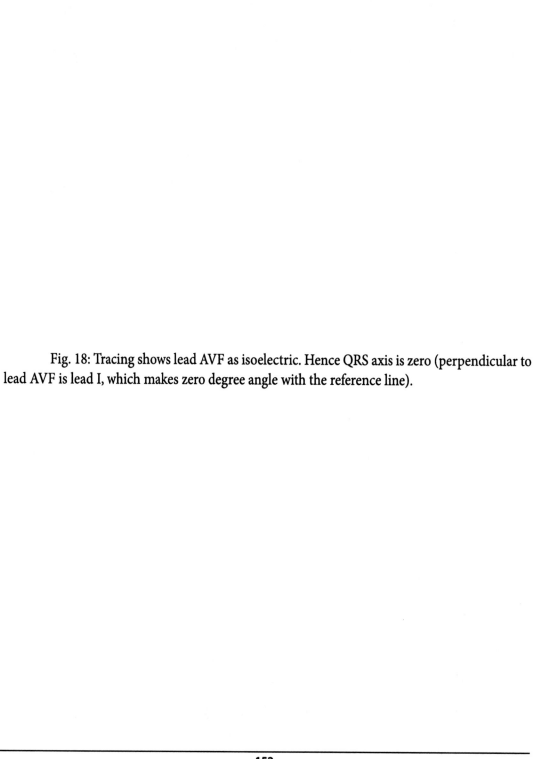

Fig. 18: Tracing shows lead AVF as isoelectric. Hence QRS axis is zero (perpendicular to lead AVF is lead I, which makes zero degree angle with the reference line).

Figure 18

Conventional method:

Select the limb lead with isoelectric or closest to isoelectric QRS complexes. Then imagine the lead perpendicular to it, and visualize the angle of QRS axis with the help of the lead AVF. Then shift this angle to the positive or negative end of the selected lead, to find the angle of QRS axis. The shift should be proportional to the ratio between the positive vs. negative components of the biphasic QRS complex. For example, if lead II is the lead closest to being isoelectric among the limb leads and it is slightly more negative, and lead AVF is also more negative, the calculated QRS axis assuming lead II to be isoelectric would be –30 degrees, but since lead II is slightly more negative, shift the QRS vector slightly toward the negative pole of lead II and thus the QRS axis in this case is slightly more than –30 degrees, which means –35 or –45 degrees, or greater, depending upon how much more the area under the negative deflection there is in lead II in comparison to its positive deflection. If, in this case, lead II were more positive, we would shift the –30 degrees angle toward the positive pole of lead II and that means the QRS axis would be less than –30 degrees. The amount of shifting should be proportional to the difference between the area under the positive and the negative deflections of this lead. Shift only slightly for small differences and a bit more if the difference is significant. Such shifting is important because a QRS axis of less than –30 degrees is normal, whereas, an axis of –30 degrees or more is abnormal.

Comparison: Anand approach Vs. Conventional approach.

The conventional approach requires imagining of the perpendicular to the nearly isoelectric limb lead, then visualizing the appropriate angle it makes with the reference line (in accordance with lead AVF), and then shifting this angle toward the positive or the negative end of the near isoelectric lead. The Anand approach avoids the imagining, visualizing, and shifting (as the calculations are already included in the memorized numbers), and instead, goes straight to the numbers and applies Anand rule to increase or decrease the number. Thus, the Anand approach makes the process more efficient, especially when none of the limb leads is biphasic, as shown in Fig. 17B.

Normal QRS axis lies between less than –30 degrees and +90 degrees. An axis of –30 degrees or greater but less than –45 degrees is called LAD (left axis deviation). A QRS axis of –45 degrees or greater up to –180 degrees indicates LAHB (left anterior hemiblock). A QRS axis of more than +90 degrees is called RAD (right axis deviation) up to +110 degrees. A right axis deviation of greater than + 110 degrees indicates LPHB (left posterior hemiblock). It should be noted that in the presence of left bundle branch block (LBBB), a QRS axis of –30 degrees or greater is interpreted as left axis deviation (LAD) and not as LAHB when it is greater than –45 degrees. Similarly, a QRS axis of greater than +110 degrees in the presence of RBBB or RVH is called RAD, not LPHB.

Recommended steps:

Having understood the above approach, now it is time to implement the basics into a practical format to follow. If you want to know the precise location of the QRS axis, you can follow the steps mentioned above. However, if the only purpose is to find out whether the QRS axis is normal or there is LAD, RAD, LAHB or LPHB, I would suggest looking at lead AVF first. If this lead is isoelectric, the QRS axis is zero degree. If this lead is more negative, we know that the QRS axis lies in the negative field of lead AVF, which means that the QRS axis is going to be a minus number, i.e. –30, –60, – 90 degrees and so on. Similarly, if lead AVF is more positive, the QRS axis lies in the positive field of lead AVF, which means that the QRS axis is going to be a plus number, i.e. +30, +60, +90, +120 degrees and so on. Therefore, if lead AVF is negative, the next step would be to go to lead II. If lead II is isoelectric, the QRS axis is –30 degrees and hence it is LAD. If lead II is more positive, the QRS axis is less than –30 degrees and hence it is normal. If lead II is a little more negative, QRS axis is slightly more than –30 degrees but less than –45 degrees and hence, again it is LAD. If lead II is a lot more negative with only a small positive deflection, the QRS axis is –45 degrees or greater and therefore it indicates LAHB (left anterior hemi-block). If you are not sure whether lead II is negative enough to be –45 degrees, then look at lead AVR and if lead AVR is isoelectric or close to being isoelectric, that means QRS axis is –60 degrees or close to it but definitely greater than –45 degrees and hence it indicates LAHB. Thus, between leads II and AVR one can be reasonably certain whether we are dealing with LADor LAHB. Looking at lead AVF and then leads II and AVR should be enough to distinguish between a normal QRS axis, LAD and LAHB when lead AVF is more negative. When lead AVF is more positive, go to lead I. If lead I is more positive or isoelectric, it is a normal QRS axis (because, an isoelectric lead I means a QRS axis of + 90 degrees in the presence of positive lead AVF and that is normal; a more positive lead I means an axis of less than + 90 degrees in the presence of positive AVF lead, and that is also normal). If lead I is more negative, it is RAD or LPHB. To differentiate, go to lead AVR. If lead AVR is isoelectric (it means + 120 degrees) or more positive (it means greater than +120 degrees), it is LPHB, otherwise RAD.

To summarize, if lead AVF is more negative, go to lead II and then to lead AVR if needed; if lead AVF is more positive, go to lead I and then to lead AVR if needed, and you will have your diagnosis. However, one should remember that LBBB (left bundle branch block) can produce a QRS axis of greater than –45 degrees; therefore, in the presence of LBBB and QRS axis ≥–30 degrees, always call it LAD even when QRS axis is greater than –45 degrees. Similarly, RVH as well as RBBB can produce a QRS axis greater than +110 degrees; therefore, in the presence of RBBB or RVH and a QRS axis > +90 degrees, always call it RAD even when the QRS axis is greater than +110 degrees, instead of calling it LPHB.

Pattern reading:

This approach involves simply reading the QRS morphology to find QRS axis. If the QRS complexes in lead AVF are negative (or more negative than positive), go to lead II. If lead II is positive or more positive than negative, it is a normal QRS axis. If lead II is isoelectric or more negative, it is left axis deviation (LAD). If lead II is mostly negative and shows very little or no positive deflection, it is left anterior hemiblock (LAHB). When lead AVF is positive (or more positive than negative), go to lead I. If lead I is positive, more positive than negative, or isoelectric, it is a normal QRS axis. If lead I is more negative than positive, it is either right axis deviation (RAD) or left posterior hemiblock (LPHB). Now, go to lead AVR and if that lead is isoelectric or more positive, it is left posterior hemiblock (LPHB), otherwise it is RAD. LAHB pattern should be interpreted as LAD in the presence of LBBB, and LPHB pattern should be interpreted as RAD in the presence of RBBB or RVH.

NOTE:

When QRS complexes are nearly isoelectric in all of the limb leads, the QRS axis is considered indeterminate (see figure 17A).

Some examples of quick diagnostic QRS axis reading are as follows. Just remember to go straight to lead II when lead AVF is negative, and to lead I when lead AVF is positive. It is that simple.

Fig. 19: Tracing shows a predominantly negative lead AVF (the QRS axis is going to be with the minus sign). Therefore, next go to lead II. It is more positive. Therefore, the axis is less than –30 degree, which is normal. QRS axis is normal.

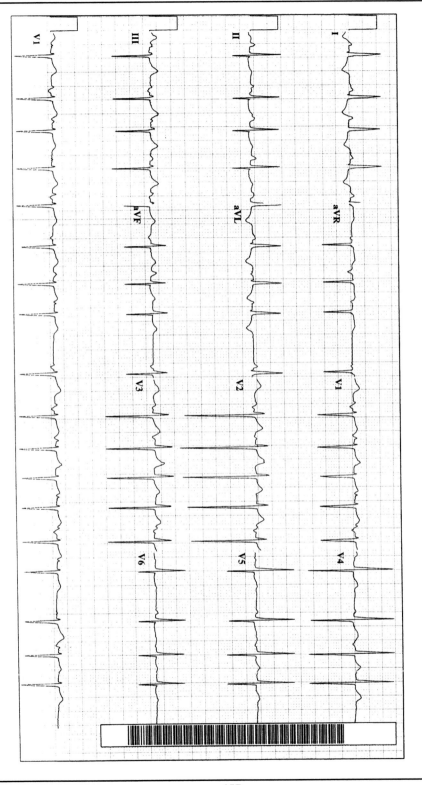

Figure 19

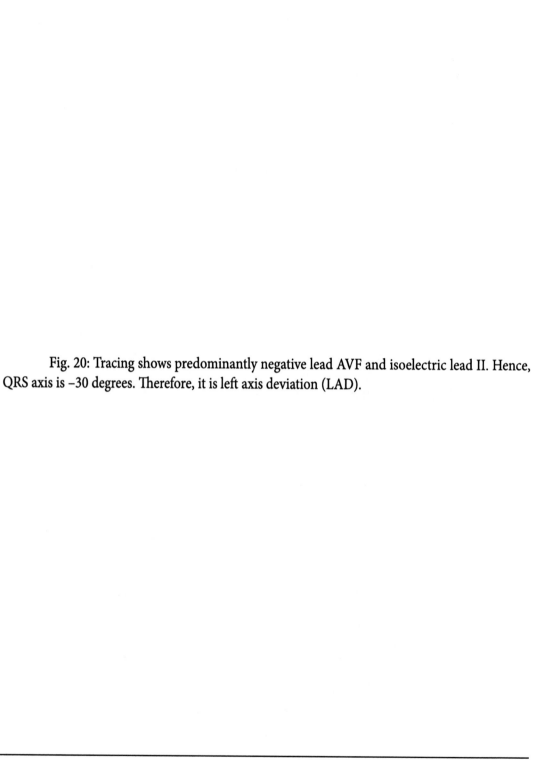

Fig. 20: Tracing shows predominantly negative lead AVF and isoelectric lead II. Hence, QRS axis is –30 degrees. Therefore, it is left axis deviation (LAD).

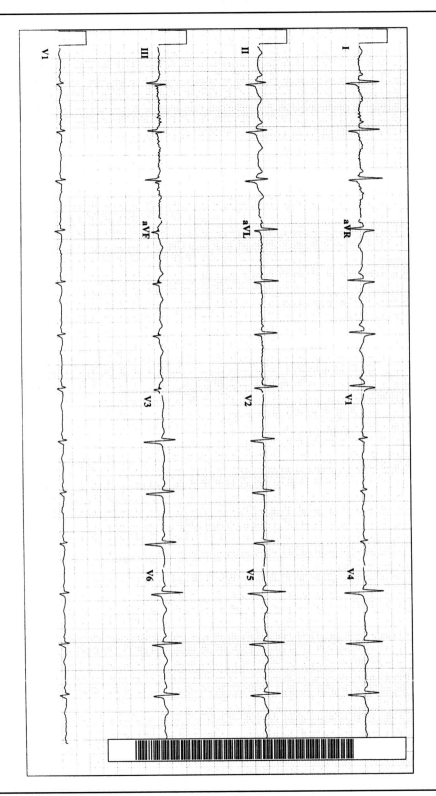

Figure 20

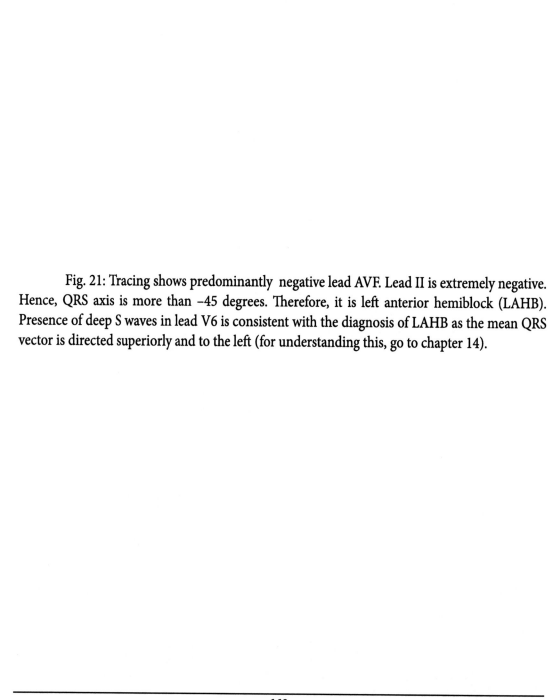

Fig. 21: Tracing shows predominantly negative lead AVF. Lead II is extremely negative. Hence, QRS axis is more than −45 degrees. Therefore, it is left anterior hemiblock (LAHB). Presence of deep S waves in lead V6 is consistent with the diagnosis of LAHB as the mean QRS vector is directed superiorly and to the left (for understanding this, go to chapter 14).

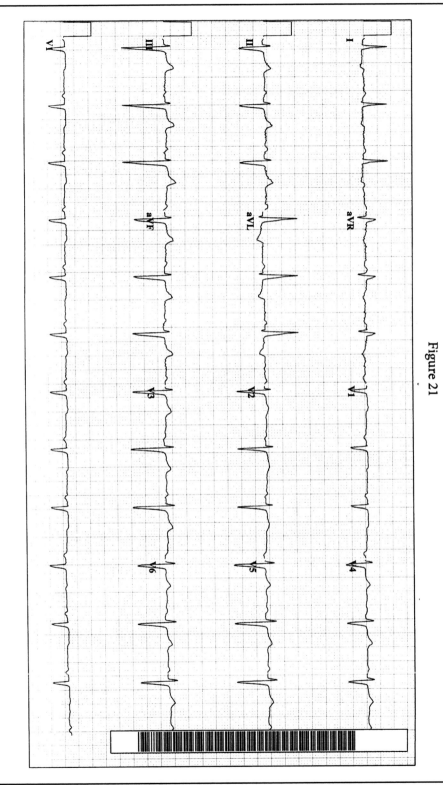

Figure 21

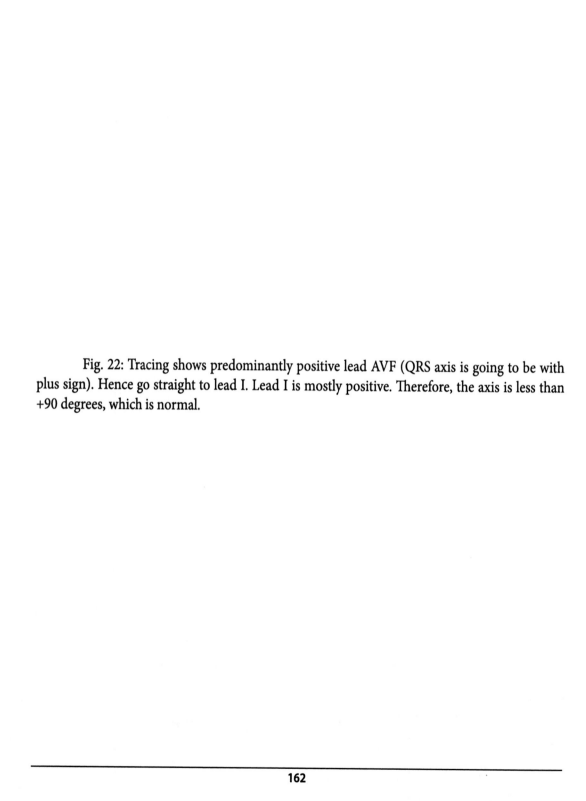

Fig. 22: Tracing shows predominantly positive lead AVF (QRS axis is going to be with plus sign). Hence go straight to lead I. Lead I is mostly positive. Therefore, the axis is less than +90 degrees, which is normal.

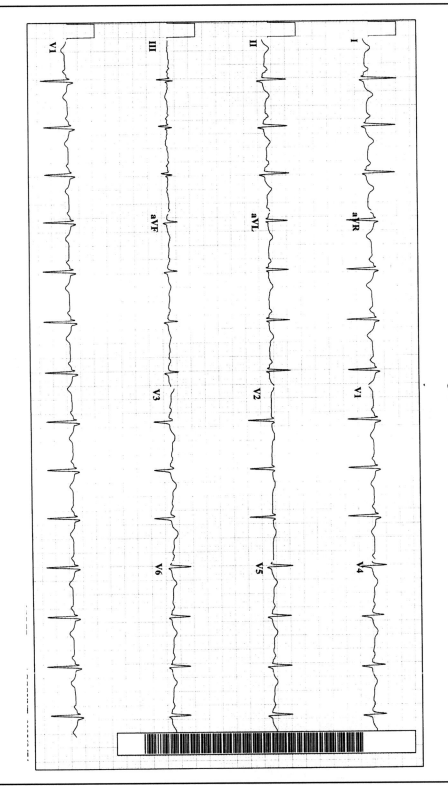

Figure 22

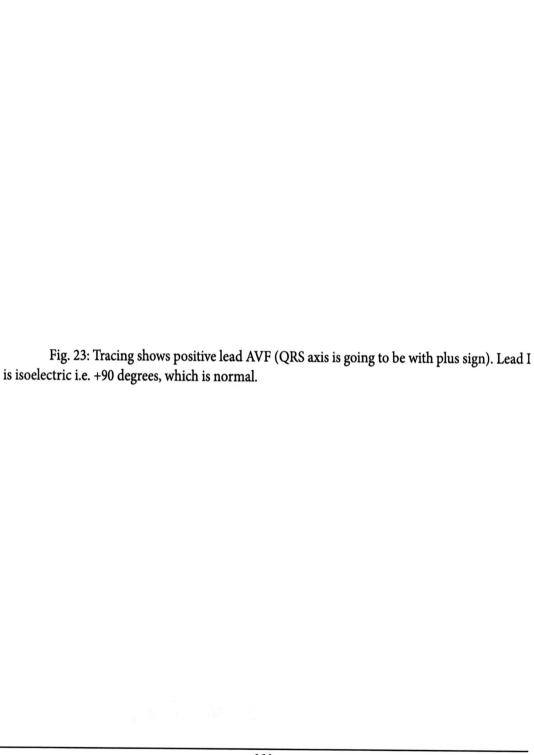

Fig. 23: Tracing shows positive lead AVF (QRS axis is going to be with plus sign). Lead I is isoelectric i.e. +90 degrees, which is normal.

Figure 23

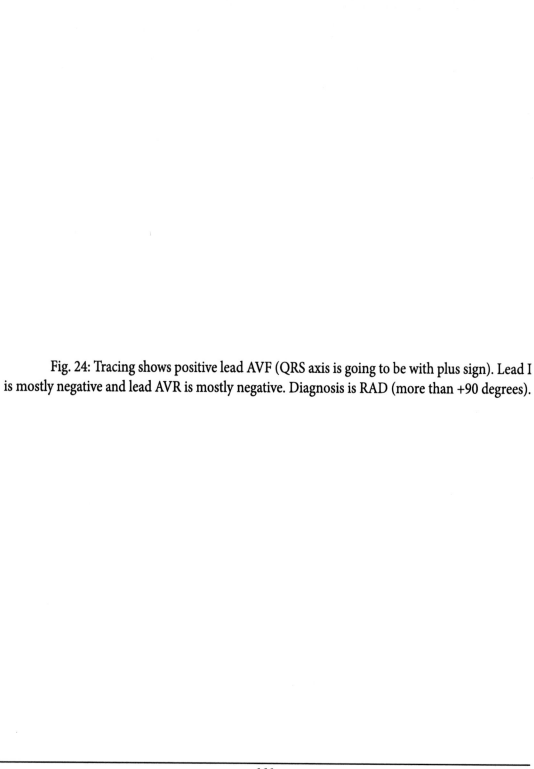

Fig. 24: Tracing shows positive lead AVF (QRS axis is going to be with plus sign). Lead I is mostly negative and lead AVR is mostly negative. Diagnosis is RAD (more than +90 degrees).

Figure 24

Fig. 25: Tracing shows positive lead AVF (QRS axis is going to be with plus sign). Lead I is mostly negative and lead AVR is isoelectric. Therefore, the QRS axis is +120 degrees. Diagnosis is Left posterior hemiblock (LPHB).

Conclusions (see Summary Chart on page 170):

When lead AVF is negative, go to lead II. If lead II is more positive, the QRS axis is normal; if lead II is isoelectric or a bit more negative, it is LAD; if it is mostly negative, it is LAHB.

When lead AVF is positive, go to lead I. If lead I is more positive or isoelectric, the QRS axis is normal; if lead I is more negative, it is RAD; if lead I is mostly negative, it is RAD or LPHB. If lead AVR is isoelectric (+120 degrees) or more positive, it is LPHB, otherwise it is RAD.

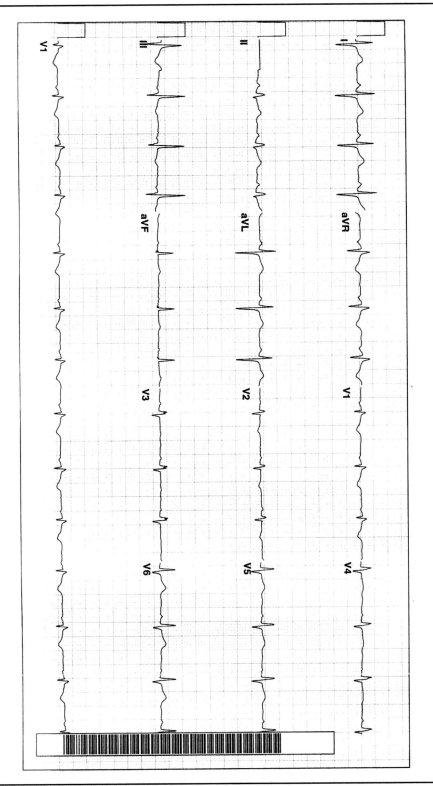

Figure 25

Summary Charts

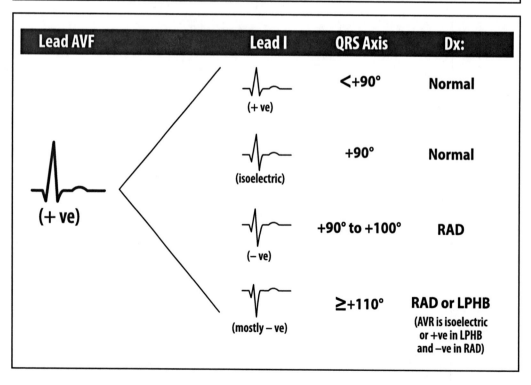

12 Lead Scanning

During this exercise, we look at each lead separately, one by one, while paying attention to the following.

Lead I:

ST segment depression or T wave inversion in this lead is always abnormal.

Inverted P and inverted T waves with negative QRS complexes indicates arm leads interchange or Dextrocardia.

Precordial leads will remain unchanged in the case of arm leads interchange, but will be abnormal in the case of Dextrocardia (Read chapter 20 for details).

Lead II:

ST segment depression or T wave inversion in this lead is always abnormal.

A peaked P wave with amplitude of greater than 2.5 mm suggests right atrial enlargement (RAE).

A notched P wave (≥ 0.12 sec. in duration) with two tops being at least 0.04 sec. apart (see page 222) suggests left atrial enlargement (LAE).

Lead III:

T wave inversion in this lead is not always abnormal.

Q wave which decreases in depth and width with inspiration is benign.

Lead AVR:

P and T waves are normally inverted in this lead, and QRS complexes are predominantly negative.

In case of arm lead interchange, lead AVR becomes lead AVL on the EKG tracing.

Lead AVL:

An upright T wave is normally expected. An inverted T wave would be considered normal only if P wave in this lead is also inverted. It is called inverted T with concordant P wave. If T wave is inverted with discordant P wave, i.e. P wave is upright, that T wave is abnormal according to David Littmann.

In case of arm lead interchange, lead AVL becomes lead AVR on the EKG tracing.

Lead AVF:

An upright T wave is normally expected. Inverted T waves in this lead are abnormal until proven otherwise.

ST depression is always abnormal.

A Q wave of 0.04 second duration or greater should suggest the possibility of an inferior myocardial infarction. However, a decrease in depth and width of Q wave with inspiration indicates that it is normal.

Leads V1 – 6:

A biphasic P wave in lead V1 with deep (≥ 1.0mm) and wide negative component with total duration of 0.12 second or greater indicates left atrial enlargement.

RSR´ or rsr´ in lead V1 in the presence of an S wave in lead I or lead V6, or both, indicates right bundle branch block. In the absence of such S wave, this morphology is considered normal. QRS interval of 0.09 – 0.11 second is consistent with incomplete RBBB, whereas a QRS interval of 0.12 second or greater suggests complete RBBB. QRS interval of <0.09 sec. suggests normal morphology.

The height of R wave should progressively increase from lead V1 to lead V6. A lack of progression of height of R wave from lead V1 to V3 is normal in a tall and thin person, but may otherwise indicate presence of anterior myocardial infarction. Absence of R wave in lead V2 indicates possible anteroseptal myocardial infarction.

T wave inversion in lead V1 is normal. T wave inversion in lead V2 may be normal in women. T wave inversion in leads V4 – 6 should be regarded as abnormal. Tall and peaking T waves in precordial leads or limb leads suggest hyperkalemia. Presence of prominent U waves (details on page 242) suggests hypokalemia.

ST segment depression in any lead indicates ischemia or digitalis effect. ST elevation in any lead suggests early repolarization, injury, or pericarditis.

Diffuse concave ST elevation, without reciprocal changes, with PR segment depression is diagnostic of acute pericarditis.

Check for any other abnormalities such as delta waves (see page 257), Osborn waves (J waves) of hypothermia (see page 244), or electronic pacemaker artifacts (spikes).

Chapter 13

Myocardial Infarction

If you put a string around a coronary vessel supplying blood to the live myocardial tissue, and make a single knot around it, and then start tightening the knot gradually, you will soon find that the T wave of the EKG becomes inverted (Fig. 1A), suggesting ischemia of the myocardium. At this point, if you undo the knot, the inverted T wave reverts back to normal, indicating reversible nature of the ischemia and the associated T wave changes. Now, if you restart tightening the knot, and continue to tighten after the T wave inversion has appeared, you will notice that the elevation of the ST segment appears in addition to the T wave inversion (Fig. 1B). This indicates injury to the myocardium with release of intracellular enzymes into the blood stream. This change in ST-T morphology is reversible, if the knot is untied quickly. Otherwise, continuing the tightening of the knot will lead to loss of R wave and appearance of Q wave, suggestive of myocardial necrosis, which is irreversible. It is called myocardial infarction (Fig. 1C). It should be noted that the presence of an injury pattern (ST elevation) in the EKG of a patient is always associated with some degree of underlying myocardial necrosis. It is called ST elevation myocardial infarction (STEMI). In the case of subendocardial injury, there is depression of ST segment (Fig. 1D), which, if associated with elevation of serum enzymes (CPK, Troponin), is referred to as non-ST elevation myocardial infarction.

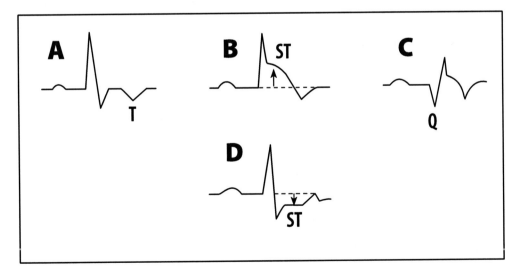

Figure 1

An injury to the myocardium on the inferior surface of the heart is associated with the above mentioned changes in inferior leads (leads II, III, AVF). The changes of injury to the interventricular septum appear in leads V1 and V2, and injury to the anterolateral surface of the heart results in above changes in leads V3, V4, V5 and V6. A lateral wall injury will be witnessed in leads V5, V6, and leads I and AVL. ST depression in leads V1 and V2 associated with tall R waves suggests acute posterior infarct. Since, the infarction is on the posterior surface of the left ventricle, an electrode placed posteriorly on the chest wall will reveal ST elevation and loss of R wave, whereas, the electrodes placed anteriorly (V1, V2) will reveal reciprocal changes (ST depression and tall R waves). Infero-posterior injury will be seen in the form of ST elevation in inferior leads and ST depression in leads V1 and V2. ST elevation of 1.0 mm or greater in leads V1 – V2 in the presence of ST elevation in inferior leads suggests possible right ventricular infarct. In such cases, additional lead V4R is very helpful. ST elevation of 1.0 mm or greater in lead V4R is diagnostic of RV infarct. However, absence of such ST elevation does not exclude this possibility. It is therefore prudent to check lead V4R in patients with ST elevation in inferior leads and abnormal neck vein pulsations ('A' and 'V' waves) and/or engorged jugular veins to evaluate the possibility of RV infarct, even when the precordial leads appear to be normal.

NOTE:

Loss of "r" waves in leads V1 and V2 indicates anteroseptal myocardial infarction. However, LBBB is also associated with diminution or loss of "r" waves in these leads, because the septal activation occurs from right to left in LBBB, and therefore the instantaneous mean vector is directed away from the right Precordial leads. It is for this reason that the diagnosis of anteroseptal myocardial infarction cannot be made in the presence of LBBB.

Some examples of different infarctions are illustrated on the following pages.

Fig. 2: The tracing shows inverted T waves in inferior leads (II, III, AVF) and anterolateral leads (V2 – 6). Findings suggest inferior and anterolateral ischemia.

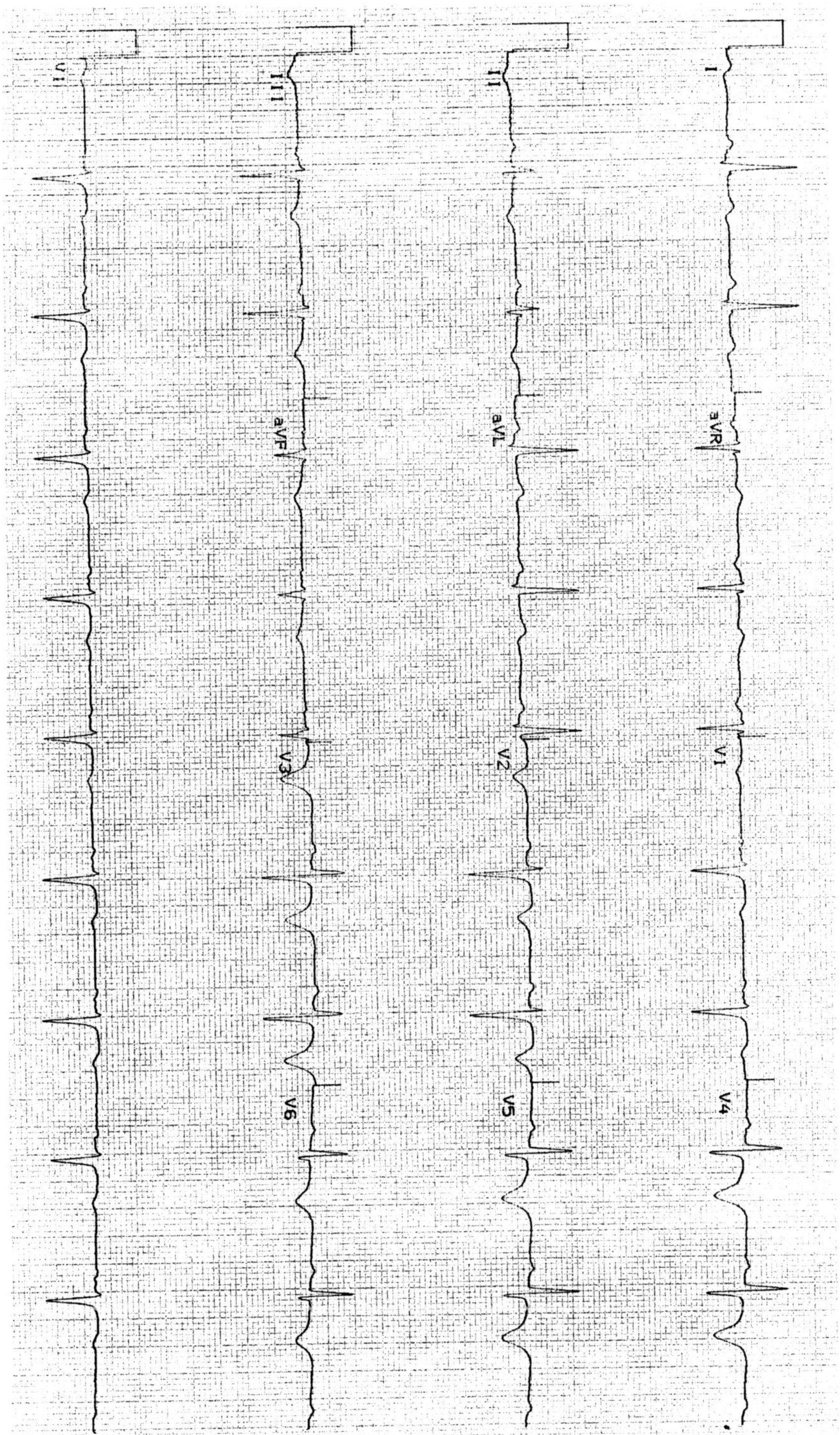

Figure 2

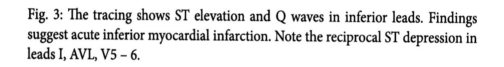

Fig. 3: The tracing shows ST elevation and Q waves in inferior leads. Findings suggest acute inferior myocardial infarction. Note the reciprocal ST depression in leads I, AVL, V5 – 6.

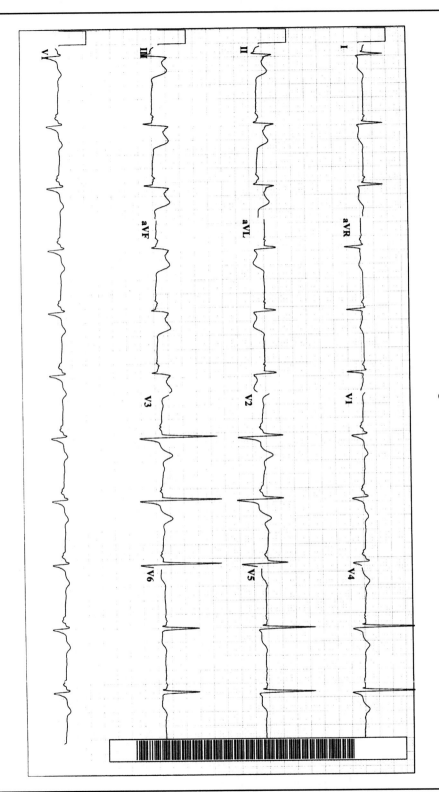

Figure 3

Fig. 4: The tracing shows ST elevation in leads V2 - 3, loss of R wave in V2, and Q waves in V3. These findings suggest acute anteroseptal myocardial infarction. There is ST depression in inferior leads and V4 – 6, suggesting inferior and lateral ischemia. ST elevation in leads I and AVL is reciprocal to ST depression in inferior leads.

Figure 4

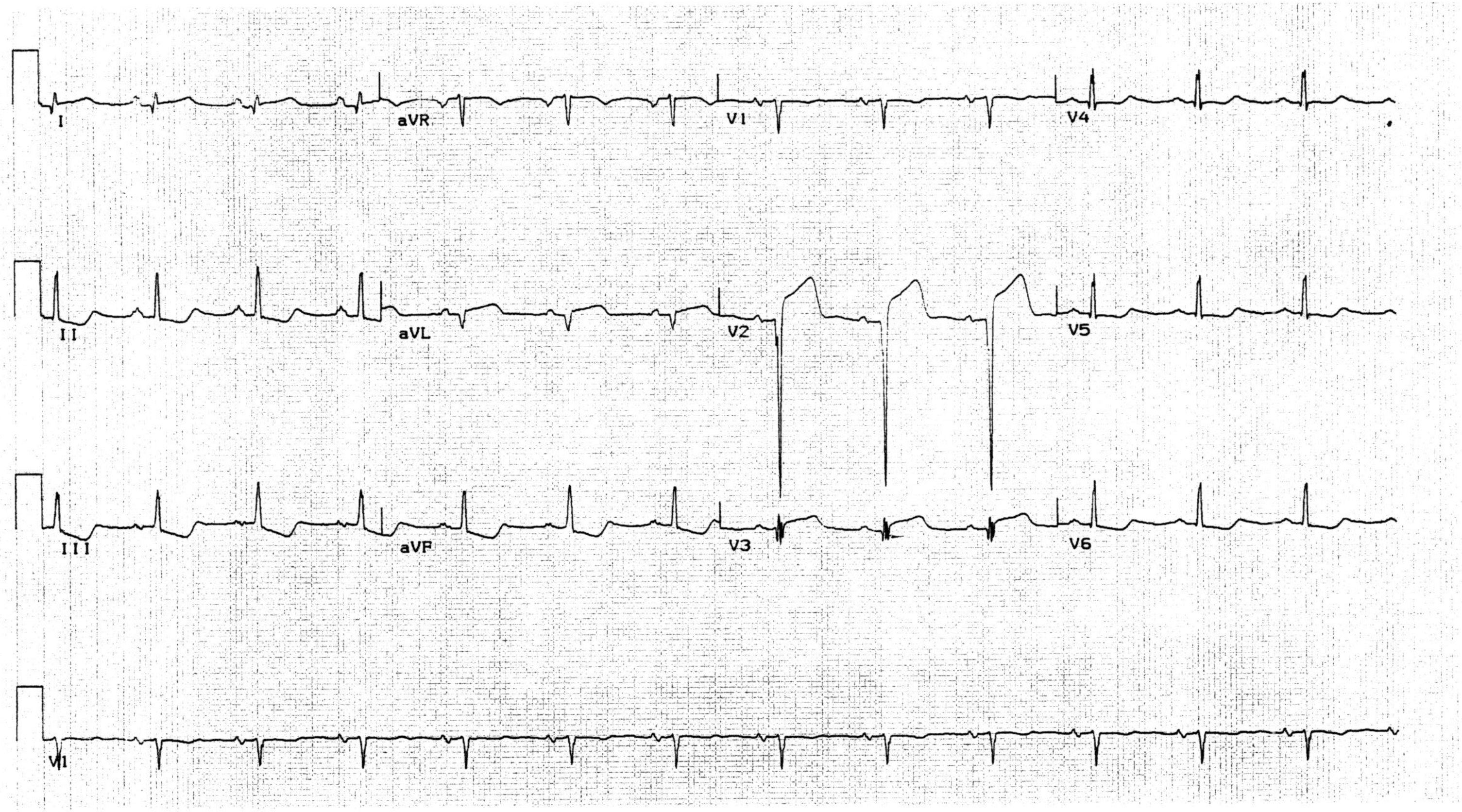

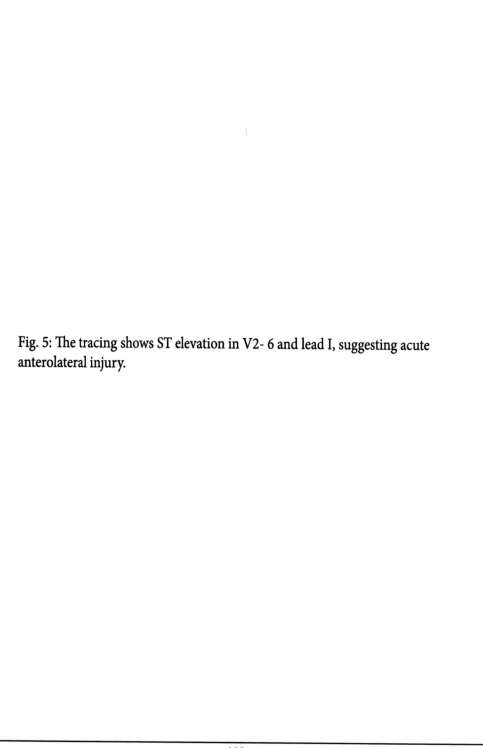

Fig. 5: The tracing shows ST elevation in V2- 6 and lead I, suggesting acute anterolateral injury.

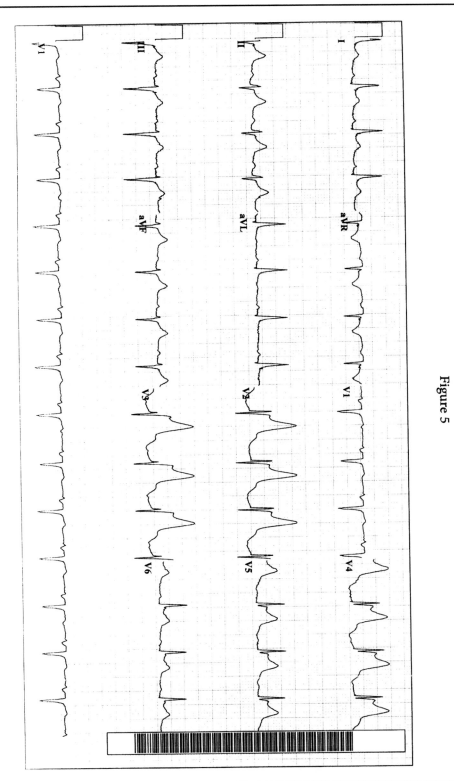

Figure 5

Fig. 6: The tracing shows ST elevation in inferior leads and leads V4 – 6, consistent with acute inferior and lateral injury. ST depression in V1 -2 suggests posterior wall injury as an extension of the inferior injury. Thus, the diagnosis is acute infero-posterior and lateral injury. ST depression in lead AVL is a reciprocal change against ST elevation in inferior leads.

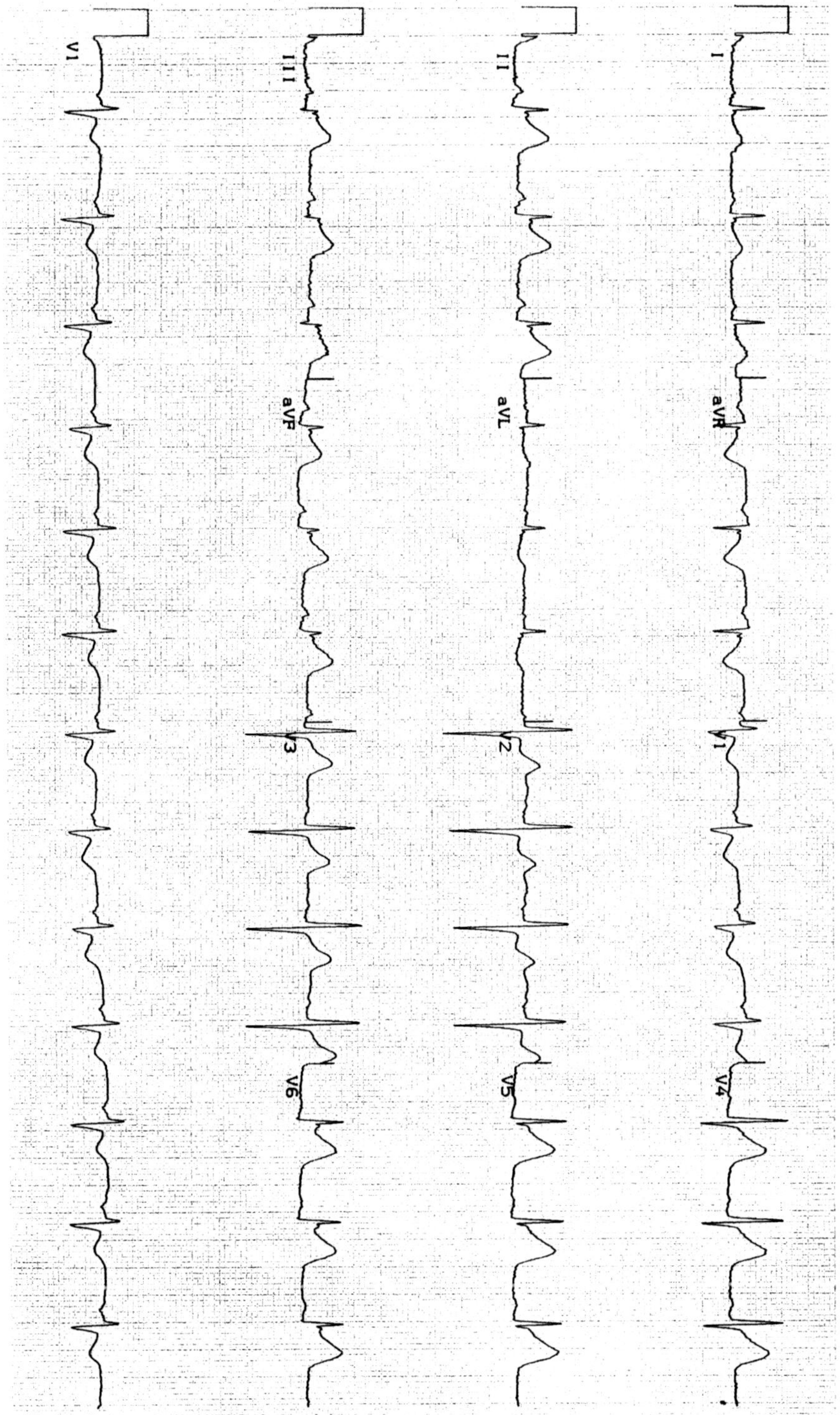

Figure 6

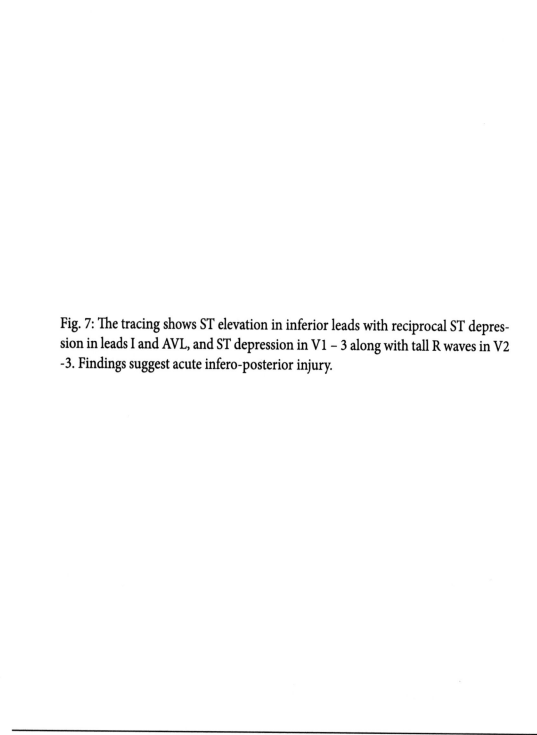

Fig. 7: The tracing shows ST elevation in inferior leads with reciprocal ST depression in leads I and AVL, and ST depression in V1 – 3 along with tall R waves in V2 -3. Findings suggest acute infero-posterior injury.

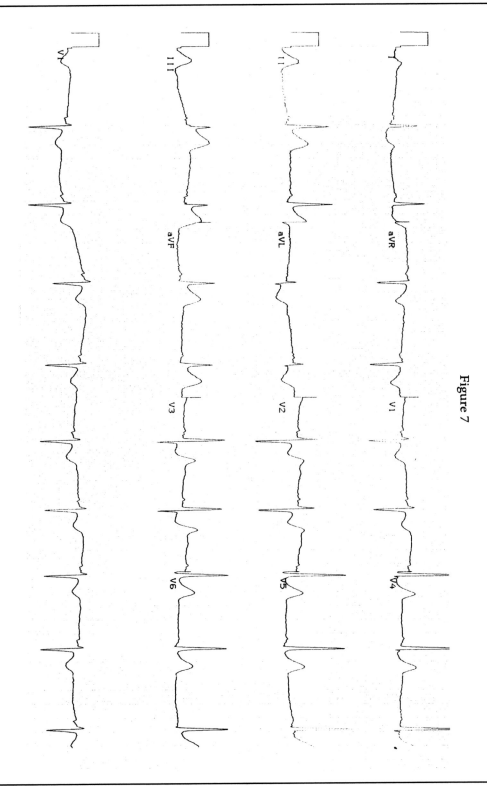

Figure 7

Fig. 8: The tracing shows ST elevation in V2 – 4, loss of R in V2 – 3, Q in V4, and abnormal T wave inversion in inferior and lateral precordial leads (V5 – 6), consistent with acute anterior myocardial infarction and infero-lateral ischemia.

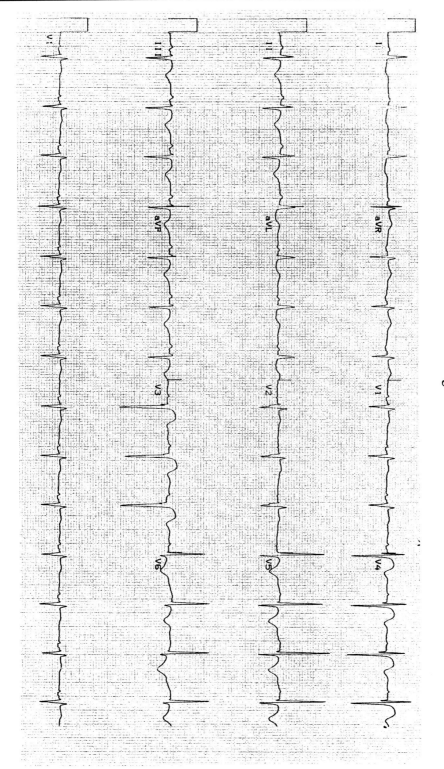

Figure 8

Fig. 9: The tracing shows ST elevation in leads I and AVL and ST depression in leads III, AVF, and V3 – 6. Findings suggest antero-lateral and inferior ischemia. ST elevation in leads I and AVL is a reciprocal change to ST depression in inferior leads, because lateral Precordial leads show ischemic changes and leads I and AVL are also lateral leads with higher location.

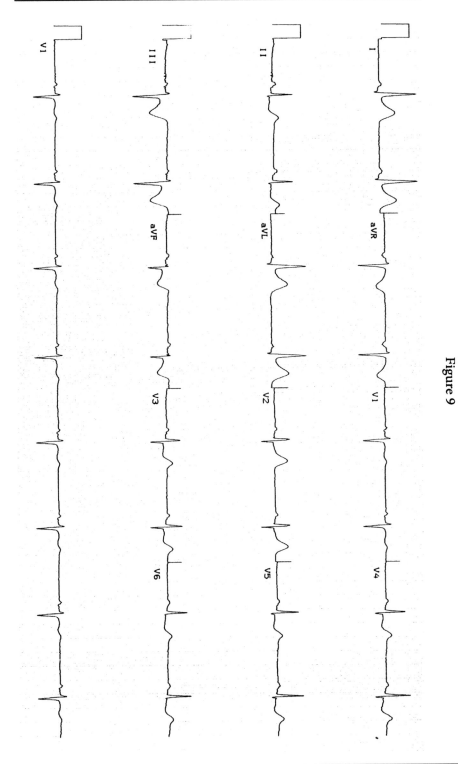

Figure 9

Fig. 10: The tracing shows loss of R wave in right precordial leads (V1 -3). Diagnosis is anteroseptal myocardial infarction, age unknown.

Figure 10

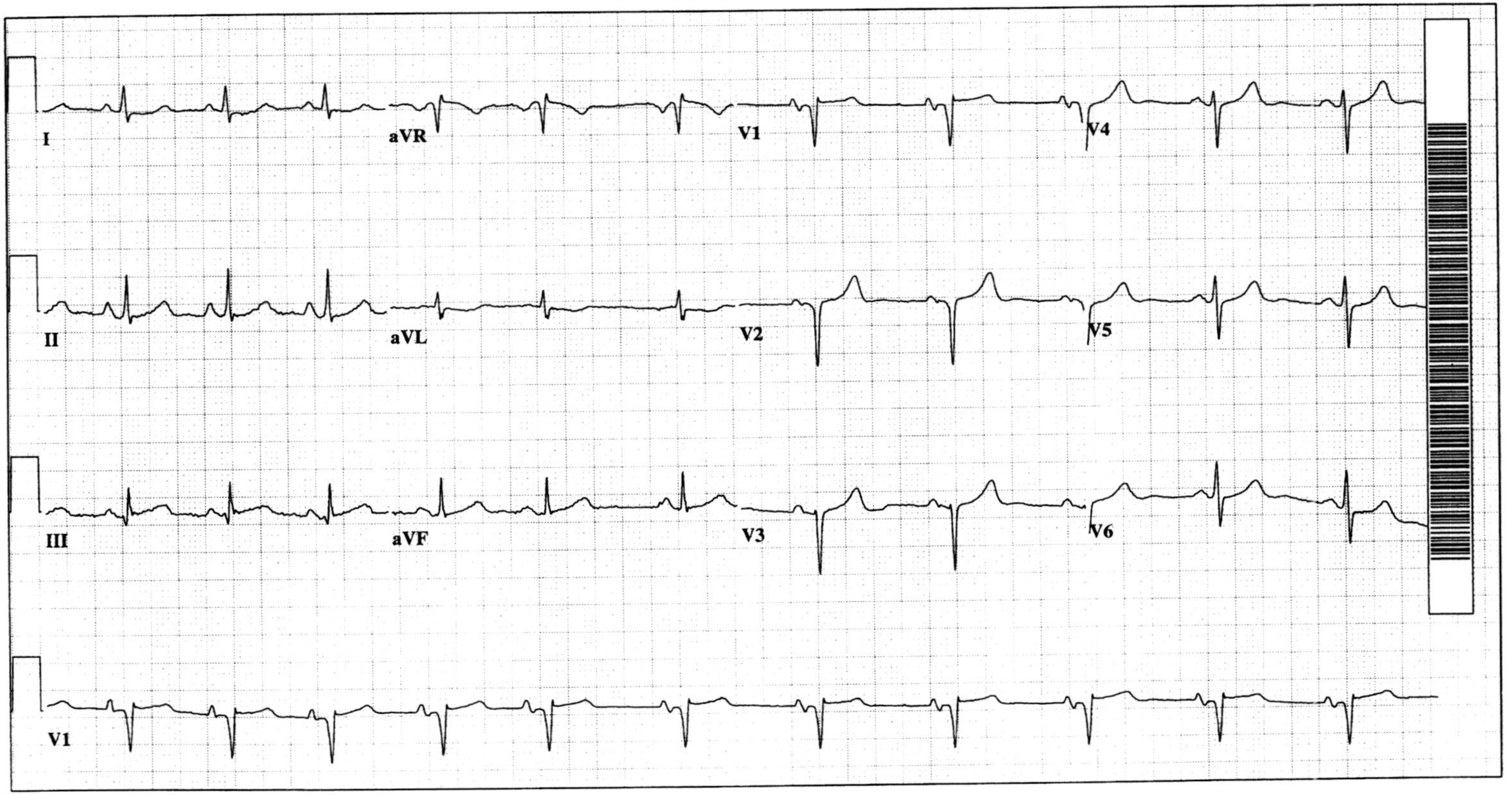

Fig. 11. : The tracing shows a "W" pattern QRS complex in lead AVF. It is always highly suspicious of inferior myocardial infarction. Since, there is no ST elevation, the age of infarction is unknown.

Figure 11

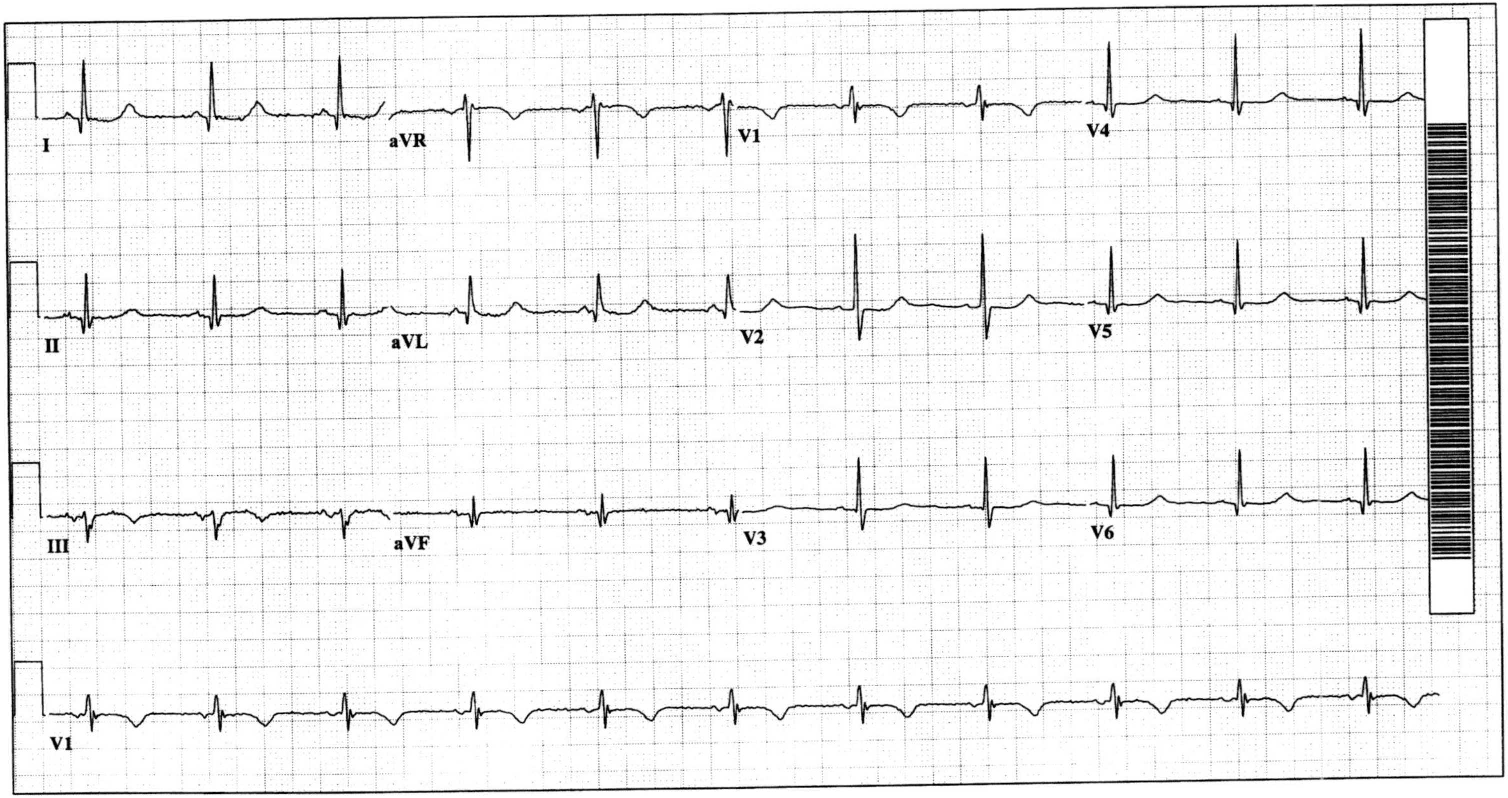

Fig. 12: The tracing shows loss of R wave in leads V1 – 4. Diagnosis is anterior myocardial infarction, age unknown.

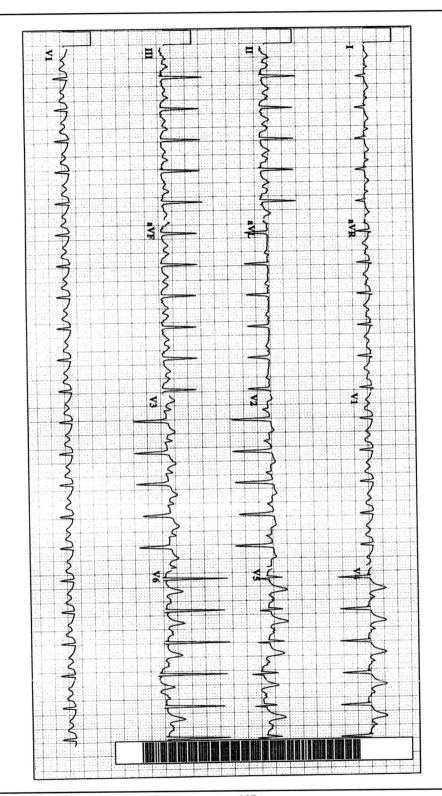

Figure 12

Chapter 14

Bundle Branch Blocks and Hemiblocks

Just like heart block at the AV node, the conduction of the impulse may be delayed or blocked at the right bundle branch (called right bundle branch block or RBBB) or at the left bundle branch (called left bundle branch block or LBBB). A complete block at both bundle branches will lead to a complete heart block.

Right bundle branch block (RBBB):

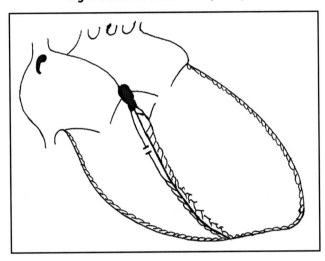

Figure 1

When an impulse gets blocked at the right bundle branch (Fig. 1), it travels along the left bundle branch in normal fashion to activate the left ventricle in antegrade manner. While traveling along the anterior division of the left bundle branch, the impulse activates the interventricular septum from left ventricle toward the right ventricle, pointing anterior and to the right, (left ventricle lies posterior and to the left of the right ventricle). The impulse continues anteriorly through the septum and activates the right ventricle. Due to slower intramuscular conduction, the QRS complexes become wide. This type of antegrade infra nodal conduction is called aberrant conduction. Since, the right ventricle is the last to be activated, and this activity is directed anteriorly and to the right, the terminal portion of the QRS complex in lead V1 is a positive deflection (called an R-prime, or r-prime if it is smaller), and the lateral leads show an S wave. Absence of S wave in lateral leads, in the presence of r-prime in lead V1, is against the diagnosis of RBBB. Various types of RSR-prime (written as RSR′) morphology in lead V1 are shown in Fig. 2. The appearance is sometimes referred to as looking like two rabbit ears. If QRS interval is 0.12 second or more, it is called complete RBBB; if it is 0.09 – 0.11 second, it is referred to as incomplete RBBB. QRS duration of less than 0.09 second indicates normal morphology. It must be noted that the typical changes in QRS morphology in RBBB must be present in lead V1. If they are seen in lead V2 and are not present in lead V1, it is not RBBB. If they are present in both the V1 and V2 leads, it is alright to call it RBBB.

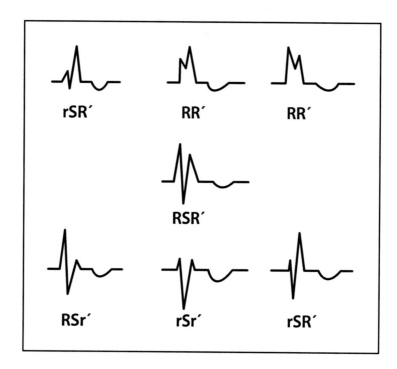

Figure 2

Above illustration shows various forms of QRS deflections seen in RBBB in Lead V1.

Following are the four examples of RBBB. Figures 3 and 4 show incomplete RBBB, and Figures 5 and 6 show complete RBBB.

Figure 3: Tracing shows incomplete RBBB. There is rSr′ in lead V1, and S wave in leads I and V6. QRS duration is 0.10 second.

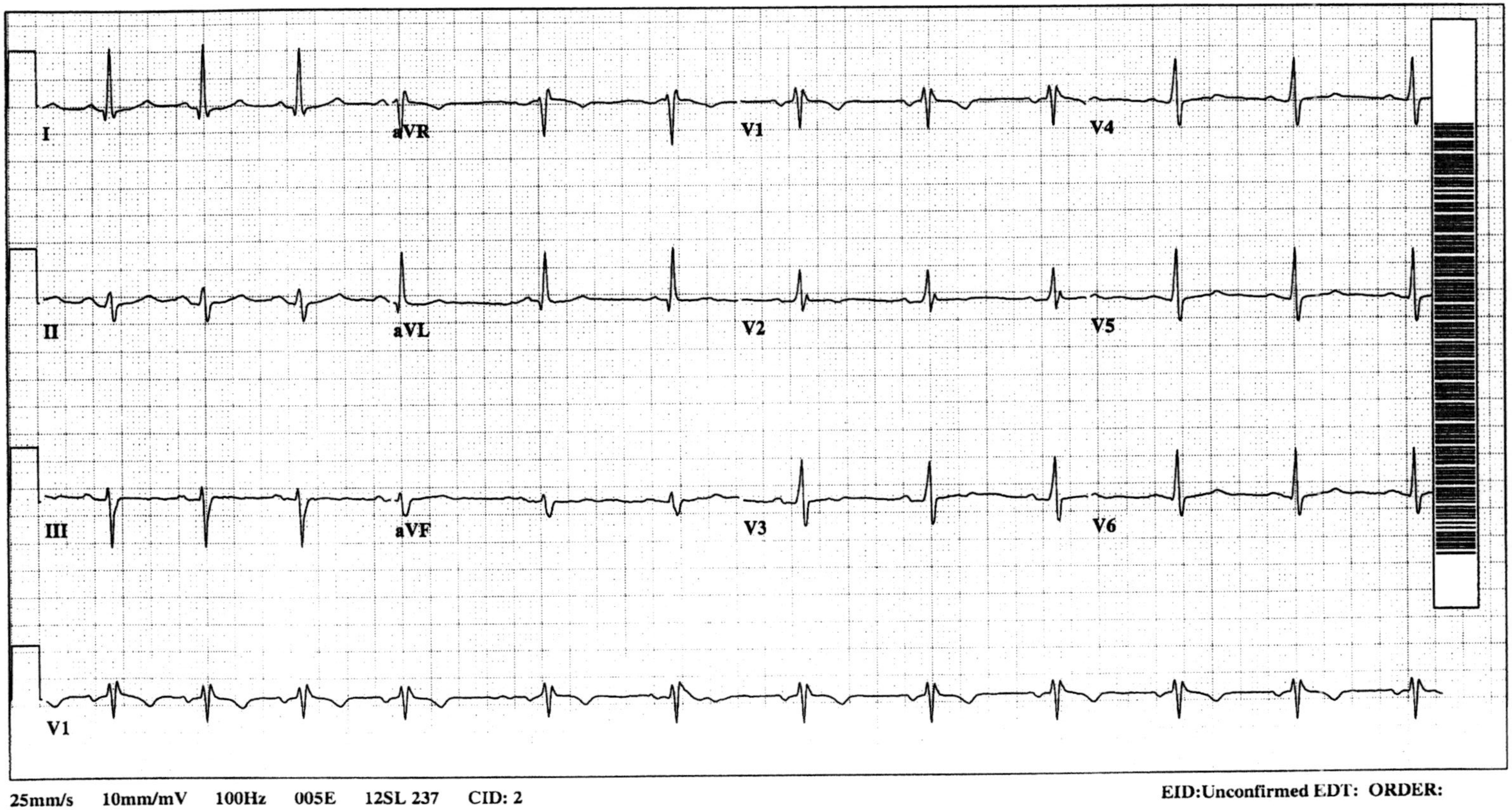
I
aVR
V1
V4
II
aVL
V2
V5
III
aVF
V3
V6
V1
25mm/s 10mm/mV 100Hz 005E 12SL 237 CID: 2
EID:Unconfirmed EDT: ORDER:

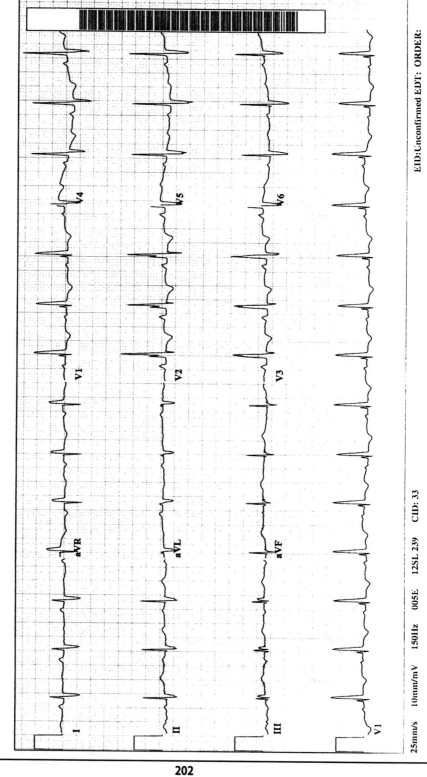

Figure 4: Tracing shows incomplete RBBB. There is rSR´ in lead V1, and S wave in leads I and V6. QRS duration is 0.10 second.

25mm/s   10mm/mV   150Hz   005E   12SL 239   CID: 33   EID:Unconfirmed EDT: ORDER:

Figure 5: Tracing shows RBBB. There is rSR´ in lead V1 and S wave in leads I and V6. QRS interval is 0.14 second.

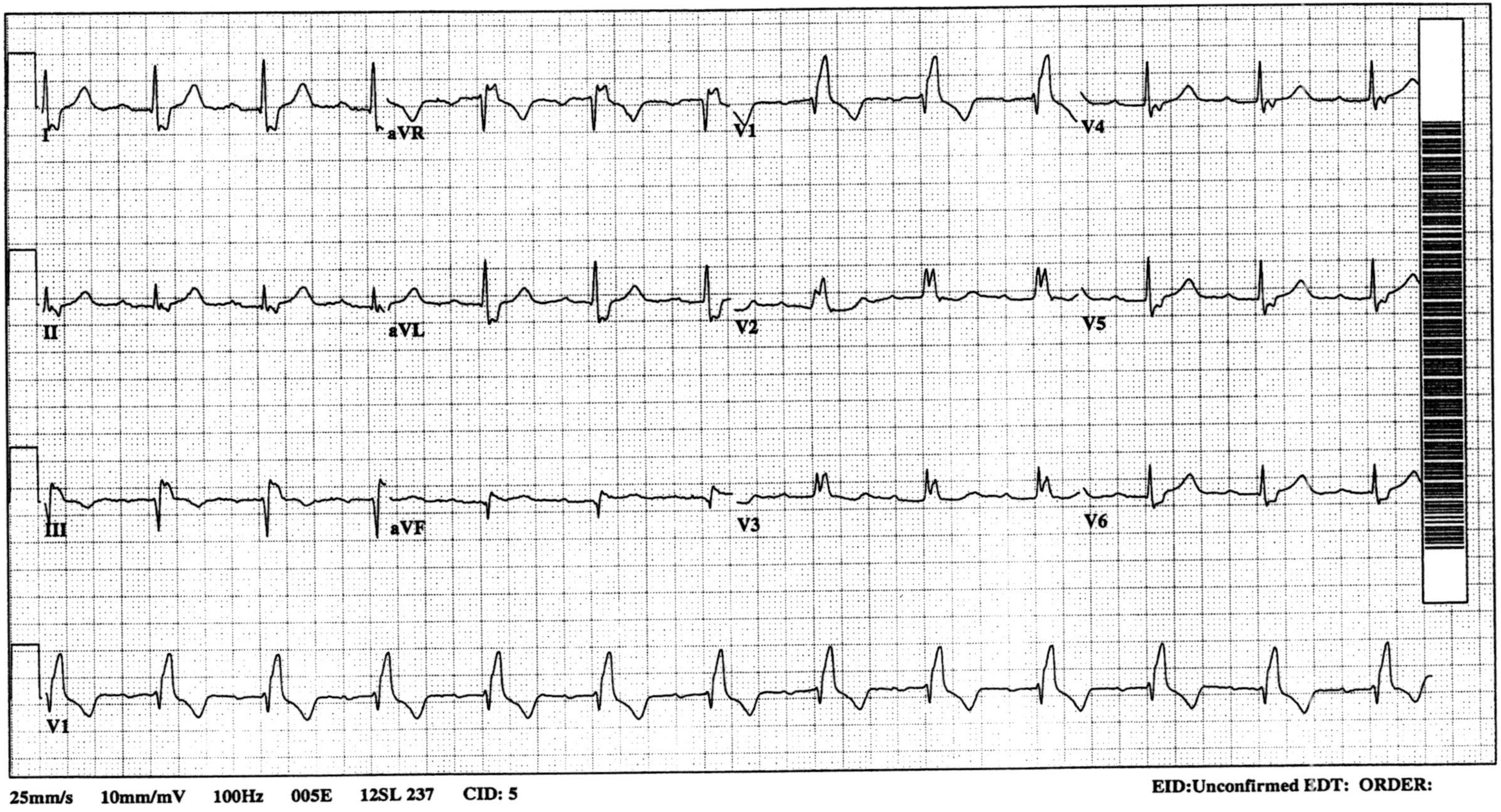

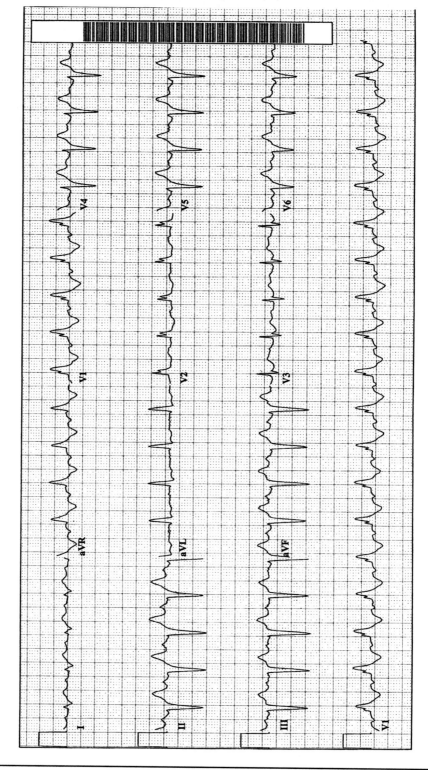

Figure 6: Tracing shows RBBB. There is rR' in lead V1 and S wave in leads I and V6. QRS duration is 0.12 second.

Left bundle branch block (LBBB):

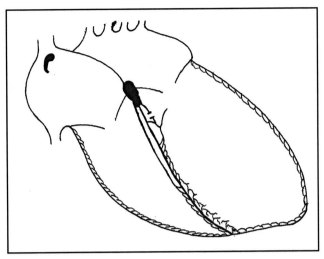

Figure 7

Above illustration shows an example of LBBB (Fig. 7). In this situation, the conduction of the impulse gets blocked at the left bundle branch, before it divides into anterior and the posterior divisions. The impulse travels in normal fashion along the right bundle branch, and activates the interventricular septum and the left ventricle from right to left. This leads to diminution or loss of initial r-waves (septal activation) in right precordial leads, as the mean instantaneous vector moves away from these leads. Due to slow intramuscular conduction of the impulse, from right to left, the QRS deflection would be wide and positive in lateral leads, and wide and negative in right precordial leads.

Following are the two examples of LBBB (Figures 8 and 9).

Figure 8: The tracing shows wide and bizarre looking positive QRS complexes in leads 1 and V6, and deep, wide, and negative QRs complexes in leads V1 – 3, along with small "r" waves in leads V1 – 3. Diagnosis is LBBB.

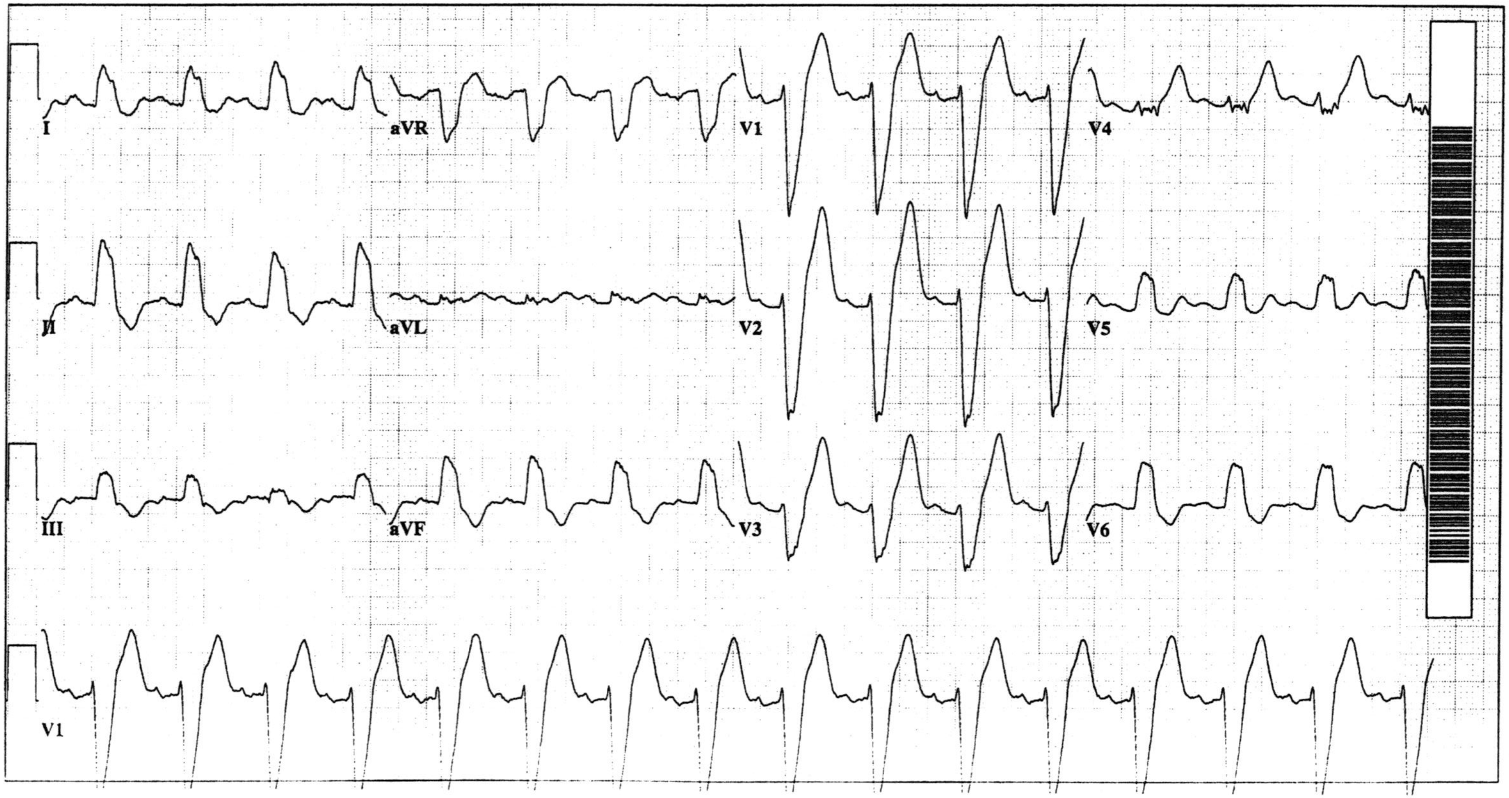

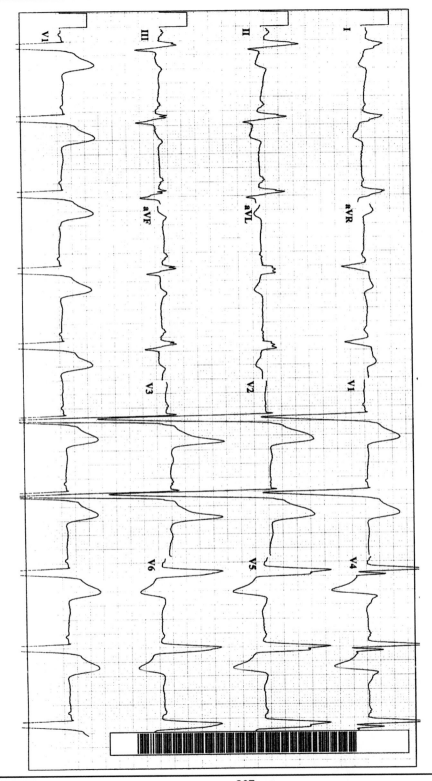

Figure 9: The tracing shows wide and bizarre looking positive QRS complexes in leads 1 and V6, and deep, wide, and negative QRS complexes with small "r" waves in right precordial leads. Diagnosis is LBBB.

Hemiblocks:

A delay or a block in the conduction of an impulse in one of the subdivisions (also called fascicles) of the left bundle branch is called a hemiblock. It could be anterior or the posterior subdivision, as shown in Figures 10 and 11 respectively. If it is the anterior subdivision which is blocked, it is called left anterior hemiblock (LAHB), also known as left anterior fascicular block; if it is the posterior subdivision, it is called left posterior hemiblock (LPHB), also known as left posterior fascicular block. It is important to note that the inferior surface of the left ventricle is normally activated by the right bundle branch. The anterolateral surface of the left ventricle is activated by the left anterior fascicle of the left bundle branch, and the base of the heart (the posterior surface) is activated by the posterior fascicle of the left bundle branch. Thus, a delay or a block in conduction through the left anterior fascicle will not affect the activation of the inferior and the posterior surface of the left ventricle. However, there will be some delay in activation of the anterolateral surface, resulting in shift of the mean QRS vector to left and superiorly, causing a QRS axis of –45 degrees or greater. There will be some delay in QRS duration, but not as much as in LBBB. Due to superior orientation of the mean QRS vector, lead V6 would show mostly negative QRS complexes. In the case of delay or a block in the posterior fascicle of the left bundle branch, the inferior and the anterolateral surface of the left ventricle would be activated normally, and only the activation of the posterior surface will be delayed. This will pull the mean QRS vector to the right, resulting in a QRS axis of more than +120 degrees. There will be only a minor delay in QRS duration.

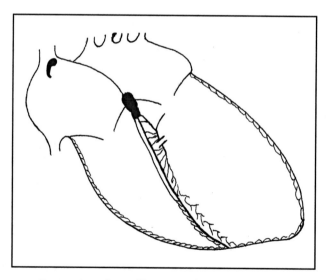

Figure 10: Above illustration shows the site of
left anterior hemiblock.

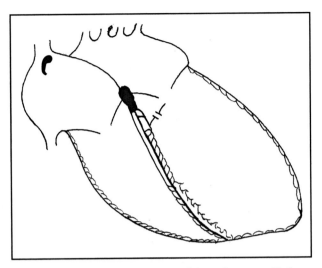

Figure 11: Above illustration shows the site of left
posterior hemiblock.

LAHB and LPHB are discussed in detail in chapter 11, along with the corresponding
EKG tracings.

Chapter 15

Nodal Rhythm
(Also called Junctional Rhythm)

When the electrical impulse originates from the AV node, it spreads upward to activate the atria, and at the same time it spreads downward to activate the ventricles. Since, the spread of the impulse occurs simultaneously in two different directions, there is always some overlap of electrical activity depolarizing two different tissues at the same time. The impulse may originate at the upper end of the AV node and spread upward to activate the atria and at the same time spread downward through the AV node, thus depolarizing at least some portion of the AV node, while retrograde spread of impulse occurs through the atrial muscle. Similarly, the impulse may originate in the middle of the AV node and spread simultaneously up and down the nodal tissue before depolarizing atria and the ventricles. The impulse may originate at the lower end of the AV node and spread upward through the AV node while depolarizing the ventricles with the downward spread at the same time.

When the impulse originates at the upper end of the AV node, the time during which it travels upward through the atria (causing P wave), it simultaneously spreads downward, depolarizing part of the AV node, causing an overlap and thus leading to a short PR interval, along with an inverted P wave in lead AVF, as seen in the EKG tracing in Fig. 1. It is the retrograde nature of the P wave which leads to an inverted P in lead AVF. An inverted P wave in inferior leads along with a short PR interval, therefore, indicates a nodal rhythm. The electrical impulse, in this case, originates from the upper end of the AV node.

When the impulse originates at the middle of the AV node, the time taken to travel upward to reach the upper end of the AV node coincides with the time during which the impulse travels downward to reach the lower end of the AV node, and then as the impulse travels through the atria, it travels through the ventricular muscle at the same time ,which means that the P wave gets buried into the QRS complex, and you see only QRS-T complexes at regular intervals without any P waves, as seen in the EKG tracing in Fig. 2.

When the impulse originates at the lower end of the AV node, it spreads quickly through the ventricular muscle (QRS) while simultaneously it spreads upward to reach the upper end of the AV node and thus the P waves occur after the QRS complexes, as shown in the EKG tracing in Fig. 3. Since it is a retrograde P wave, it is inverted in lead AVF. In the tracing in Fig. 3, the P waves are better seen in lead V1 following the QRS (see arrows).

To summarize: In the case of high nodal rhythm, there is an inverted P with short PR interval in inferior leads, and the P wave precedes the QRS complex. In the case of mid nodal rhythm, there are no P waves (they are buried within the QRS), and all you see is QRS-T complexes at regular intervals. In the case of low nodal rhythm, there are QRS complexes followed by inverted P waves in inferior leads; the P appears immediately after the end of the QRS complex and before the ST segment.

NOTE:

1. An inverted P in lead AVF with short PR is referred to as nodal rhythm (junctional rhythm) up to a heart rate of 60 BPM. When heart rate is > 60 to 100 BPM, it is called accelerated nodal rhythm. With a heart rate of 101 – 115 BPM, it is called nodal (junctional) tachycardia. A heart rate of more than 115 BPM with inverted P wave preceding QRS in AVF makes it ectopic atrial tachycardia. In case of slow atrial flutter with atrial rate of <250/minute, the sawtooth appearance of atrial waves in lead V1 will help differentiate it from ectopic atrial tachycardia, in which the P waves are abnormal, but not sawtooth in appearance in lead V1.

2. Narrow QRS complexes without P waves, with regular R–R interval, indicates nodal rhythm (up to a heart rate of 60 BPM), accelerated nodal rhythm (H.R. of > 60 – 100 BPM), or nodal tachycardia (H.R. of > 100 – 115 BPM). A heart rate of > 115 BPM is referred to as SVT (supraventricular tachycardia) or AVNRT (AV nodal re-entrant tachycardia).

Fig. 1: The tracing shows nodal rhythm, originating at the upper end of the AV node.

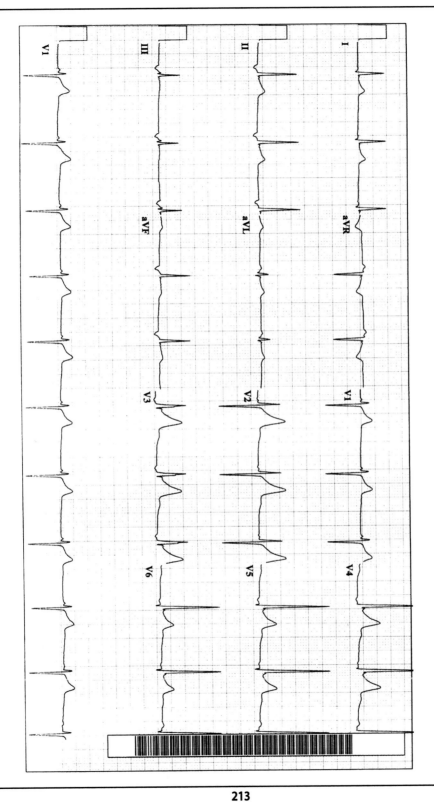

Figure 1

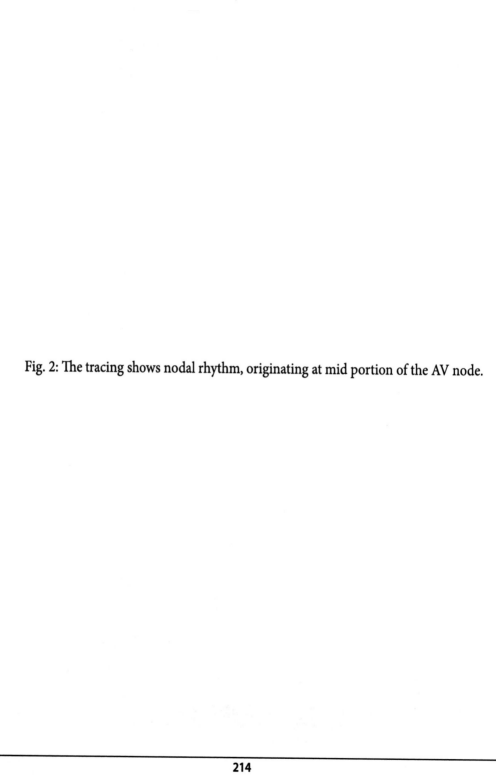

Fig. 2: The tracing shows nodal rhythm, originating at mid portion of the AV node.

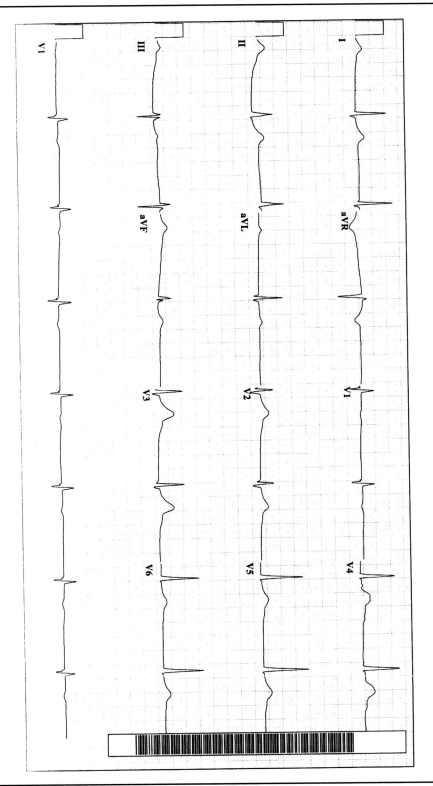

Figure 2

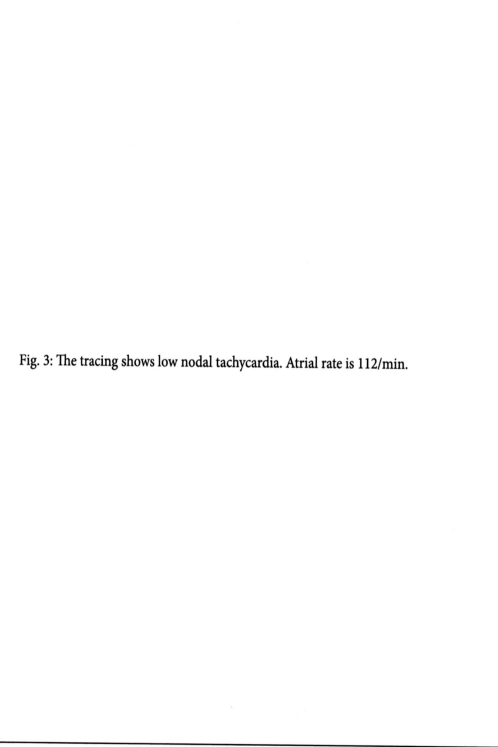

Fig. 3: The tracing shows low nodal tachycardia. Atrial rate is 112/min.

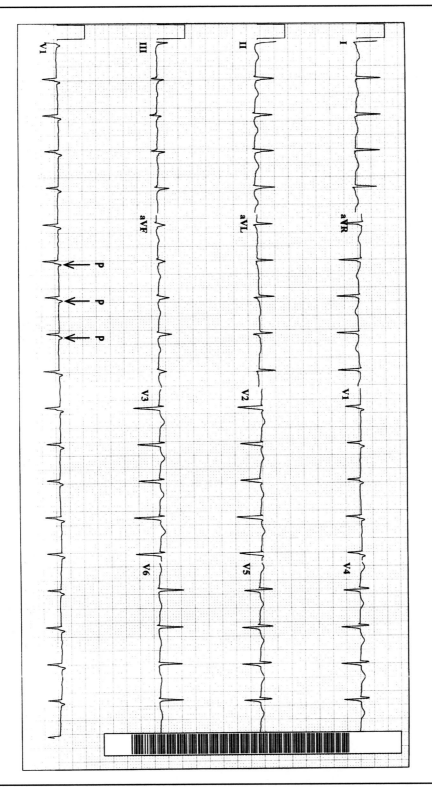

Figure 3

Atrioventricular Nodal Re-entrant Tachycardia (AVNRT) and
Atrioventricular Re-entrant Tachycardia (AVRT):

A narrow QRS tachycardia with heart rate of greater than 115/minute and regular, without P waves, is referred to as atrioventricular nodal re-entrant tachycardia (AVNRT), also called supraventricular tachycardia. The retrograde P waves are buried within the QRS complexes. Sometimes, the retrograde P wave is buried into the terminal portion of the QRS complex, and appears as pseudo S wave in inferior leads and/or pseudo r- prime in lead V1. In case of atrioventricular re-entrant tachycardia (AVRT), the P waves appear after the QRS complex (see Figure 4). However, the latter phenomenon can rarely be seen in AVNRT as well, due to slow retrograde AV node conduction. The presence of delta waves in a previous EKG with sinus rhythm suggests the diagnosis of AVRT, also called reciprocal tachycardia.

In case of AVRT, there is an accessory pathway between atria and the ventricles, outside the AV node. The impulse travels down the AV node and, during ventricular activation, enters the accessory pathway and moves upward in clockwise manner to activate the atria in retrograde fashion, and re-enters the AV node. This repetitive clockwise movement of the impulse precipitates the arrhythmia. The retrograde P wave is inscribed after the QRS on the ST segment, and QRS complexes remain narrow. This is referred to as orthodromic AVRT. Rarely, the impulse may enter the accessory pathway from the atria to activate the ventricles, and enter the lower end of the AV node to travel upward counterclockwise, and then re-enter the accessory pathway during retrograde activation of the atria. This form is referred to as antidromic AVRT. The P wave is located on the ST segment after the QRS complex due to conduction delay in the AV node, and the QRS complexes are wide and bizarre in antidromic AVRT. In case of AVNRT, the impulse travels down and up within the AV node in circular fashion, and the P wave is buried within the QRS complex.

Fig.4: The tracing shows AVRT (atrioventricular tachycardia, also called reciprocal tachycardia). Note, the P waves in lead V1 are located on the ST segments after the QRS complexes.

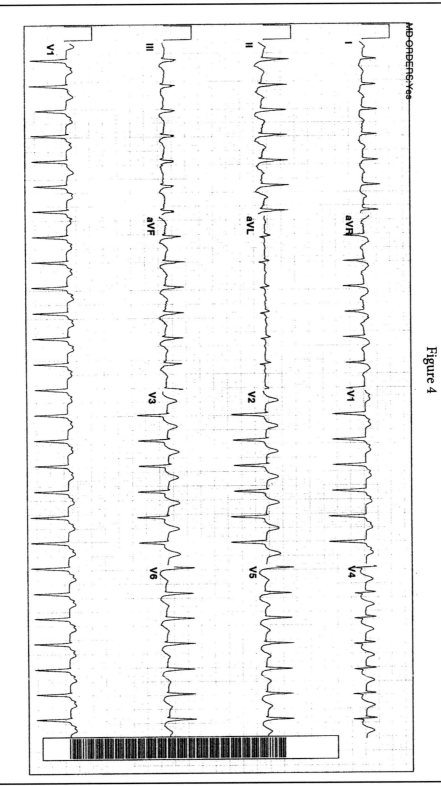

Figure 4

Chapter 16

Hypertrophy

Left Ventricular Hypertrophy (LVH):

EKG diagnosis of LVH is difficult. There are voltage criteria and repolarization criteria for the diagnosis. Voltage criteria are unreliable when used alone.

Voltage criteria:

The sum of the voltage of S wave in lead V1 and R wave in lead V5 or V6 is 35 mm or greater.

Voltage of S in V1 or V2 is 30 mm or greater.

Amplitude of R in V5 or V6 is 30 mm or greater.

R wave amplitude in lead AVL is 12 mm or greater.

R wave amplitude in lead I is 14 mm or greater.

Repolarization criteria:

Down sloping ST segment with inverted T wave in lateral leads (I, AVL, V5 and V6), and tall R (greater than 30 mm) in leads V5 – 6.

When above ST – T changes are present in lateral leads without tall R waves, it should be interpreted as ST – T changes suggestive of LVH and / or ischemia.

Figure 1 illustrates EKG changes of LVH.

Fig.1: The tracing shows tall R in lateral leads and ST – T abnormality in anterior and lateral leads. Findings are consistent with LVH with repolarization abnormality. A biphasic P wave in lead V1 with deep and wide negative component, and total duration of 0.12 second suggests left atrial enlargement.

Right Ventricular Hypertrophy (RVH):

EKG findings of RVH are as follows:

Amplitude of R wave in lead V1 is 7mm or greater, T wave is inverted in V1, and right axis deviation (see Fig.2). Amplitude of R greater than voltage of S (R/S = >1.0) in V1 with inverted T wave and right axis deviation is also consistent with RVH.

Right Atrial enlargement (RAE):

A peaked P wave with amplitude of greater than 2.5 mm in lead II suggests right atrial enlargement (see Fig. 8 in chapter 17).

Left Atrial Enlargement (LAE):

A biphasic P wave with deep ($\geq$ 1.0mm) and wide negative component in lead V1 with total duration of 0.12 sec. or more is consistent with left atrial enlargement (LAE), as shown in Fig. 1. A notched P wave in lead II ($\geq$ 0.12 sec. in duration) with the two tops being $\geq$ 0.04 sec. apart is suggestive of LAE (see below).

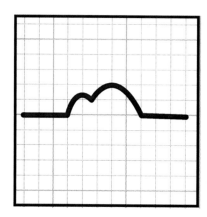

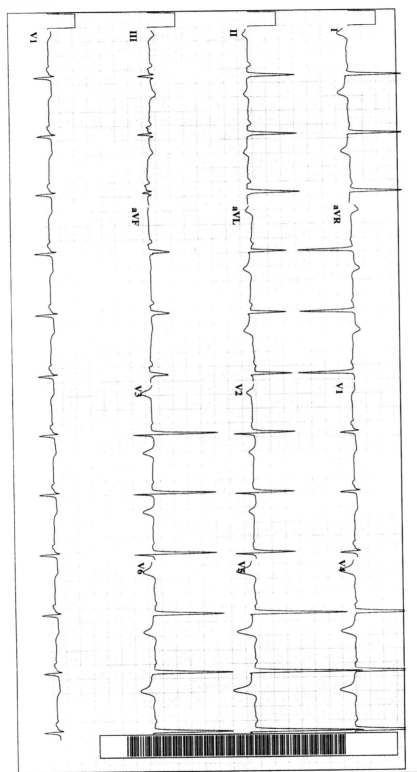

Figure 1

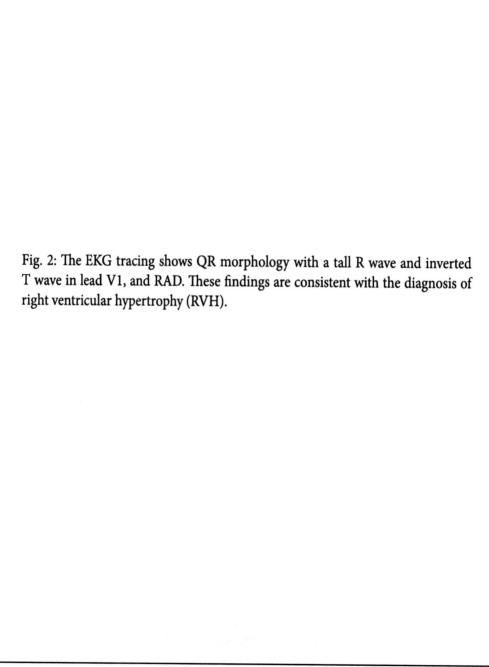

Fig. 2: The EKG tracing shows QR morphology with a tall R wave and inverted T wave in lead V1, and RAD. These findings are consistent with the diagnosis of right ventricular hypertrophy (RVH).

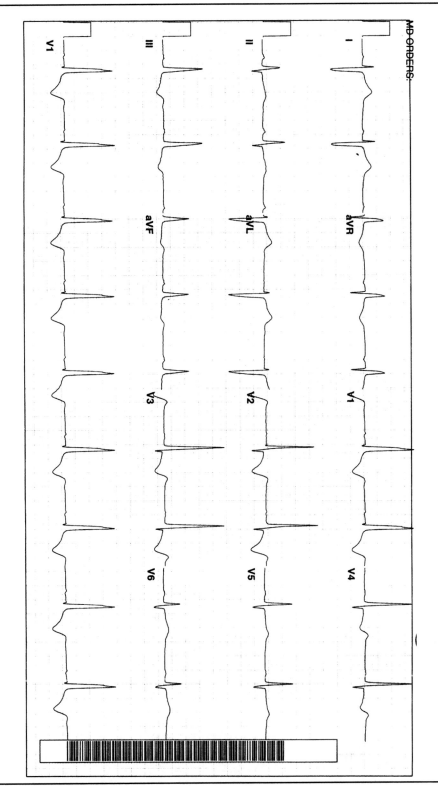

Figure 2

Chapter 17

Repolarization Abnormalities

ST Depression:

ST segment depression, whether horizontal or down sloping, is suggestive of ischemia. A down sloping ST segment with T wave inversion in lateral leads is seen also in left ventricular hypertrophy. A hammock shaped ST depression is consistent with digitalis effect and / or ischemia. Fig. 1 illustrates horizontal ST depression in leads V4 – 6. Fig. 2 illustrates down sloping ST segments with T wave inversion in inferior leads (II, III, and AVF) and leads V4 – 6.

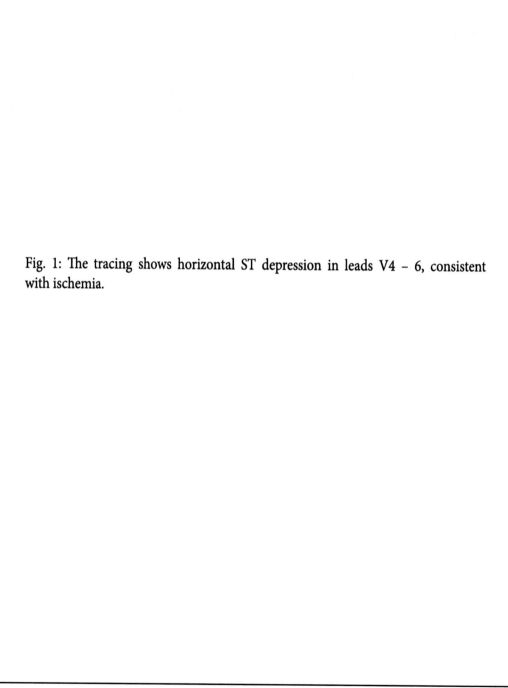

Fig. 1: The tracing shows horizontal ST depression in leads V4 – 6, consistent with ischemia.

Figure 1

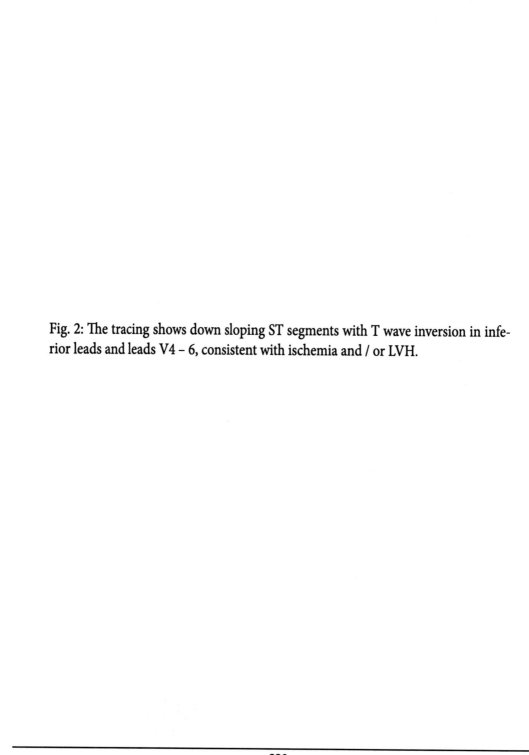

Fig. 2: The tracing shows down sloping ST segments with T wave inversion in inferior leads and leads V4 – 6, consistent with ischemia and / or LVH.

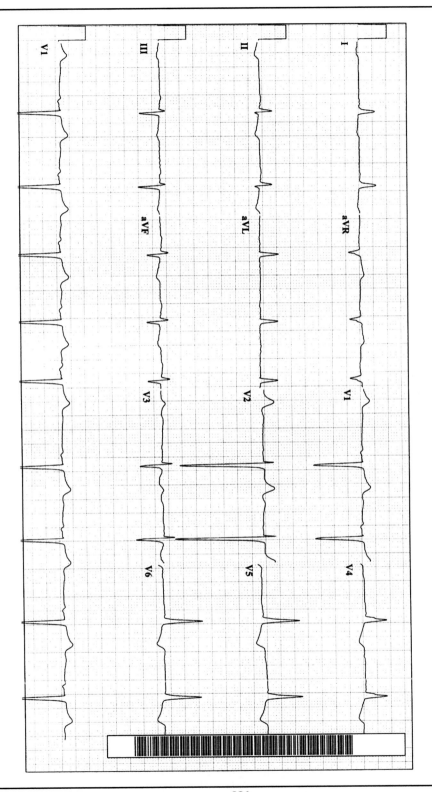

Figure 2

ST Elevation:

ST elevation in the presence of narrow QRS complexes is suggestive of early repolarization, injury or pericarditis. A convex upward ST elevation always suggests myocardial injury. A concave upward ST elevation is seen in early repolarization, injury or pericarditis. Fig. 3. shows convex upward ST elevation in leads V3 – 4 (T waves are inverted in inferior leads and leads V5 – 6 without ST elevation, indicating infer-olateral ischemia). Fig. 4 illustrates concave upward ST elevation. Fig. 5 shows diffuse concave ST elevation.

Following would help reach the diagnosis when concave ST elevation is present.

Localized concave ST elevation suggests early repolarization or injury. Diffuse concave ST elevation favors pericarditis, but consistent with early repolarization, injury or pericarditis.

Presence of reciprocal ST segment changes, i.e. ST depression in lead AVL when there is ST elevation in lead AVF and vice versa, is consistent with injury. Leads I and III are reciprocal to each other. Absence of reciprocal changes does not rule out injury.

Diffuse concave ST elevation with PR segment depression, without reciprocal ST segment changes is diagnostic of pericarditis. Height of ST/T ratio is >0.25. PR segment depression is demonstrated by advancing the PR segment to the left, and comparing the level with that of the preceding TP segment. It is usually seen in lead II and / or leads V3 – 6.

Tall T waves with appearance of a fish hook at 'J' point (Fig.4, leads V3 – 4), called Marriott sign, without reciprocal ST segment changes is consistent with early repolarization. Height of ST/T ratio is <0.25.

Sometimes, it may not be possible to pinpoint a single diagnosis, and one may be forced to call the EKG changes as consistent with "injury or early repolarization" or consistent with "injury, pericarditis or early repolarization."

Fig. 3: Tracing shows acute anterior myocardial infarction (loss of R wave in V1 – 3, and convex ST elevation in V3 – 4) and ST – T changes of inferior and lateral ischemia.

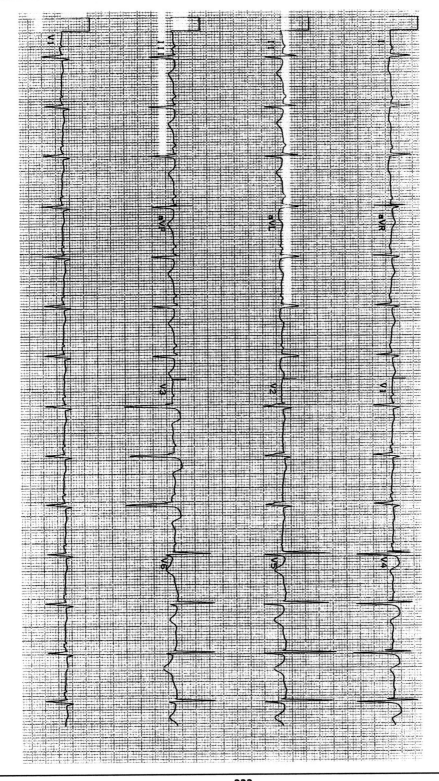

Figure 3

Fig. 4: Tracing shows diffuse concave ST elevation. There is no PR depression, and no reciprocal ST depression in lead AVL or lead I. Fish hook is seen in leads V3 – 4, and tall T waves are present. Height of ST/T ratio is <0.25. Findings are consistent with early repolarization.

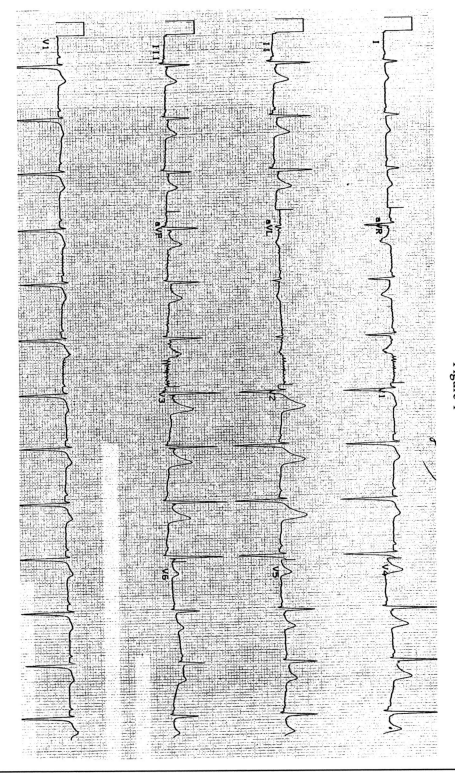

Figure 4

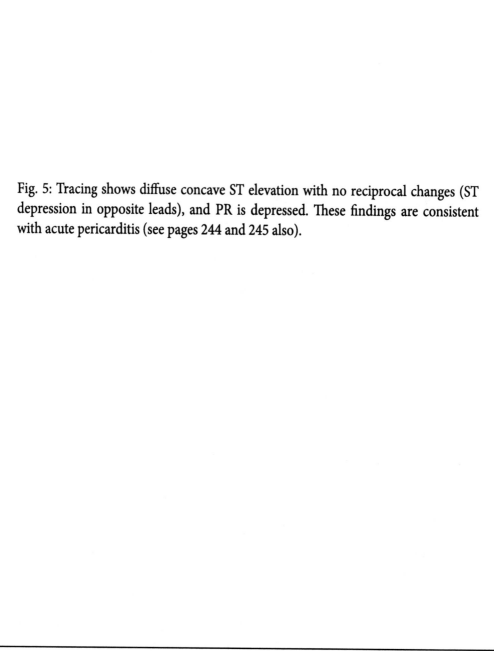

Fig. 5: Tracing shows diffuse concave ST elevation with no reciprocal changes (ST depression in opposite leads), and PR is depressed. These findings are consistent with acute pericarditis (see pages 244 and 245 also).

Figure 5

T Wave Abnormality:

Deep T wave inversion in leads other than leads III, AVR and V1 is suggestive of ischemia. T waves are normally inverted in lead AVR, usually inverted in V1, and may be inverted in lead III. Minor T wave inversion of 1.0 mm or less in anterolateral leads is usually considered non-specific, but may be associated with acute coronary syndrome. T wave inversion in lead AVL is normal if P wave is also inverted. Figure 6 reveals deep T wave inversion in anterolateral leads, consistent with ischemia and/or LVH.

Fig. 6: Tracing shows ST – T abnormality, suggestive of anterolateral ischemia and/or LVH.

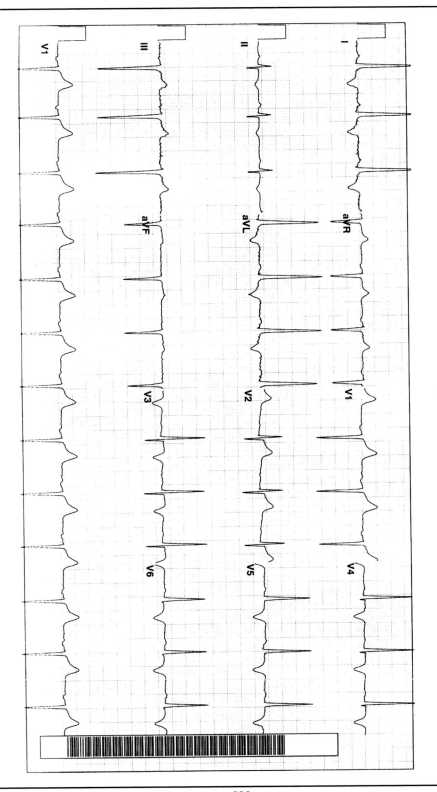

Figure 6

Tall peaked T waves are suggestive of hyperkalemia, as seen in Fig. 7.

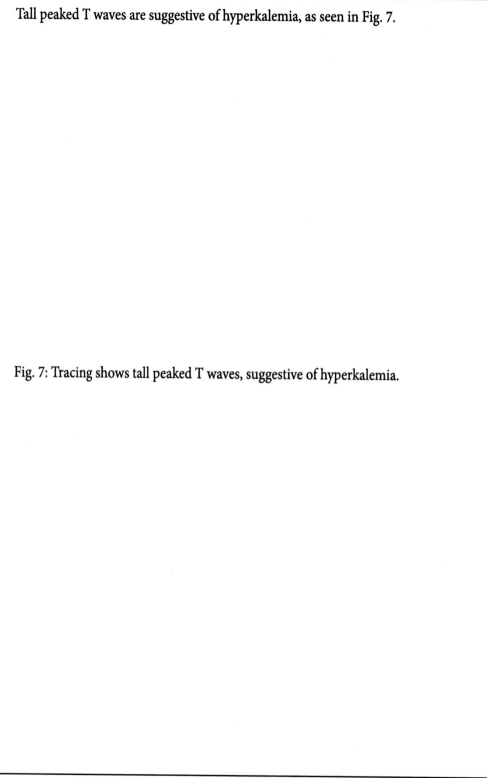

Fig. 7: Tracing shows tall peaked T waves, suggestive of hyperkalemia.

Figure 7

U Waves:

Prominent U waves which follow the T waves are seen in hypokalemia, as illustrated in Fig. 8. Pathophysiology of U waves is not clearly understood.

Fig. 8: Tracing shows prominent U waves following the T waves, consistent with hypokalemia. Tall peaked P waves in inferior leads are consistent with right atrial enlargement.

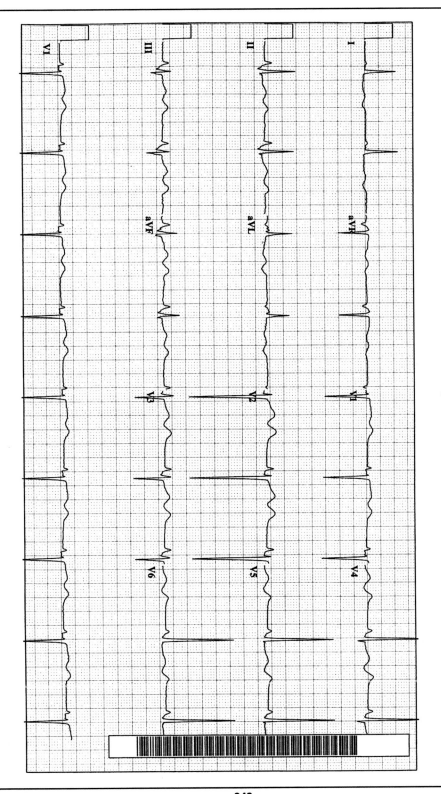

Figure 8

Hyper and Hypo Calcemia:

QT is prolonged in hypocalcemia, and shortened in hypercalcemia.

J Waves:

A round elevation of J point, giving appearance of a hump, is called J wave. J waves are usually seen in lateral and inferior leads, and called Osborn waves. Osborn waves, however, can be present in right Precordial leads in addition to their presence in lateral leads. When J waves are present only in right Precordial leads in the presence of RBBB, they are called Brugada syndrome (see details in chapter 21). Osborn waves are considered to be characteristic of hypothermia, especially when associated with wide QRS, prolonged QT, prolonged PR, and sinus bradycardia or atrial fibrillation, along with shivering artifacts on an EKG tracing. But Osborn waves have also been reported in cases of hypercalcemia, pericarditis, subarachnoid hemorrhage, brain injury, vasospastic angina, cardiopulmonary arrest from oversedation, idiopathic ventricular fibrillation, and some normal individuals with early repolarization. The underlying mechanism may be different for J waves in Brugada syndrome and Osborn waves. The vector in Osborn waves is directed to the left and infero-posteriorly, thus giving rise to J waves in these leads, whereas, the direction of the vector is anterior and to the right in Brugada syndrome. Fatal ventricular arrhythmias are seen with both of these conditions. Figure 9 demonstrates Osborn waves. The EKG tracings in Figures 9 and 5 belong to the same patient (with pericarditis); the tracing in Fig. 5 was taken 15 hours earlier than the tracing in Fig. 9. Please note the presence of Osborn waves in lateral leads in Fig. 9; they are absent in Fig. 5, especially leads V4 – 6.

Fig. 9: EKG tracing of a 47 year old lady with acute pericarditis and normal temperature with J waves (Osborn waves) seen in lateral leads.

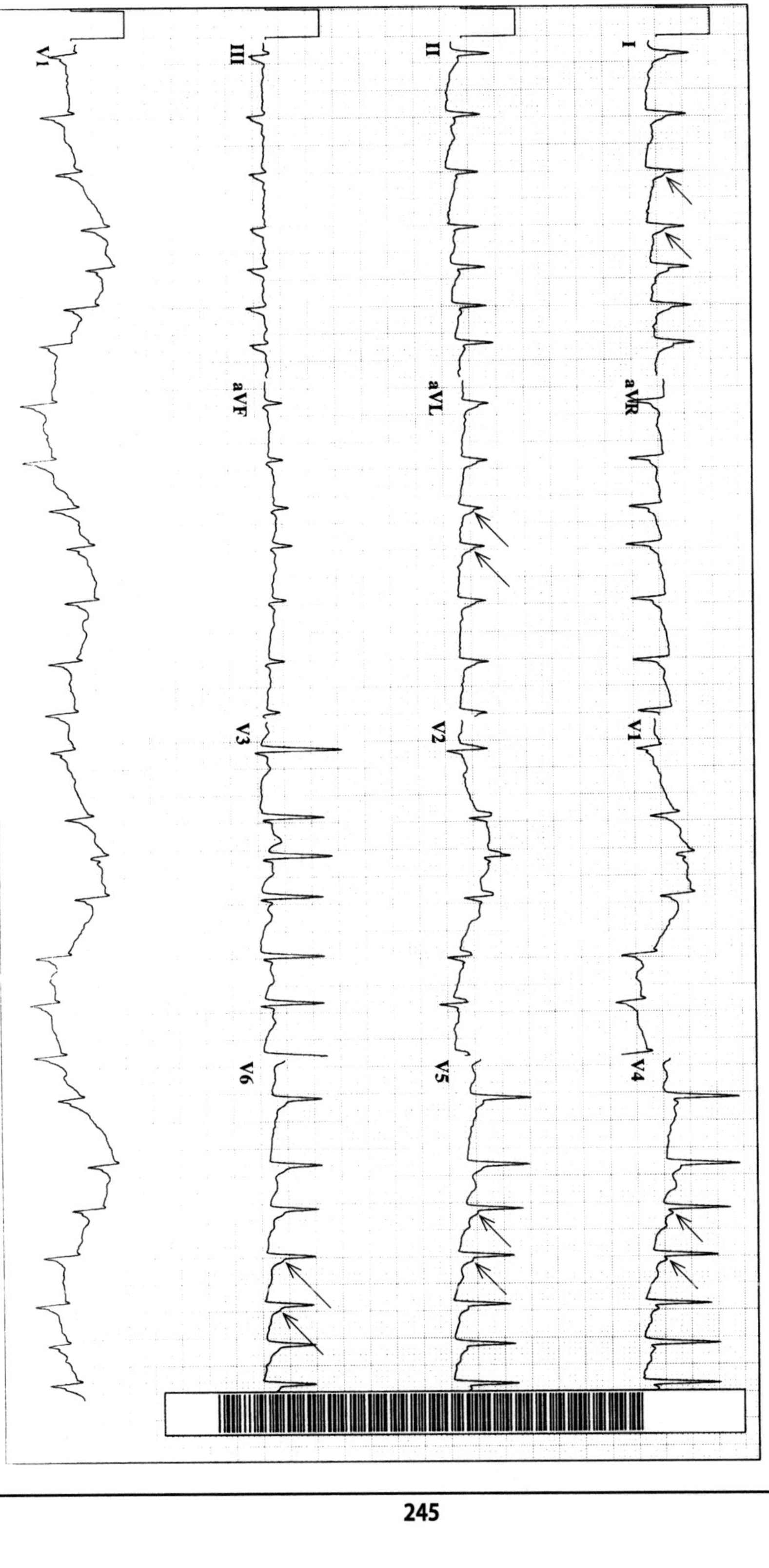

Figure 9

Chapter 18

Pacemakers

A Pacemaker is a device which generates electrical impulses to stimulate the atria and/or the ventricles. It consists of a pulse generator which has battery in it, and a pulse delivery mechanism called the catheter. The catheter consists of an insulated wire with teflon coating. The catheter is either unipolar or bipolar. The unipolar catheter has one electrode at the distal end which is in contact with the myocardium and serves as the negative electrode; the positive electrode being the metal plate attached to the pulse generator. The proximal end of the catheter is connected to the pulse generator during the procedure when pacemaker is implanted. The bipolar catheter has two electrodes at the distal end, the distal of the two serving as the negative electrode.

The pacemakers can be temporary or permanent. Temporary pacemakers utilize bipolar catheters whereas permanent pacemakers may utilize unipolar or bipolar catheters. Unipolar pacemakers create a bigger artifact due to the long distance between the negative and the positive electrodes, which is easily visible on the EKG tracing. The catheter is inserted through a vein and it is called transvenous pacing. Subclavian vein, or superficial or deep jugular vein is usually preferred for permanent as well as temporary pacing. However, median cubital or superficial femoral vein can be used for temporary pacing. Pacing of the heart can also be achieved through transcutaneous approach, where the electrode pads are applied directly over the chest, and this type of pacing is very useful during an emergency while waiting for transvenous pacing. Epicardial pacing during surgery, with chest already open, is also another approach. The permanent pulse generator is usually implanted in the pectoral area below the lateral part of the clavicle under the skin. The catheter electrode is implanted into the ventricle for ventricular pacing, and into the right atrium for atrial pacing.

There are two types of pacing mechanisms. One is called the fixed rate pacing and the other a demand pacing to avoid competition with heart's own pacing mechanism. A fixed rate pacemaker continues to pace the heart at a predetermined rate regardless of patient's own heart beat. Therefore, there is always a danger that the electronic ventricular pacemaker may discharge an impulse when T wave is being inscribed on the EKG and thus lead to ventricular tachycardia. For this reason, the fixed rate pacemakers are not preferred these days, even though they are relatively cheaper to implant. The demand pacemakers have a sensing mechanism in the pulse generator which senses the patient's own heart beat and recalculates the interval after which it is supposed to discharge its impulse, thus avoiding the competition. The ventricular pacemaker generates a spike just before the QRS is inscribed, and the atrial pacemaker inscribes a spike at the time of atrial pacing followed by a wide negative deflection in lead V1, which coincides with atrial depolarization. This negative deflection is not always visible in the EKG tracing.

The pacing can be purely ventricular with the pacing electrode in the ventricle, or only atrial with pacing electrode in the right atrium, or a dual chamber pacing with one electrode in the ventricle and one in the right atrium. The ventricular electrode is usually in the right ventricle, but biventricular pacing is occasionally necessary. A dual chamber pacing is preferred as it preserves the relationship between atrial and ventricular systole, thus preserving the cardiac output which would otherwise decrease if this harmony was lost. Such pacing is demand pacing and therefore the atrial and the ventricular contractions are sensed by the pacemaker generator to allow it to readjust the firing of the next impulse to avoid competition.

Following are some examples of electronic pacing.

Fig. 1: The tracing shows electronic ventricular pacing. Note the electronic pacing spike just before the ventricular QRS complexes.

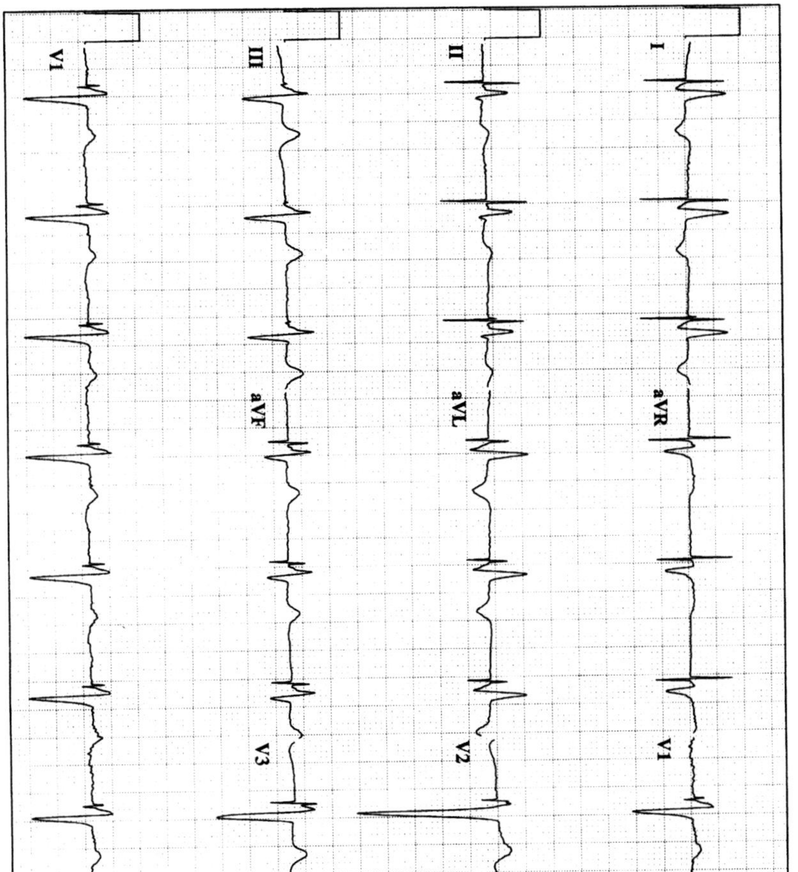

Figure 1

Fig. 2: The tracing shows electronic atrial pacing. Note the electronic pacing spike followed by a wide negative deflection in lead V1, which represents atrial depolarization. The interval between the spike and the start of the QRS complex is PR interval.

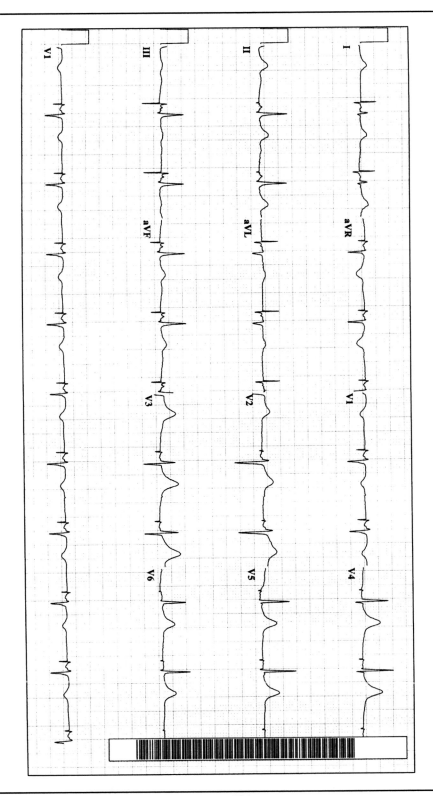

Figure 2

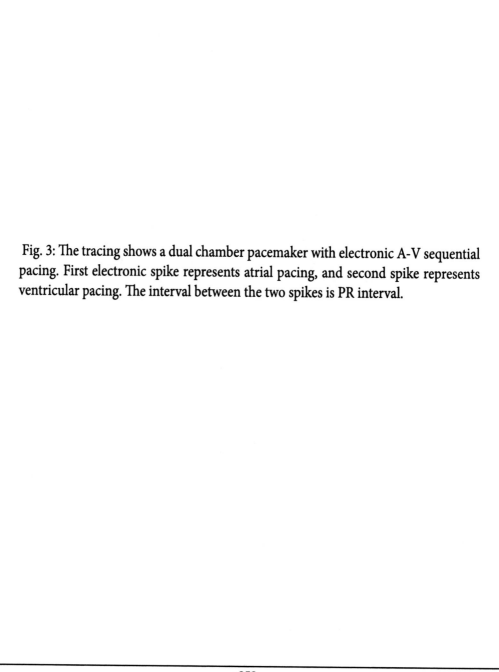

Fig. 3: The tracing shows a dual chamber pacemaker with electronic A-V sequential pacing. First electronic spike represents atrial pacing, and second spike represents ventricular pacing. The interval between the two spikes is PR interval.

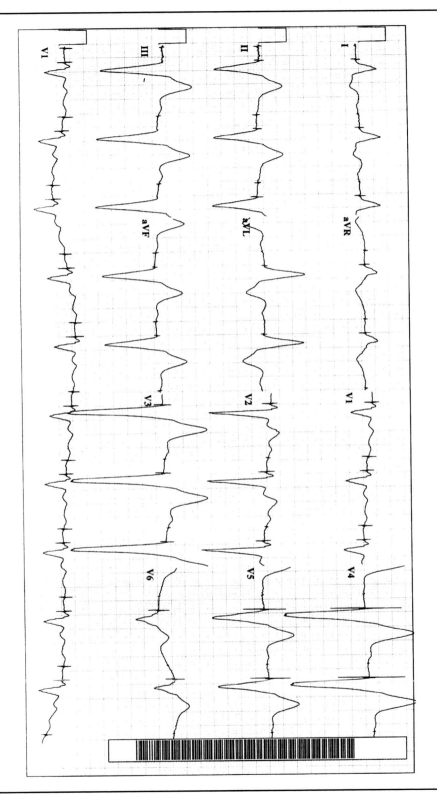

Figure 3

Fig. 4: The tracing shows a dual chamber pacemaker in VAT mode. The letter V stands for ventricular pacing; the letter A stands for atrial sensing; the letter T stands for " R wave triggered" which means that there is an electronic spike preceding each QRS complex indicating that the R wave has been triggered by the pacemaker and not from antegrade AV conduction (this spike can be electronically suppressed so that there would be QRS complexes resulting from electronic pacing but without an electronic spike – this phenomenon is called "R wave inhibited"). Note that there is a normal P wave from sinus node before each each QRS complex. This P is being sensed by the atrial electrode, and this electrode sends information to the pulse generator which then does not fire its impulse to stimulate the atrium but fires ventricular impulse after a predetermined PR interval to stimulate the ventricular systole resulting in electronic spike followed by QRS complex.

Fig. 5: The tracing shows a large electronic pacemaker spike on the left side with successful ventricular capture. The P wave before the capture is being sensed appropriately. Small electronic atrial pacemaker spikes on the right (see arrows) fail to capture. The electronic atrial rate is set at 60/minute (1500/number of vertical lines between 2 consecutive spikes).

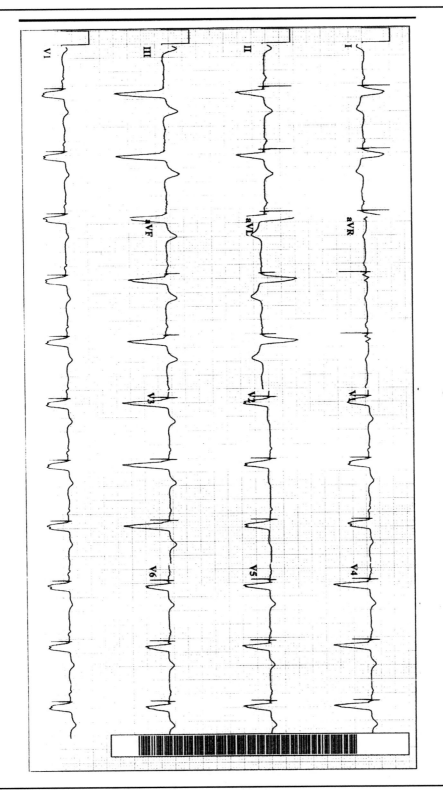

Figure 4

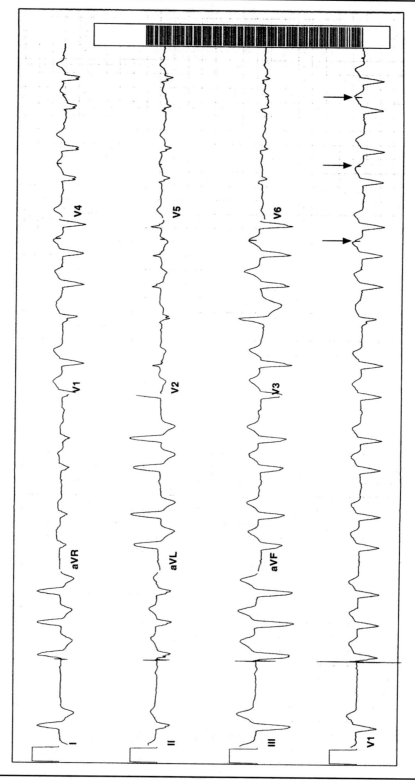

Figure 5

Chapter 19

Wolf Parkinson White Syndrome

(WPW Syndrome)

EKG characteristics of WPW syndrome are short PR interval, slurred R wave upstroke (called delta wave), and wide QRS (0.12 sec. or greater) complex. This is called WPW pattern. A combination of WPW pattern and a history of palpitations is called WPW syndrome. Short PR is due to delta wave, the PJ interval (from the start of P wave to the J point) remains unchanged. The delta wave is caused by rapid conduction of the impulse through a strand of fibers of conduction tissue connecting atria directly with the ventricular muscle, bypassing the AV node. This strand of accessory fibers is called bundle of Kent or an accessory pathway. The ventricles are activated initially by the impulse conducted through the accessory pathway creating delta wave, and then by the antegrade conduction through the AV node (see diagram below). There are two types of WPW pattern, type A and B. In type A, the delta wave is directed anteriorly and therefore gives rise to an upward initial deflection in lead V1 along with positive RS deflection (Fig.1). In type B, the initial deflection is to the left and posterior, giving rise to QS complex or rS complex in lead V1 and upward delta deflection in lateral leads (Fig.2). Fig.3 shows intermittent WPW pattern, type B.

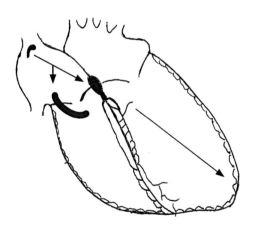

Lown-Ganong- Levine syndrome (LGL syndrome) is a variant of WPW syndrome. The accessory pathway (bundle of Kent) in LGL syndrome is connected to the bundle of His instead of the ventricular muscle. Therefore, there is no delta wave or widening of the QRS complexes. PR is short (0.12 sec. or less) and QRS complexes are normal.

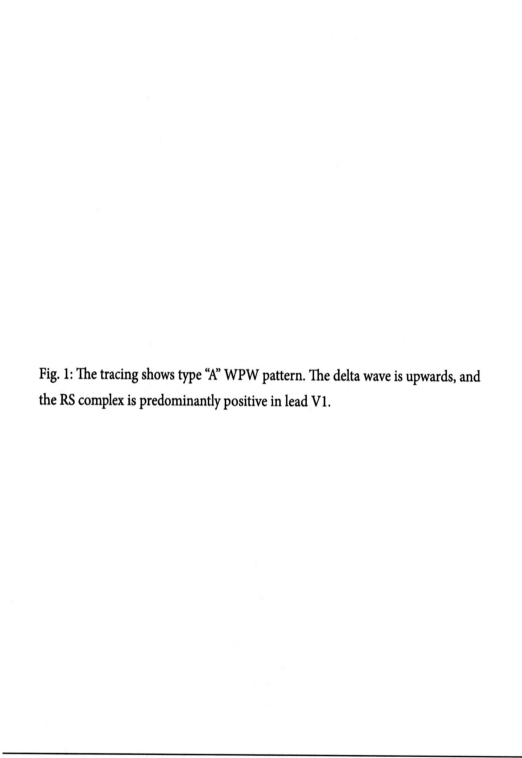

Fig. 1: The tracing shows type "A" WPW pattern. The delta wave is upwards, and the RS complex is predominantly positive in lead V1.

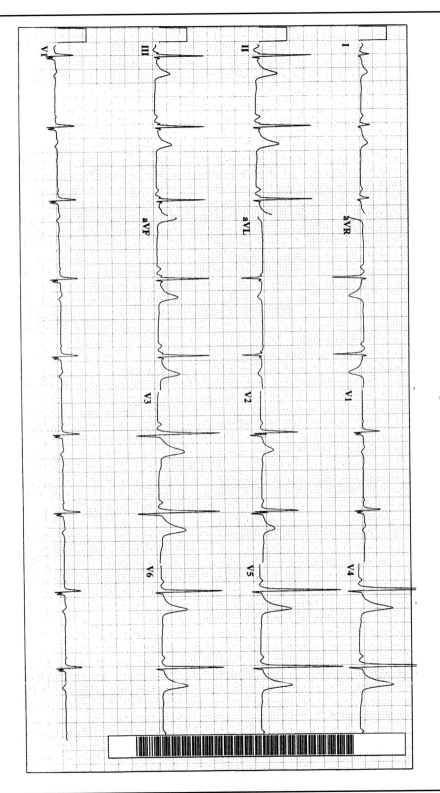

Figure 1

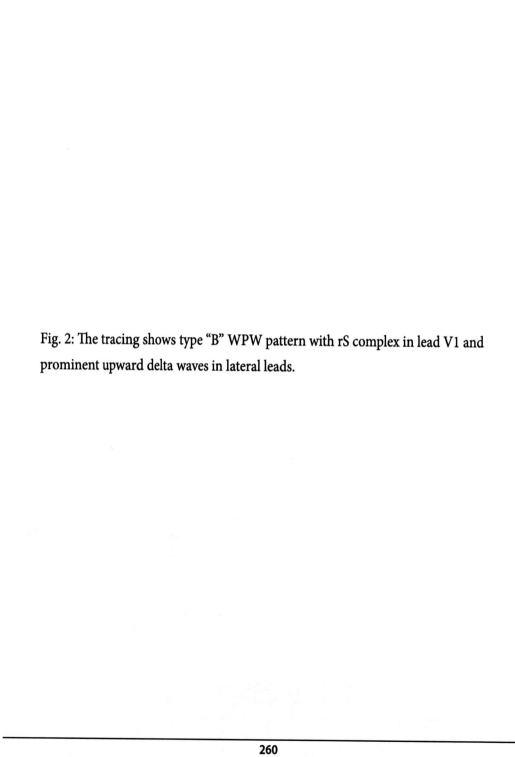

Fig. 2: The tracing shows type "B" WPW pattern with rS complex in lead V1 and prominent upward delta waves in lateral leads.

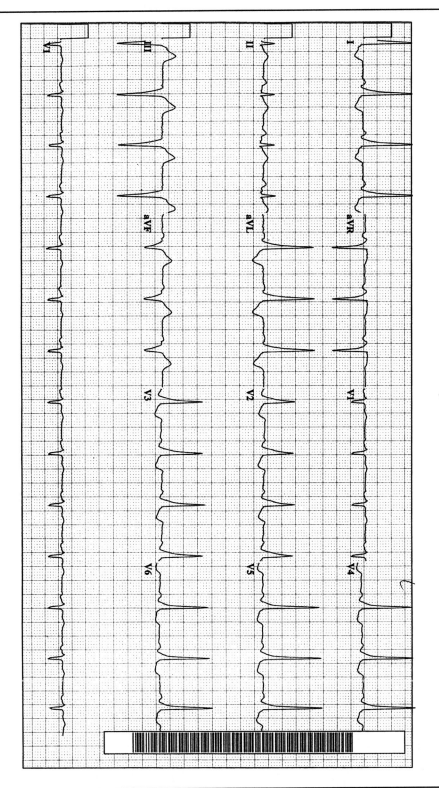

Figure 2

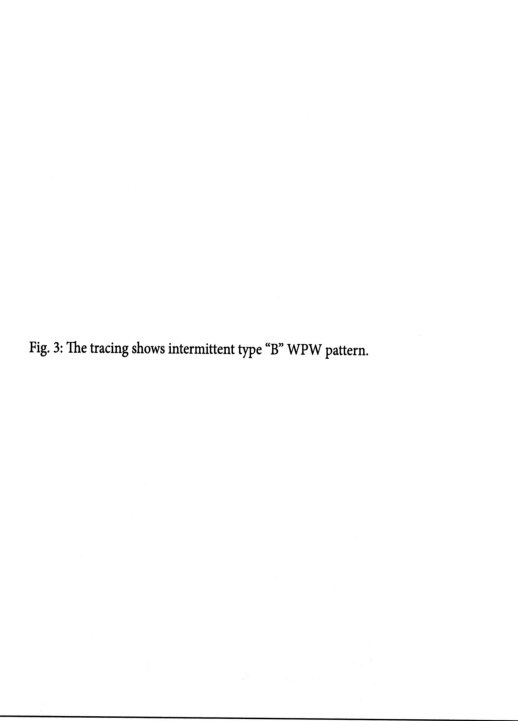

Fig. 3: The tracing shows intermittent type "B" WPW pattern.

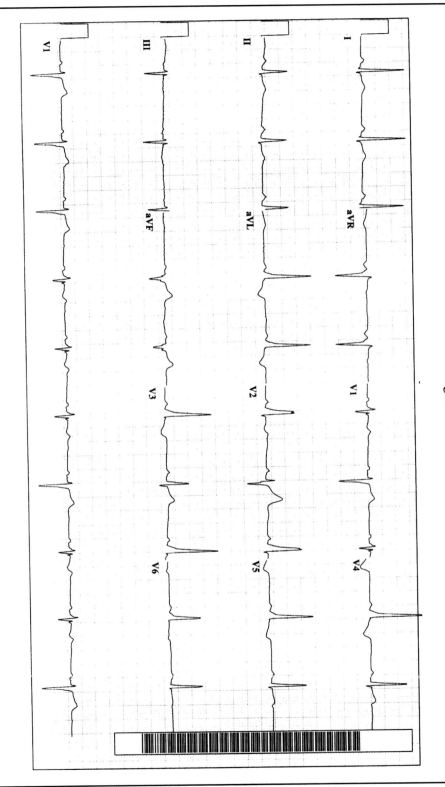

Figure 3

Chapter 20

Dextrocardia

Dextrocardia or right sided heart is mirror image of the normal heart. It is characterized on the EKG by inverted P, QRS and T waves in lead I. Leads V1 and V2 are reversed ("r" wave in V1 is taller than in V2), and there is progressive regression of "r" wave from lead V2 to V6, instead of normal progression. The above changes in lead I are also seen if arm leads are reversed, but in that case, the Precordial leads will remain unchanged. Leads AVR and AVL are interchanged in both conditions. EKG appearance in dextrocardia is illustrated in Fig. 1. The appearance with arm leads interchange is shown in Fig. 2.

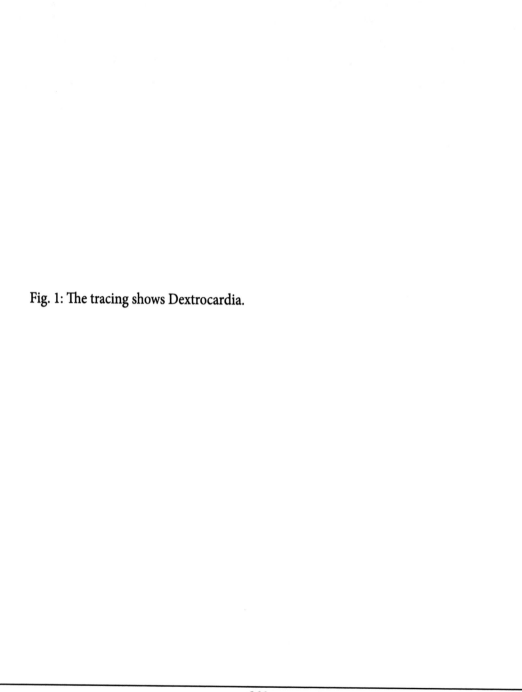

Fig. 1: The tracing shows Dextrocardia.

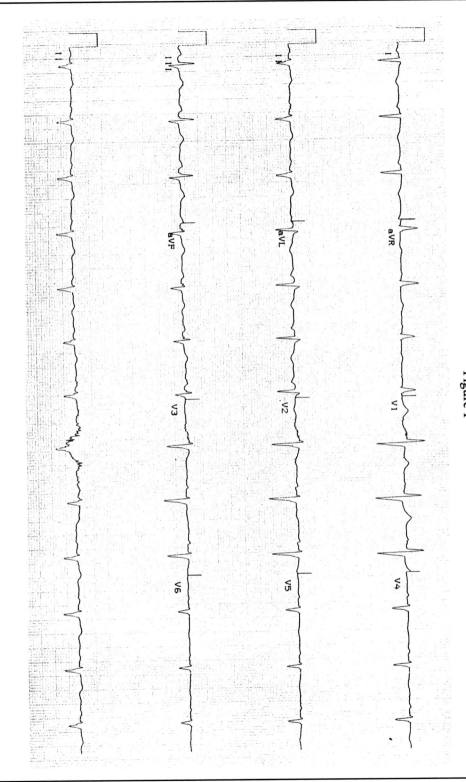

Figure 1

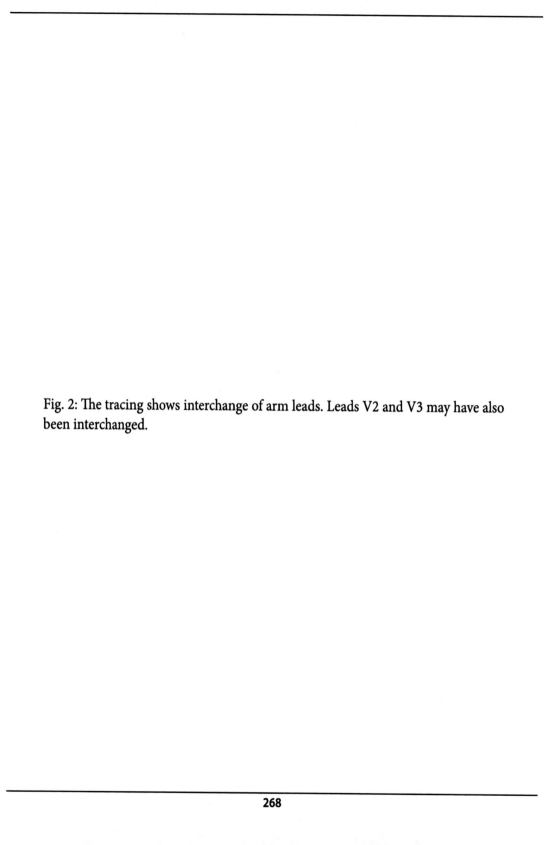

Fig. 2: The tracing shows interchange of arm leads. Leads V2 and V3 may have also been interchanged.

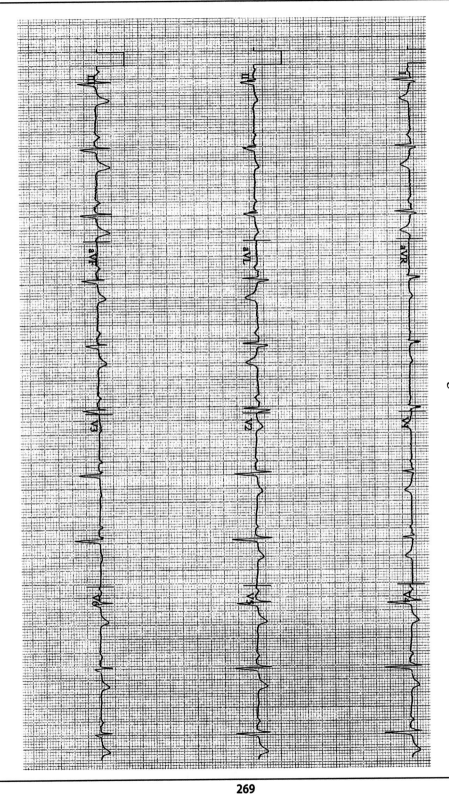

Figure 2

Chapter 21

Brugada Syndrome

It is a hereditary disorder with potential for sudden death. History of aborted sudden death, syncope, presyncope, dizziness, palpitations, or family history of sudden death, along with EKG pattern of ST elevation in more than one of right Precordial leads (V1 – 3) in the presence of right bundle branch block should raise the suspicion of Brugada syndrome. There are 3 types of EKG patterns in Brugada syndrome. Type 1 is characterized by J point or ST segment elevation of 2.0 mm or more, coved ST segment, and T inversion. Type 2 is characterized by J point elevation of 2.0 mm or more, saddleback shaped ST elevation of greater than 1.0 mm, and upright or biphasic T wave. Type 3 is characterized by coved or saddleback ST elevation of less than 1.0 mm. Type 1 is illustrated in Fig.1. Type 2 is illustrated in Fig.2. It should be noted that type 1 is the only true diagnostic pattern for Brugada syndrome. Type 2 and 3 are suggestive but not diagnostic of this syndrome.

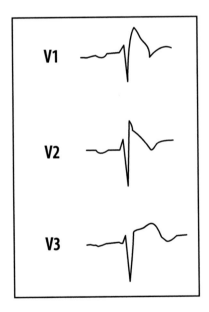

Figure 1

Fig.1: Above diagram is an illustration of Brugada syndrome, type 1.

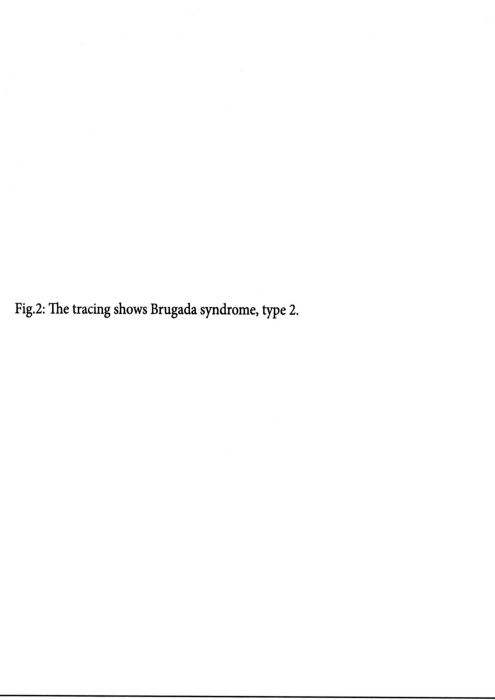

Fig.2: The tracing shows Brugada syndrome, type 2.

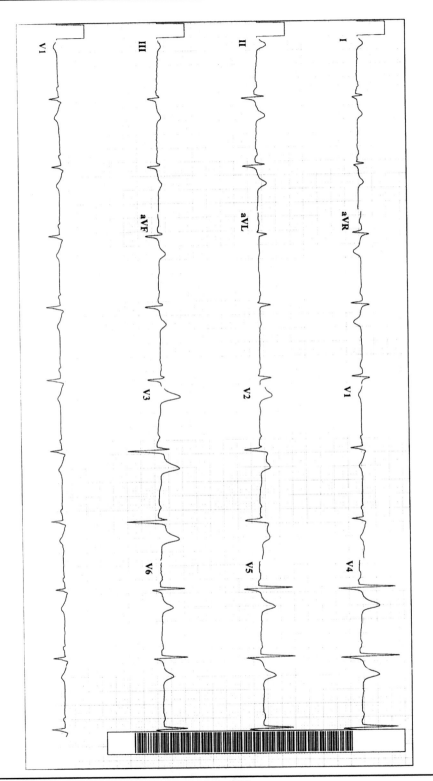

Figure 2

Chapter 22

Ashman Phenomenon

Gouaux and Ashman reported an observation in 1947 in atrial fibrillation. They found some aberrantly conducted QRS complexes with the morphology seen in right bundle branch block (Fig. 1). These wide QRS complexes can be confused with premature ventricular complexes. Sometimes there could be several such abnormal complexes in succession, and have to be differentiated from bursts of ventricular tachycardia. Ashman complexes are quite benign and represent antegrade AV conduction of supraventricular arrhythmia - atrial fibrillation. The explanation for this phenomenon lies in electrophysiology of infra nodal conduction tissue. When a long R – R cycle is preceded by a short R – R cycle, it increases the refractory period of the next following R – R cycle. Therefore, if the supraventricular impulse gets conducted too soon through the AV node following the long R – R cycle, it finds the conduction tissue refractory, thus resulting in aberrant conduction. Normally, the refractory period of the right bundle branch is longer than the refractory period of left bundle branch. Hence, the QRS complex shows morphology of RBBB. Conduction through the left bundle branch is not affected. When you look at the rhythm strip of the EKG, the R – R interval which precedes the first abnormal QRS complex – with RBBB pattern – is shorter than the preceding R – R interval, which, itself is preceded by a short R – R interval. Thus starting with the abnormal QRS complex and going to the left, there is a sequence of short, long, short R – R cycles in succession. It is this sequence which helps differentiate Ashman phenomenon from ventricular premature beats. The EKG tracing (Fig. 1) illustrates this clinical entity. You will note that the tracing shows atrial fibrillation with irregular R – R intervals. The rhythm strip at the bottom (lead V1), shows 14th QRS complex from the left as abnormal with RBBB morphology. The R – R interval between this complex and the preceding QRS complex is shorter than the preceding R – R interval, which in turn is longer than the R – R interval which precedes it. Thus, starting with the abnormal QRS complex and going to the left, there is a sequence of short, long, short R – R cycles. This sequence tells us that we are dealing with Ashman phenomenon in the presence of atrial fibrillation, and not a premature ventricular complex (PVC). This phenomenon can also be seen in atrial flutter with varying AV block, because the heart rate is irregular, which creates a potential for aberrant conduction, if an impulse gets conducted too soon after a long R – R cycle, when the long R – R cycle is preceded by a short R – R cycle.

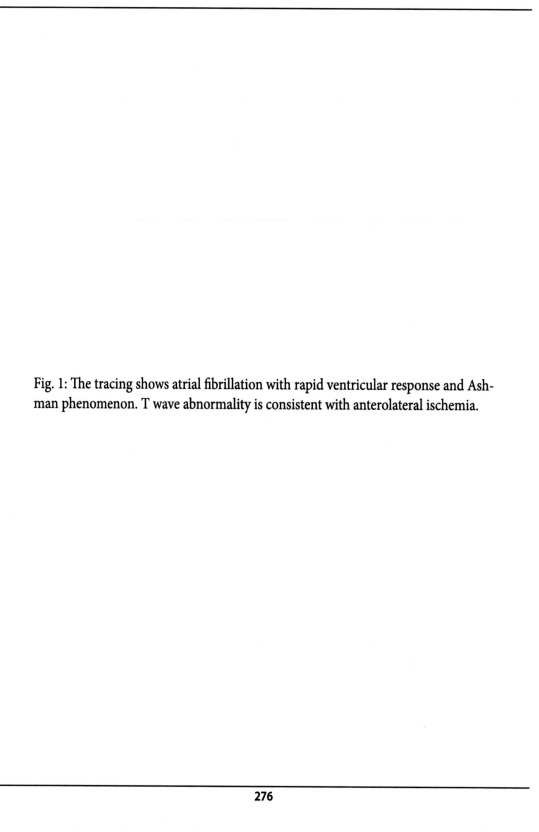

Fig. 1: The tracing shows atrial fibrillation with rapid ventricular response and Ashman phenomenon. T wave abnormality is consistent with anterolateral ischemia.

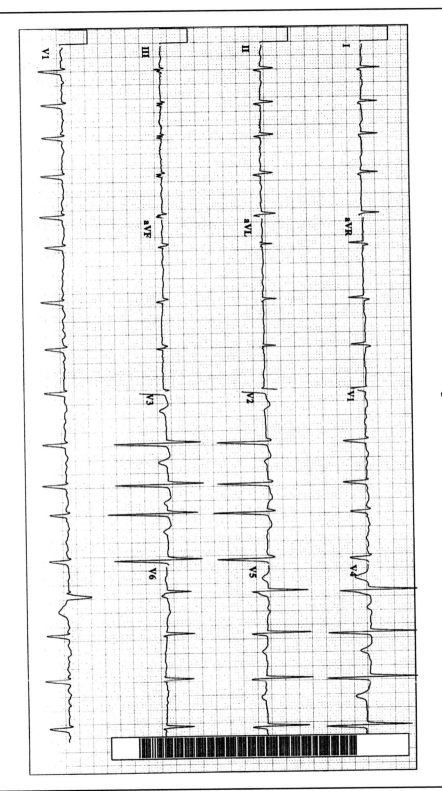

Figure 1

Artifacts

EKG tracing is a graphic recording of the signal (potential) generated over the skin by electrical activity within the heart. However, shivering, tremors (e.g. Parkinsonism), simple body movements like combing of hair or brushing teeth, skeletal muscle contractions, or stretching of the skin near the electrode can generate more powerful signal than the cardiac potential, thus causing interference in the EKG tracing. An increase in impedance to conduction due to poor contact between the surface of the skin and the electrode, or a broken lead wire can also cause abnormalities in the EKG tracing. Such abnormalities are called artifacts. Electronic devices attached to or implanted in the body of a patient, or medical electronic equipment in the vicinity may also lead to such artifacts through its electromagnetic field (60 HTZ noise). Some examples of commonly seen artifacts are shown on the following pages.

Figure 1: The tracing shows chicken scratch appearance in the rhythm strip (lead V1) and in leads I, II and AVR. This is also referred to as fuzzy appearance or 60 HTZ noise. This artifact usually indicates a poor contact between the electrode and the surface of the skin, but can also be caused by shivering, tremors, muscular contractions or stretching of the skin near the electrode. Electromagnetic field generated by medical equipment or devices implanted inside or attached to the body can also result in 60 HTZ noise.

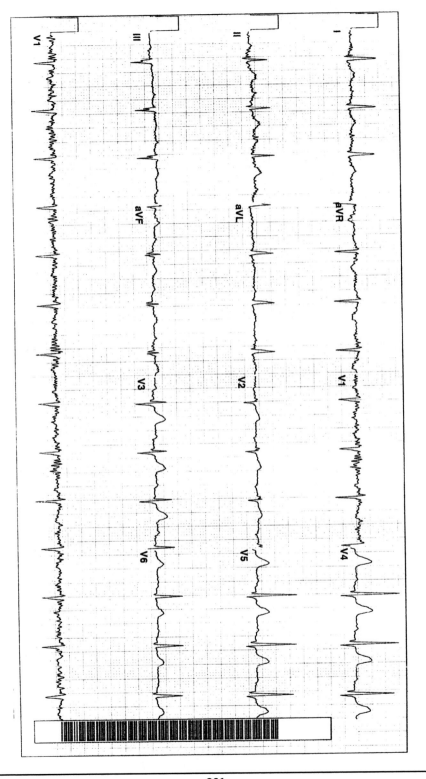

Figure 1

Figure 2: The tracing shows baseline drifting in Precordial leads and in the rhythm strip. This results from simple body movements. Respiratory movements of the chest may sometime result in this abnormality. Significant baseline drifting can occur with major body movements or during DC cardioversion.

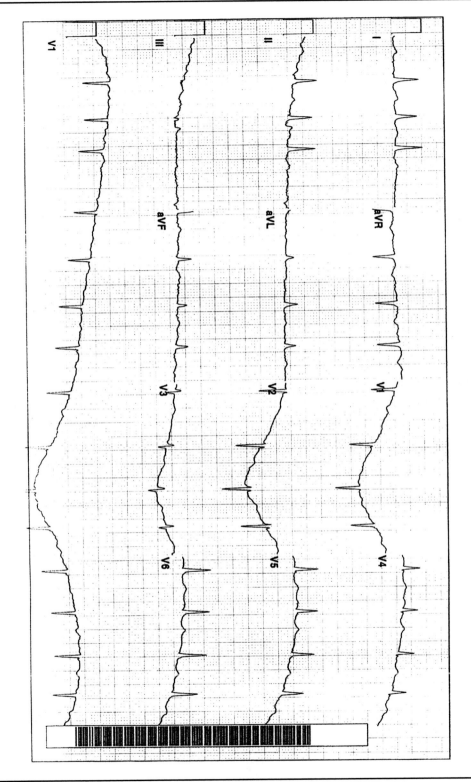

Figure 2

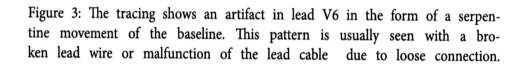

Figure 3: The tracing shows an artifact in lead V6 in the form of a serpentine movement of the baseline. This pattern is usually seen with a broken lead wire or malfunction of the lead cable due to loose connection.

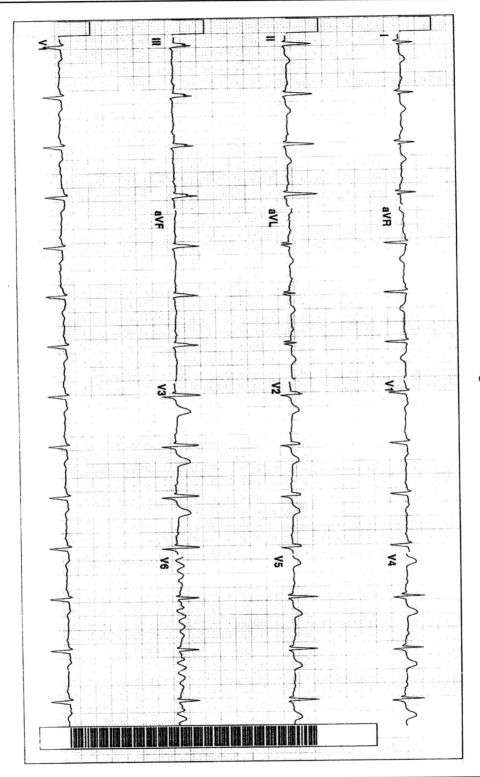

Figure 3

285

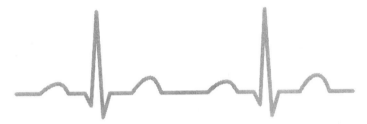

Step by Step
Guided
Interpretation
of EKGs

EKG Tracing # 1

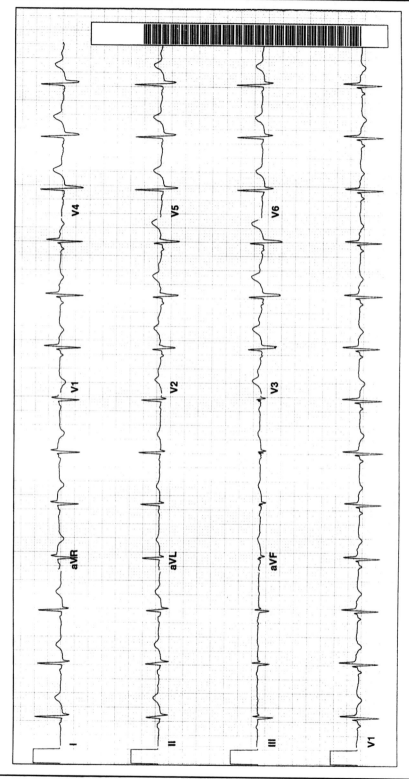

EKG Tracing #1

Heart rate is 78/min. and regular.

RHYTHM:

QRS complexes are narrow, indicating a supraventricular rhythm (sinus, atrial, or nodal) with normal infranodal conduction. P wave is upright (antegrade) in lead AVF @ 78/min., indicating normal sinus rhythm activating the atria. PR is constant and normal, indicating normal antegrade AV conduction. In summary, Sinus is activating the atria at normal rate, there is normal antegrade AV conduction, and normal infranodal conduction, leading to the ventricular activation, i.e. sinus node is activating the atria as well as the ventricles and the conduction is normal. Therefore, it is a normal sinus rhythm.

QRS AXIS:

Lead AVF is negative, and Lead II is closest to being isoelectric. If it were isoelectric, the axis would be –30 degrees. Since lead II is lot more positive than negative, the QRS axis,according to Anand rule, is lot less, i.e. 15 to 20 degrees less. Therefore, it is –10 to –15 degrees or approximately –12 degrees, which is normal. If you are not sure whether to choose lead II or lead AVR as closest to being isoelectric, always choose one with smaller number, e.g. –30 is smaller than –60 degrees; therefore, we will start with lead II.

PR interval is 0.12 second. QRS interval is 0.09 second. QTc is 0.46 second.

SCANNING:

There is r prime in lead V1. If QRS interval is less than 0.09 sec., r prime in V1 is normal. If QRS interval is 90 msec. or greater but less than 0.12 sec., it is incomplete RBBB. If QRS interval is 0.12 sec. or greater, it suggests complete RBBB. There must be "S" wave in lead I and/or V6 along with r prime (or R prime) in V1 to make the diagnosis of IRBBB or RBBB.

INTERPRETATION:
Normal sinus rhythm
Incomplete RBBB

Note: The presence of incomplete RBBB by itself does not make an EKG abnormal.

EKG Tracing # 2

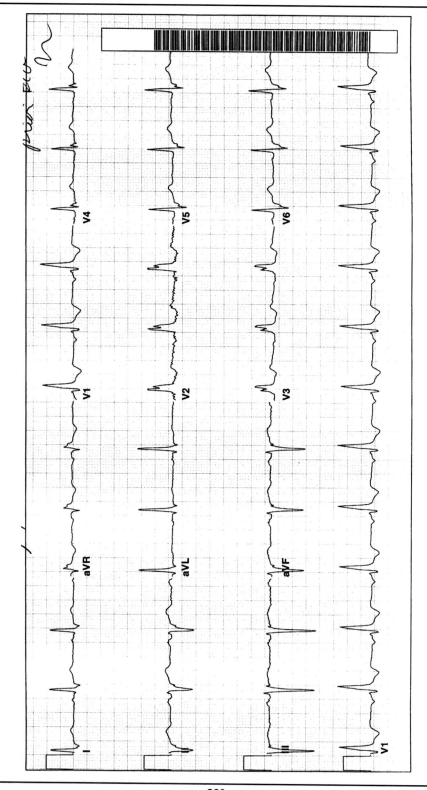

Heart rate is 72/min. and regular.

RHYTHM:

QRS complexes are wide, indicating a supraventricular rhythm with aberrancy or a ventricular rhythm. The shape of the P wave in lead AVF is upright (antegrade) @ 72/min., indicating normal sinus rhythm activating the atria. PR interval is constant and normal, indicating normal antegrade AV conduction. Since, AV conduction is antegrade, the impulse must be conducted down the right and the left bundle branches with aberrancy. If there was a complete block at the AV node (called complete AV block) instead of antegrade AV conduction, it would indicate ventricular rhythm in the presence of wide QRS complexes. So, we have sinus rhythm activating the atria, antegrade AV conduction, and aberrant conduction in the ventricles in this EKG. The question now is whether aberrant conduction is due to RBBB, LBBB, or IVC delay. The presence of rabbit ears in lead V1 suggests RBBB. S wave is present in lead 1. Therefore, the diagnosis is NSR (normal sinus rhythm) with RBBB.

QRS AXIS:

Lead AVF is predominently negative, indicating minus axis. Lead AVR is closest to being isoelectric. If it were isoelectric, the axis would be –60 degrees. But it is a little more positive. Therefore, according to Anand rule, add 5 to 10 degrees. Thus, the QRS axis is –65 to –70 degrees, i.e. approximately –68 degrees. A QRS axis of –45 degrees or greater suggests left anterior hemiblock.

PR = 0.i2 sec.; QRS = 0.12 sec., QTc = 0.486 sec.

SCANNING:

ST depression in leads V2 and V3 is a part of RBBB due to wide QRS complexes. When QRS is wide, the ST – T moves in opposite direction to the QRS.

INTERPRETATION:

Normal Sinus Rhythm

RBBB

LAHB (left anterior hemiblock)

Abnormal EKG

EKG Tracing # 3

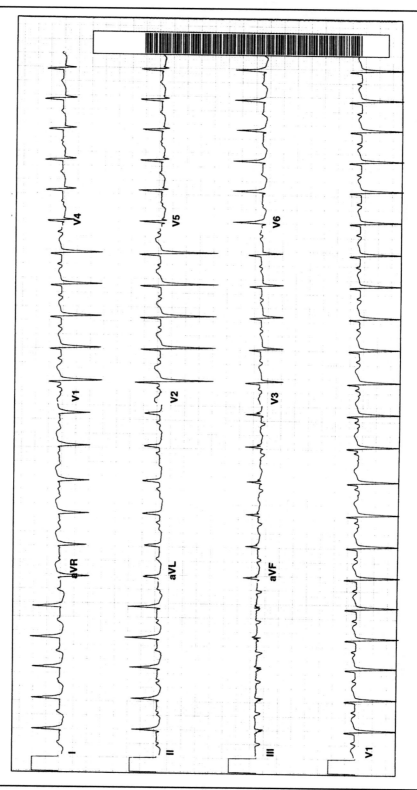

EKG Tracing #3

Heart rate is 132/min. and irregular.

RHYTHM:

QRS complexes are narrow, indicating supraventricular rhythm with normal infranodal conduction. The rate and shape of the P wave in lead AVF shows a retrograde P @ 132/min., indicating ectopic atrial tachycardia (nodal tachycardia does not go above 115/min.; nodal rhythm is below 60/min.; accelerated nodal rhythm is between 60 and 100/min.; nodal tachycardia is 100 – 115/min.). PR is varying, indicating varying AV block or complete AV block. R – R is irregular in varying AV block and regular in complete AV block. Here in above EKG, the R – R is irregular. This favors the diagnosis of varying AV block. In case of varying AV block, each P must be followed by a QRS and each QRS must be preceded by a P wave and PR segment. Above EKG tracing satisfies this criterion also. Hence, it is varying AV block. In summary, we have ectopic atrial tachycardia with varying AV block and normal infranodal conduction. Diagnosis, therefore, is ectopic atrial tachycardia with varying AV block.

QRS AXIS:

Lead AVF is positive. There is no lead with biphasic QRS complexes. We know that the QRS axis is with the plus sign due to positive AVF lead. Therefore, let us start with +30, where lead III should be isoelectric. But lead III is negative, which means the QRS axis is less than +30 degrees. Moreover, lead III is actually entirely negative, which means it is lot less than +30 degrees, i.e. 15 – 20 degrees less than +30 degrees. Therefore, QRS axis is +10 to +15 degrees or approximately +12 degrees. If lead AVF were to be negative in above EKG, we would have chosen lead II to work with because –30 is the smallest minus number, just as +30 is the smallest plus number to work with.

PR = varying; QRS = 0.08 sec.; QTc = 0.453 sec.

SCANNING:

ST – T abnormality in lateral leads (leads I, AVL, V5 – 6) consistent with lateral ischemia and/or LVH.

INTERPRETATION:

Ectopic atrial tachycardia with varying AV block

ST – T abnormality consistent with lateral ischemia and/or LVH

Abnormal EKG

EKG Tracing # 4

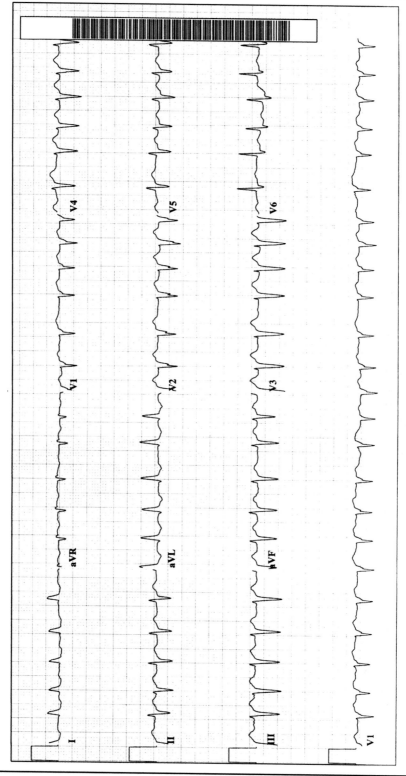

EKG Tracing #4

Heart rate is 144/min. and irregular.

RHYTHM:

QRS complexes are narrow, indicating supraventricular rhythm with normal infranodal conduction. There are no P waves in lead AVF or in the rhythm strip at the bottom of the EKG tracing. Since, there are no P waves, the question of PR is muted. Therefore, we look at R – R instead, which is irregular. Whenever, R – R is irregular, always think of atrial fibrillation until proven otherwise. Absence of P waves, irregular R – R, and narrow QRS is consistent with the diagnosis of atrial fibrillation with antegrade AV conduction. If QRS complexes were wide with irregular R – R and no visible P waves, the diagnosis would have been atrial fibrillation with aberrant conduction.

QRS Axis:

QRS complexes in lead AVF are predominantly negative. Therefore, the QRS axis is with the minus sign. Lead II is closest to being isoelectric. If this lead were isoelectric, the QRS axis in the presence of negative lead AVF would be –30 degrees. However, lead II is lot more negative (area under the negative deflection is more than twice the area under the positive deflection). Hence, the axis is higher by 15 – 20 degrees, i.e. it is – 45 to – 50 degrees, or it is approximately – 47 degrees. A QRS axis of – 45 degrees or more suggests left anterior hemiblock (LAHB).

QRS = 0.1 sec., QTc = 0.492 sec.

SCANNING:

There is ST – T abnormality in leads I and AVL, consistent with ischemia and/or digitalis effect. There is also poor progression of R wave in leads V1 – 4, consistent with anterior M.I., ? age, or LAHB.

INTERPRETATION:

Atrial fibrillation

LAHB

ST – T abnormality consistent with ischemia and/or digitalis effect

Anterior M.I., ? Age, masked by LAHB cannot be excluded.

Prolonged Q – Tc

Abnormal EKG

EKG Tracing # 5

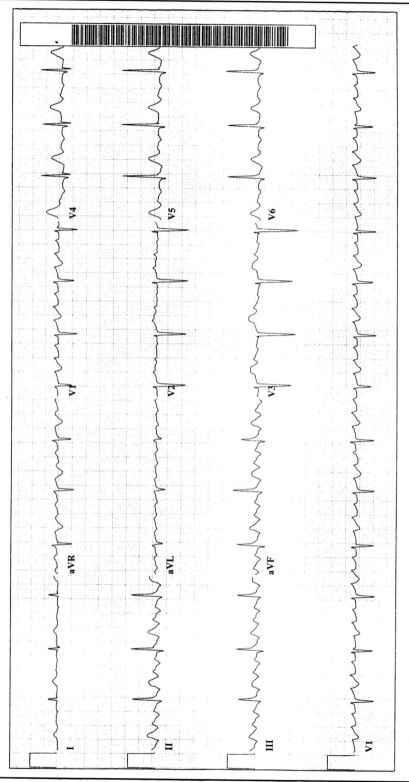

EKG Tracing #5

Heart rate is 78/min. and regular.

RHYTHM:

QRS complexes are narrow, indicating supraventricular rhythym with normal infranodal conduction. The shape of the P in lead AVF is saw-toothed, indicating atrial flutter. Since, there is no P wave, the question of PR being constant or not does not arise, and this step is replaced by R – R being regular or irregular. R – R is regular. That means, it is either a fixed 4:1 AV conduction (atrial rate is 4 times the ventricular rate) or there is complete AV block with nodal rhythm (QRS is narrow). The interval between the flutter wave preceeding each QRS complex and the corresponding following QRS would be varying if it were a complete AV block because of independent beating of ventricular and atrial chambers, but it is constant in the above EKG tracing. Therefore, it is not a case of complete AV block. Hence, there is a fixed 4:1 AV conduction. Therefore, the diagnosis is atrial flutter with 4:1 AV conduction.

QRS Axis:

Lead AVF is positive and lead AVL is closest to being isoelectric. If it were isoelectric, the QRS axis would be +60 degrees. But it is a little more negative than positive, i.e., the negative area is bigger but no more than twice the positive area. Thus, add 5 to 10 degrees. Since the bigger area is almost close to being twice the smaller area, we would add 10, i.e., the QRS axis is +70 degrees. Note: if bigger area was more than twice the smaller area, we would have called it "a lot more" instead of "a little more" and would have added 15 – 20 degrees.

QRS = 0.08 sec., Q – Tc = 0.429 sec.

SCANNING:

Poor r wave progression in leads V1 – 3, indicating possible anterior M.I., ?age.

INTERPRETATION:

Atrial flutter with 4:1 AV conduction

Possible anterior M.I., ? Age

Abnormal EKG

EKG Tracing # 6

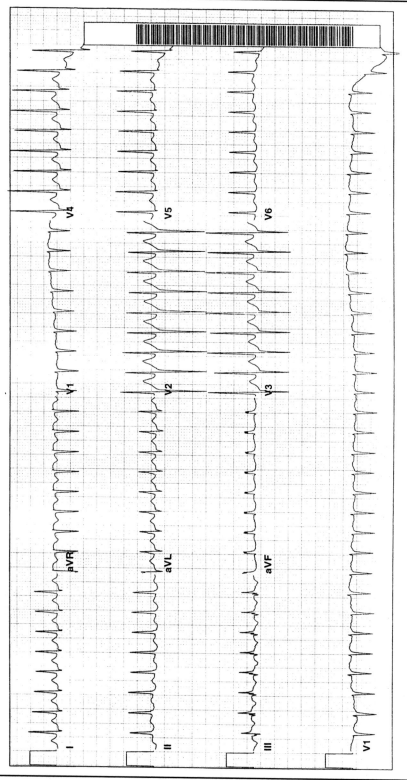

EKG Tracing #6

Heart rate is 210/min. and regular.

RHYTHM:

QRS complexes are narrow, indicating supraventricular rhythm with normal infranodal conduction. No P waves are visible in lead AVF. When rhythm is supraventricular and no P waves are visible, rhythm is atrial fib. if R – R is irregular, and nodal or SVT if R – R is regular. Above R – R is regular. Therefore, the rhythm should be nodal tachycardia or SVT. When the ventricular rate is more than 115/min., it is called supraventricular tachycardia (SVT) and not nodal tachycardia as the AV node is not supposed to discharge at a rate above 115/min. The diagnosis, therefore, is SVT.

QRS Axis:

Lead AVF is positive and lead AVL is closest to being isoelectric, If it were isoelectric, the QRS axis would be +60 degrees. But it is lot more positive than negative. Hence, decrease by 15 – 20 degrees, i.e. QRS axis is +60 minus 15 to 20 = +40 to +45 degrees, approximately +42 degrees.

QRS = 0.07 sec., Q – Tc = 0.409 sec.

SCANNING:

ST depression in leads II, V4 – 6, suggestive of ischemia. Note: In leads I and V3, there is J point depression with upsloping ST segments, which is normal.

INTERPRETATION:

Supraventricular Tachycardia

ST – T abnormality consistent with ischemia

Abnormal EKG

EKG Tracing # 7

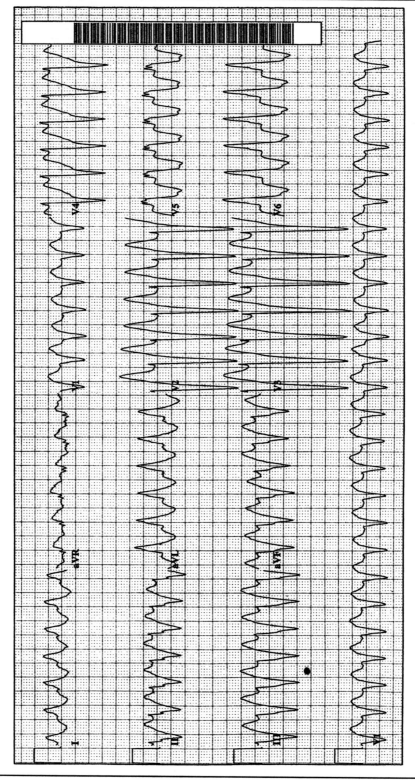

EKG Tracing #7

Heart rate is 156/min. and regular.

RHYRHM:

QRS complexes are wide, indicating that the rhythm is either supraventricular with aberrancy or it is ventricular. Lead AVF shows no P waves. When there are no P waves, the next step is to see if R – R is regular or irregular. If it is irregular, it is atrial fibrillation; if it is regular, it is nodal or SVT when QRS is narrow, and it is ventricular when QRS is wide. In the above EKG, the R – R is regular and QRS is wide. Therefore, it is Ventricular rhythm @ 156/min., i.e. ventricular tachycardia, which is also called wide QRS tachycardia.

QRS AXIS:

Leads II, III and AVF look alike and it is very difficult to find one which can be called as closest to being isoelectric. But one thing is sure that the axis is with the minus sign, as lead AVF is negative. The smallest number in that category is –30 degrees, next is –60 degrees, and the next is –90 degrees. Number –30 belongs to lead II, – 60 belongs to lead AVR, and –90 belongs to lead I. Therefore, let us try all of these three leads. According to lead II, the QRS axis is greater than – 30 degrees. According to lead AVR, it is greater than – 60 degrees. According to lead I, it is less than – 90 degrees. Therefore, the axis is between – 60 and – 90 degrees. Hence, the QRS axis is –75 degrees. It does not indicate LAHB because the rhythm is ventricular and there is no infranodal conduction along bundle branches.

QRS = 0.16 sec., Q – Tc = 0.565 sec. (it is prolonged).

SCANNING:

ST – T abnormality in lateral leads is due to wide QRS complexes.

INTERPRETATION:
Wide QRS tachycardia
Prolonged Q –Tc
Abnormal EKG

EKG Tracing # 8

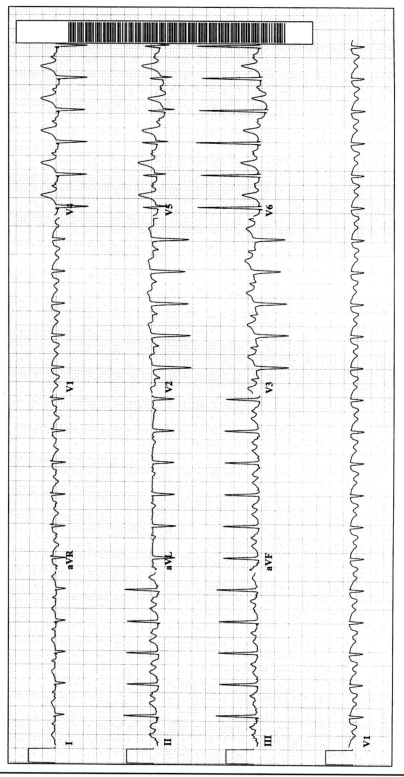

EKG Tracing #8

Heart rate is 132/min. and regular.

RHYTHM:

QRS complexes are narrow, indicating supraventricular rhythm with normal infra nodal conduction. The shape of the P wave in lead AVF is upright (antegrade) @ 132/min., indicating sinus tachycardia. PR is constant and normal, suggesting normal antegrade AV conduction. Thus, we have sinus tachycardia with normal antegrade AV conduction and normal infranodal conduction. Therefore, the diagnosis is sinus tachycardia.

QRS Axis:

Lead AVF is positive, indicating the QRS axis with plus sign. Now the question is, which lead is closest to being isoelectric? Some students will choose lead AVR, while some will prefer lead I. Let us choose both and calculate QRS axis. According to lead AVR, the axis is +120 and substract (because lead AVR is lot more negative) 15 to 20 = +100 to +105. According to lead I, the axis is +90 and add (because lead I is lot more negative) 15 to 20 = +105 to +110. Thus the Qrs axis is +105 to +110. Thus the Qrs axis is +105 degrees according to both approaches. Whether you choose lead I or lead AVR you are within 5 degrees of +105 if you happen to choose +110 or +100 respectively. If you decide that none of the limb leads is biphasic, start with the smallest plus number because lead AVF is positive, and that number is +30 which belongs to lead III. Lead III is entirely positive which means that the axis is more than +30. Next number is +60 which belongs to lead AVL which is all negative and that means that the axis is more than +60. Next is +90 and lead I is mostly negative and that means the axis is more than +90. Next is +120 and that number belongs to lead AVR which is mostly negative which means the axis is less than +120. So, we know that the axis lies between +90 and +120. Thus, the axis is +105 degrees. Again you come to the same conclusion. This last method is more accurate under above circumstances.

PR = 0.16 sec., QRS = 0.08 sec., Q – Tc = 0.419 sec.

SCANNING:

Left atrial enlargement; Loss of R in leads V1 – 4, indicating anterior M.I., ? Age

INTERPRETATION:

Sinus tachycardia
LAE (left Atrial Enlargement)
Right axis deviation (RAD)
Anterior M.I., ? Age

EKG Tracing # 9

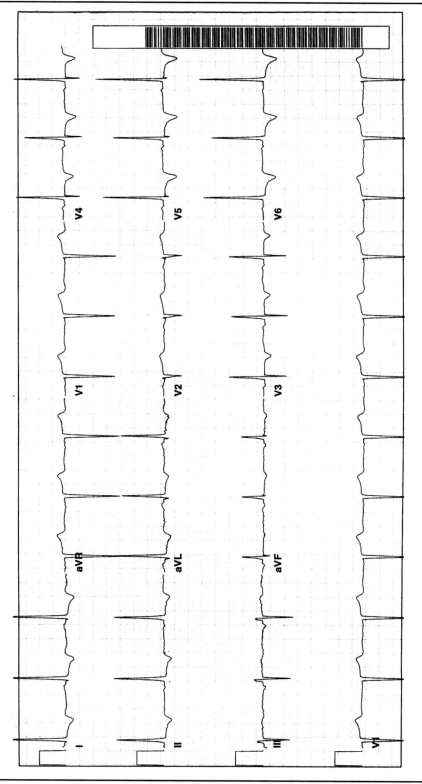

EKG Tracing #9

Heart rate is 70/min. and regular.

RHYTHM:

QRS complexes are narrow, indicating supraventricular rhythm with normal infranodal conduction. The shape of the P in lead AVF is biphasic (antegrade) @ 70/min., indicating normal sinus rhythm activating the atria. PR is constant and normal, indicating antegrade AV conduction. Thus, we have normal sinus rhythm activating the atria, antegrade AV conduction, and normal infranodal conduction. Therefore, the diagnosis is normal sinus rhythm (NSR), which means that the sinus node is activating both the atria as well as the ventrcles with antegrade AV conduction and normal infranodal conduction.

QRS Axis:

Lead AVF is positive. Therefore, the QRS axis is going to be with the + sign. Lead III appears to be a biphasic lead which is closest to being isoelectric among the limb leads. If lead III was isoelectric, the QRS axis would be +30 degrees. But it is lot more negative. Therefore, according to Anand rule, you should deduct 15 to 20 degrees,i.e. the axis is +10 to +15 degrees, which is normal.

PR = 0.12 sec., QRS = 0.09 sec., Q – Tc = 0.453 sec.

SCANNING:

There is ST depression in lateral leads (I, II, AVL, and leads V4 – 6), and T wave inversion in inferior (II, III, AVF) and anterolateral leads (V3 – 6). Tall R waves in lateral leads. Note: The ST segments in lateral leads are coved. This morphology is suggestive of ischemia and/or LVH.

INTERPRETATION:

Normal Sinus Rhythm

ST – T abnormality consistent with LVH and/or ischemia (some cardiologists read it as "ST – T abnormality consistent with LVH with repolarization abnormality; it means the same thing)

EKG Tracing # 10

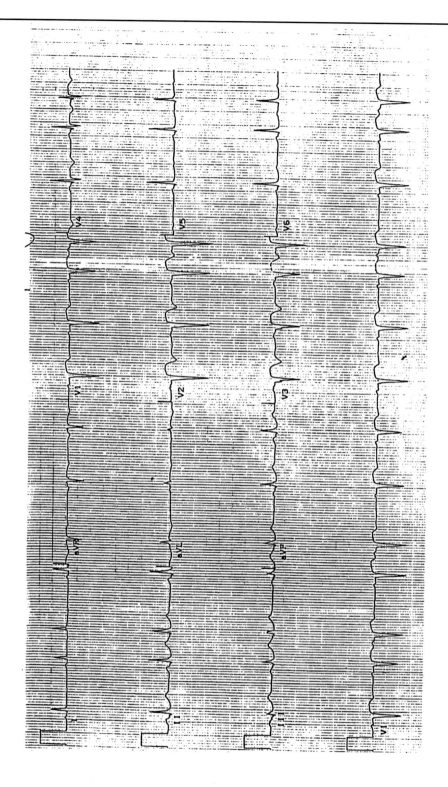

Heart rate is 84/min. with occasional irregularity. Looking at the rhythm strip at the bottom of the EKG and starting from left, the 3rd, 5th, 11th, and 14th QRS complexes are premature and narrow (supraventricular), and preceded by corresponding P waves which are also premature in P – P cycle suggestive of PACs (premature atrial contractions).

RHYTHM:

QRS complexes are narrow, indicating supraventricular rhythm with normal infranodal conduction. The shape of the P wave in lead AVF is upright and the atrial rate is normal, indicating normal sinus rhythm activating the atria. PR is constant and normal, indicating normal antegrade AV conduction. Thus, sinus is activating the atria at normal rate, AV conduction is antegrade and normal, and infranodal conduction is normal. Therefore, it is normal sinus rhythm(NSR) with occasional PACs.

QRS Axis:

Lead AVF is positive and it is difficult to pin-point a limb lead which is closest to being isoelectric. We know that the QRS axis is with the plus sign and the smallest memorized number is +30 degrees which belongs to lead III. Therefore, let us begin with lead III. Lead III is mostly positive which means that the axis is more than +30 degrees. Next memorized number is +60 degrees which belongs to lead AVL. So, let us look at lead AVL. Lead AVL is more positive which means that the QRS axis, according to Anand rule, is less than +60 degrees. Thus, we know that the QRS axis is between +30 and +60 degrees. Therefore, the QRS axis is +45 degrees. This way moving upward in stepwise fashion, we can find the QRS axis when it is difficult to locate a limb lead which is closest to being isoelectric.

PR = 0.12 sec., QRS = 0.10 sec., Q – Tc = 0.415 sec.

SCANNING:

ST – T in lead I is flat. T wave in lead AVL is inverted but the P is also inverted, which is normal. There is loss of R wave in leads V1 to V3, suggesting infarction in anteroseptal area, and the ST segments in these leads are elevated and convex upward, indicating that the infarction is acute (injury pattern). T wave inversion in leads V2 – 4 is a part of this injury.

INTERPRETATION:

Normal sinus rhythm with occasional PACs

Acute anteroseptal M.I.

Abnormal EKG

EKG Tracing # 11

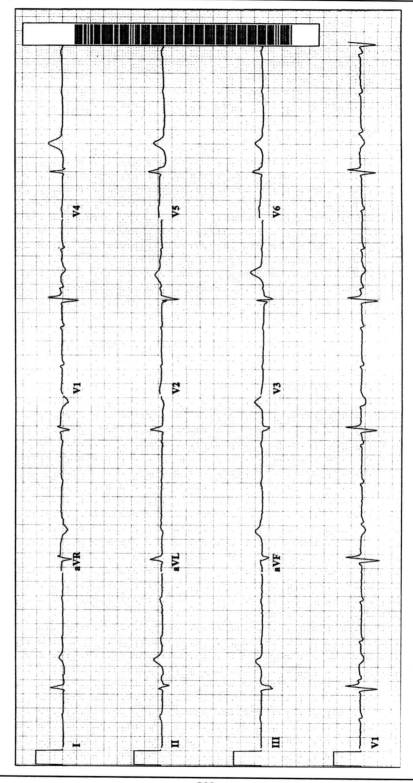

EKG Tracing #11

Heart rate is 33/min. and regular.

RHYTHM:

QRS is narrow, indicating supraventricular rhythm with normal infranodal conduction. The shape of the P in lead AVF is antegrade, indicating sinus node activating the atria @ 107/min., i.e. sinus tachycardia. It is to be noted that the atrial rate is much higher than the ventricular rate, indicating some kind of AV block. Next step is to look at the rhythm strip to see whether PR is constant or not. While we do that, it is also obvious that some P waves are followed by QRS and some P waves are not followed by QRS, and those P waves which are not followed by QRS are not premature P waves. This finding always means either second degree or third degree AV block. Always first ask yourself if it is third degree, because a third degree block is much easier to rule in or out. To qualify for third degree AV block, R – R is regular and PR is not regular (it is not constant). If these criteria are not present, it is a second degree AV block. In the above tracing, R – R is regular and PR is not, and the P waves which are not followed by QRS are not premature, therefore, it is a third degree AV block. Since, QRS is narrow, the ventricles are being activated by the AV node with normal infranodal conduction. Thus, the rhythm is sinus tachycardia with complete AV block and nodal rhythm.

QRS Axis:

Lead AVF is negative and lead II is isoelectric. Therefore, the QRS axis is –30 degrees, i.e. left axis deviation (LAD).

PR is varying; QRS interval = 0.1 sec., Q – Tc = 0.409 sec.

SCANNING:

rSR prime (suggesting incomplete RBBB); loss of R in V2 and a Q wave in lead V3 (suggesting anteroseptal M.I.). ST depression in V5 is an artifact. T wave inversion in lead AVL is concordant with P wave inversion which is normal.

INTERPRETATION:

Sinus tachycardia with complete AV block and nodal escape rhythm

LAD

IRBBB

ASMI, ? Age

Abnormal EKG

EKG Tracing # 12

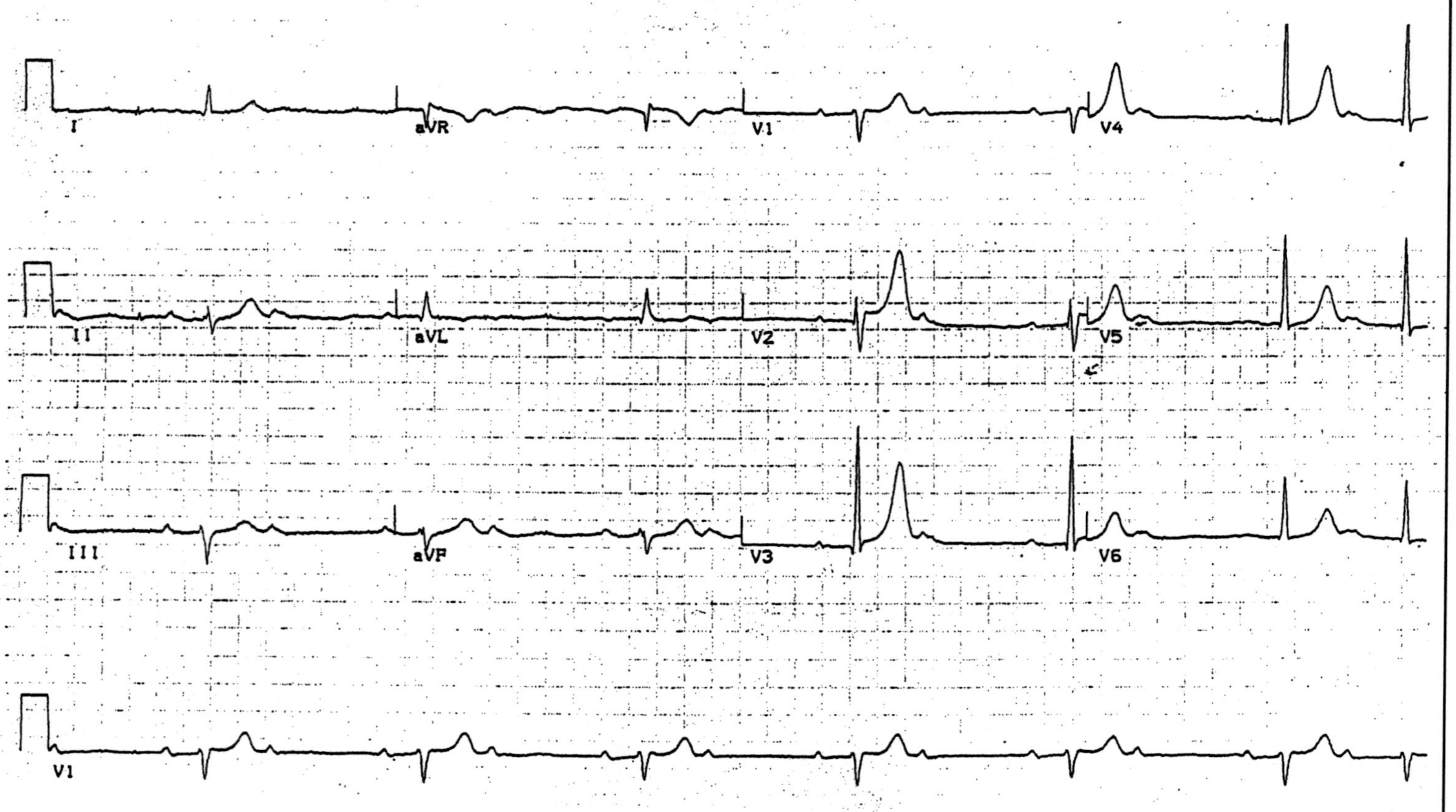

EKG Tracing #12

Heart rate is 42/min. and essentially regular except the last QRS on the right.

RHYTHM:

QRS complexes are narrow, indicating a supraventricular rhythm with normal infranodal conduction. The shape of the P wave in lead AVF is antegrade, indicating sinus node activating the atria @ 84/min. Some P waves are followed by QRS and some are not, and those that are not, are not premature P waves. Therefore, it is either a second or a third degree AV block. Is it a third degree block? To qualify for a third degree AV block, R – R should be regular and PR should not be regular. Here, R – R is not regular. Hence, it is a second degree AV block. If you ignore the last QRS on the right and call it essentially regular R – R, note that the PR then is also constant which rules out third degree AV block and makes it a second degree AV block. It is not a Mobitz type I block (also known as Wenckebach block), and it is not a high grade block; therefore, it is Mobitz type II AV block.

QRS Axis:

Lead AVF is negative, and lead II is isoelectric. Therefore, the QRS axis is –30 degrees, i.e. LAD (left axis deviation).

PR = 0.24 sec, QRS = 0.08 sec., Q – Tc = 0.40 sec.

SCANNING:

Tall T waves in precordial leads suggestive of hyperkalemia.

INTERPRETATION:

Sinus rhythm with second degree AV block with predominently 2:1 AV conduction

LAD

Tall T waves, ? Hyperkalemia

Abnormal EKG

EKG Tracing # 13

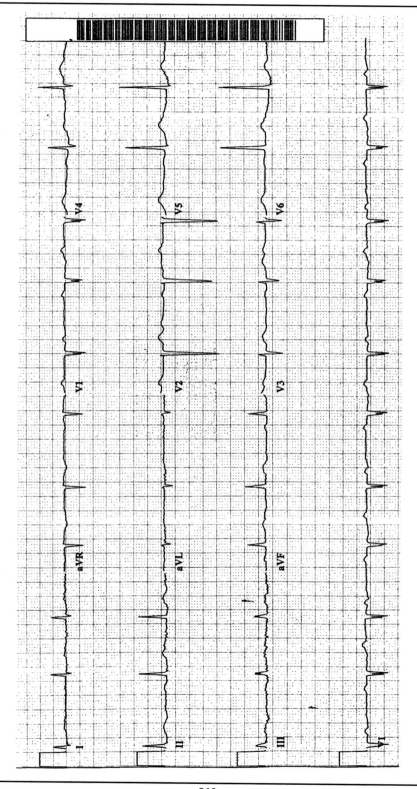

EKG Tracing #13

Heart rate is 66/min. and irregular.

RHYTHM:

QRS complexes are narrow, indicating supraventricular rhythm with normal infranodal conduction. The shape of the P wave in lead AVF is upright (antegrade) @ 100/min., indicating sinus node activating the atria. Since, the atrial rate is much higher than the ventricular rate, it indicates some kind of heart block. PR is varying and some P waves are followed by a QRS and some are not. Those P waves which are not followed by a QRS are not premature. Therefore, it is either a second degree or a third degree AV block. To qualify for a third degree AV block, R – R should be regular and PR should not be regular. Here, R – R is not regular. Therefore, it is not a third degree AV block, but a second degree AV block. There is a repetative pattern where successive PR intervals get longer until the P wave is not followed by a QRS , and the cycle starts again. Thus, it is a Mobitz type I AV block (also called Wenckebach AV block).

QRS Axis:

Lead AVF is positive and lead AVL is closest to being isoelectric, but a little more negative. Therefore, according to Anand rule, the QRS axis is +60 plus 5 – 10 degrees, i.e. +65 to +70 degrees or approximately +67 degrees.

PR = variable; QRS = 0.09 sec.; Q – Tc = 0.403 sec.

SCANNING:

No ST – T abnormality; no left atrial enlargrment; no r prime in V1; satisfactory R wave progression in precordial leads.

INTERPRETATION:

Sinus rhythm with second degree AV block (Mobitz type I).

Abnormal EKG

EKG Tracing # 14

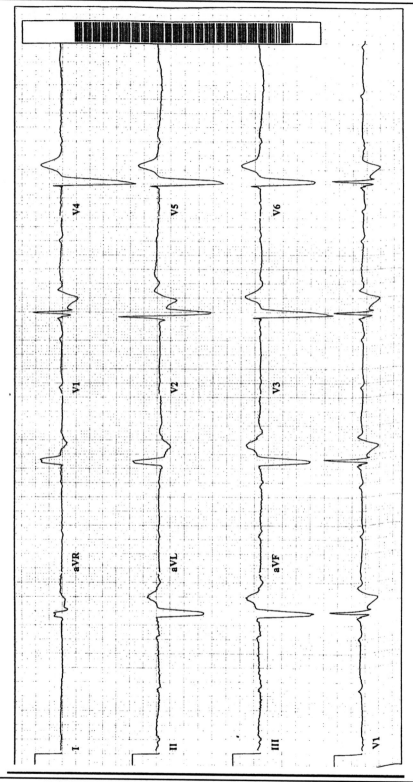

EKG Tracing #14

Heart rate is 28/min. and regular.

RHYTHM:

QRS is wide, indicating supraventricular rhythm with aberrancy or a ventricular rhythm. The shape of P in lead AVF is antegrade @ 84/min. It is obvious that the atrial rate is much higher than the ventricular rate, which indicates some kind of AV block. PR is constant but some P waves are followed by a QRS and some are not. That indicates 2nd or 3rd degree AV block. In 3rd degree AV block, the R – R is regular and PR is not regular. Here, R – R is regular but PR is also regular. Therefore, it is a second degree AV block. It is obviously not a Mobitz type I block. There are 3 P waves for each QRS complex i.e. it is a high grade 2nd degree AV block (in Mobitz type II block, there is occasional P without the QRS or P to QRS ratio is 2:1, 3:2, 4:3, 5:4 etc, i.e. there is one more P wave than the number of QRS complexes in each cycle). Thus the diagnosis is sinus rhythm with high grade second degree AV block and aberrant infranodal conduction. The appearance of rabbit ears in lead V1 (rSR prime) suggests RBBB. Therefore, it is sinus rhythm with high grade 2nd degree AV block and RBBB.

QRS Axis:

Lead AVF is negative and lead I is closest to being isoelectric but a lot more positive i.e. it is –90 decreased by 15 = –75 degrees, which is consistent with LAHB (left anterior hemi-block).

$PR = 0.28$ sec., $QRS = 0.16$ sec., $Q - Tc = 0.34$ sec.

SCANNING:

ST – T abnormality is secondary to wide QRS complexes.

INTERPRETATION:

Sinus rhythm with high grade second degree AV block.

RBBB

LAHB

Abnormal EKG

EKG Tracing # 15

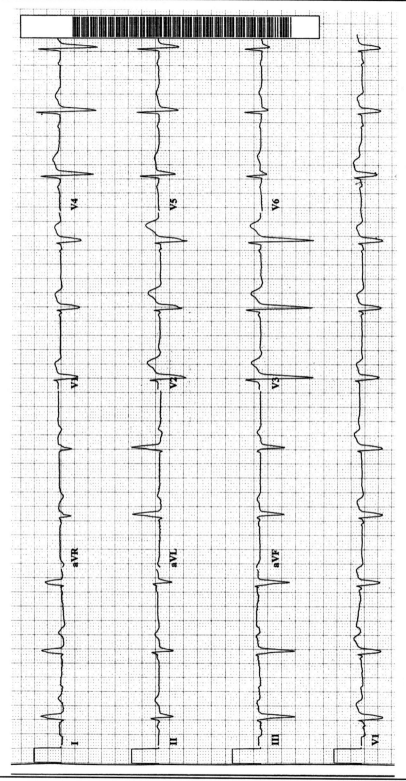

EKG Tracing #15

Heart rate is 63/min. and regular.

RHYTHM:

QRS is wide, indicating supraventricular rhythm with aberrant infranodal conduction or a ventricular rhythm. The shape of the P wave in lead AVF is antegrade @ 65/min., indicating sinus node activating the atria. It is noteworthy that the atrial and the ventricular rates are different but almost identical. PR is varying and the R – R is regular, indicating complete AV block or AV dissociation. Since, ventrcular rate is greater than 50/min., and the atrial and ventricular rates are almost identical, the diagnosis is isorhythmic AV dissociation, i.e. there is accelerated idioventricular rhythm with AV dissociation and underlying sinus rhythm.

QRS Axis:

Lead AVF is negative, and lead II is closest to being isoelectric but lot more negative than positive. Therefore, the QRS axis is –45 to 50 degrees. It does not indicate LAHB because the rhythm is ventricular and there is no infranodal conduction of the sinus impulse.

PR = varying; QRS = 0.14 sec., Q – Tc = 0.418 sec.

SCANNING:

ST elevation in leads V1 – 3 is secondary to wide negative QRS in these leads.

INTERPRETATION:

Sinus rhythm with isorhythmic AV dissociation and underlying ventricular rhythm.

Abnormal EKG

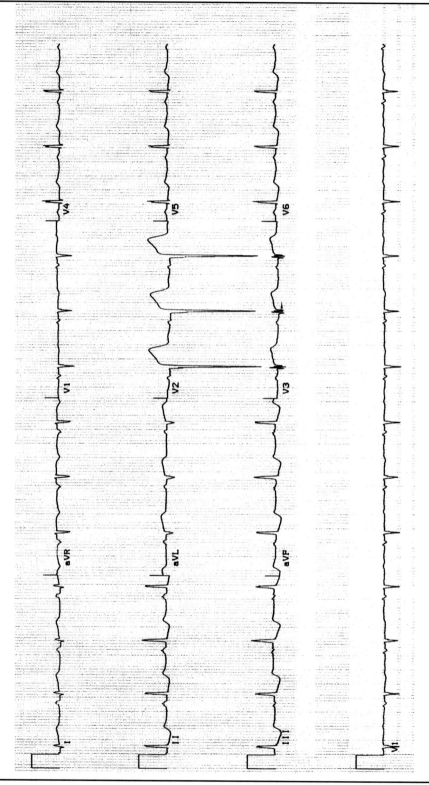

EKG Tracing #16

Heart rate is 78/min. and regular.

RHYTHM:

QRS complexes are narrow, indicating supraventricular rhythm with normal infranodal conduction. P wave in lead AVF is antegrade @ 78/min., indicating normal sinus rhythm activating the atria. PR is constant and normal, indicating normal antegrade AV conduction. Thus, there is sinus rhythm with normal antegrade AV conduction and normal infranodal conduction, i.e. normal sinus rhythm.

QRS Axis:

QRS complex is positive in lead AVF, and lead I is isoelectric. That means the QRS axis is +90 degrees, which is normal.

PR = 0.14 sec., QRS = 0.08 sec., Q – Tc = 0.438 sec.

SCANNING:

There is ST depression in inferior and lateral precordial leads (V5 – 6), suggestive of ischemis. There is ST elevation in V2 – 3, consistent with injury. There is loss of R wave in V2, and there is Q wave in V3; findings consistent with myocardial necrosis (infarction),i.e. anteroseptal M.I.

INTERPRETATION:

Normal sinus rhythm

Anteroseptal M.I., acute

ST – T abnormality consistent with inferior and lateral ischemia

Abnormal EKG

EKG Tracing # 17

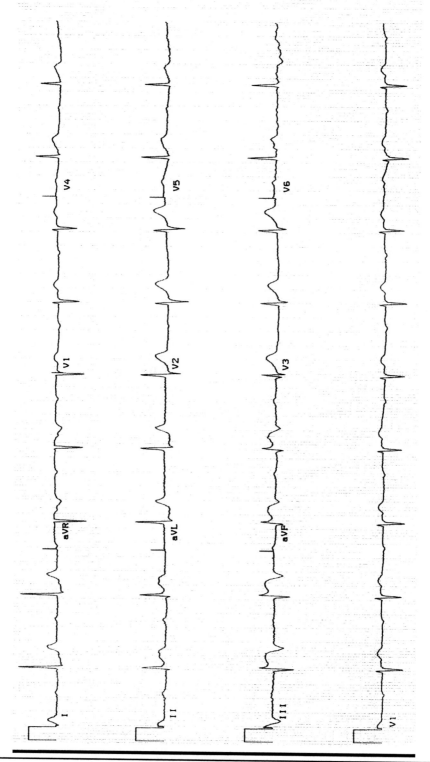

EKG Tracing #17

Heart rate is 56/min. and regular.

RHYTHM:

QRS complexes are narrow, indicating supraventricular rhythm with normal infranodal conduction. The rate and the shape of the P wave in lead AVF reveals antegrade P wave @ 56/min., suggesting sinus bradycardia activating the atria. PR is constant and prolonged, indicating antegrade AV conduction with 1st degree AV block. Therefore, it is a sinus bradycardia with antegrade AV conduction with 1st degree AV block and normal infranodal conduction. Thus, the diagnosis is sinus bradycardia with 1st degree AV block.

QRS Axis:

Lead AVF is positive, and lead III is isoelectric. Therefore, the QRS axis is +30 degrees.

PR = 0.36 sec., QRS = 0.08 sec., Q − Tc = 0.402 sec.

SCANNING:

ST is elevated in inferior leads and is convex upwards, indicating inferior injury. There is also a Q wave in lead AVF, suggesting inferior M.I. Thus, these findings suggest acute inferior M.I. ST depression in lead AVL is reciprocal to ST elevation in lead AVF.

INTERPRETATION:

Sinus bradycardia with first degree AV block

Acute inferior M.I.

Abnormal EKG

EKG Tracing # 18

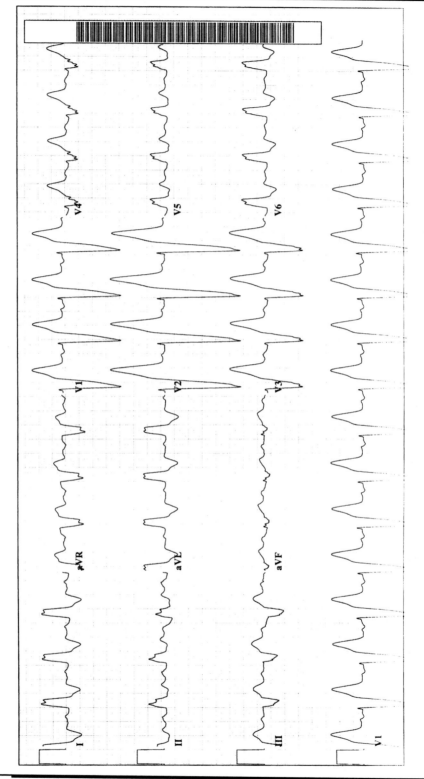

EKG Tracing #18

Heart rate is 93/min. and regular.

RHYTHM:

QRS complexes are wide, indicating supraventricular rhythm with aberrancy or ventricular rhythm. The rate and the shape of the P wave in lead AVF reveals an antegrade P @ 93/min., indicating sinus node activating the atria. The PR is constant and normal, indicating normal antegrade AV conduction. These findings suggest normal sinus rhythm with aberrant conduction. The appearance of QRS morphology in lead I is consistent with LBBB which explains the aberrant conduction. Therefore, the diagnosis is sinus rhythm with LBBB.

QRS Axis:

Lead AVF is negative and lead II is positive. According to Anand rule, the QRS axis is −30 less 20 = −10 degrees.

PR = 0.18 sec., QRS = 0.18 sec., Q − Tc = 0.514 sec.

SCANNING:

ST − T abnormality secondary to QRS widening. Poor r wave progression in leads V1 − 3 is due to LBBB resulting in right to left septal activation (left ventricle lies posteriorly).

INTERPRETATION:

Normal Sinus Rhythm

LBBB

Prolonged Q − TC

ABNORMAL EKG

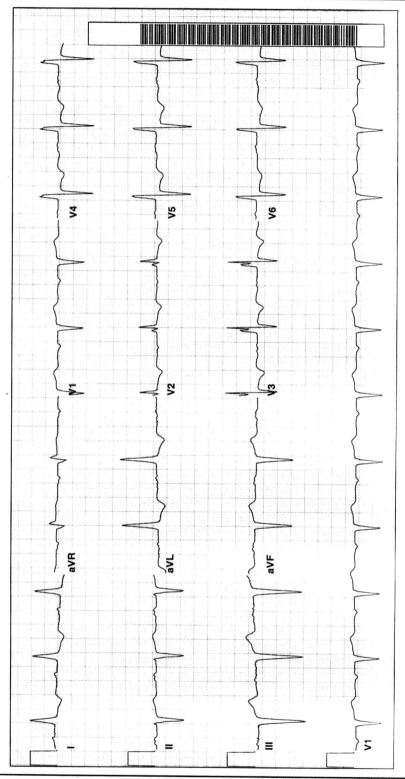

EKG Tracing #19

Heart rate is 64/min. and regular.

RHYTHM:

QRS complexes are wide, indicating supraventricular rhythm with aberrancy or ventricular rhythm. The rate and shape of the P wave in lead AVF reveals antegrade P @ 64/min., indicating sinus node activating the atria at normal rate. PR is constant and prolonged, indicating antegrade AV conduction with first degree AV block. Thus, it is sinus rhythm with first degree AV block and aberrant infranodal conduction. There is no evidence of RBBB or LBBB. Therefore, aberrancy is due to IVC delay. Hence, the diagnosis is sinus rhythm with first degree AV block and IVC delay.

QRS Axis:

Lead AVF is negative and lead AVR is isoelectric but a little more negative. These findings suggest QRS axis of –60 degrees 5 degrees less = –55 degrees, i.e. LAHB.

PR = 0.28 sec., QRS = 0.12 sec., Q – Tc = 0.468 sec.

SCANNING:

ST – T abnormality in anterolateral leads suggestive of ischemia and/or LVH. Note: QRS morphology in V2 reveals rabbit ears; this morphology must be present in lead V1 to qualify for the diagnosis of RBBB; hence, it is not RBBB.

INTERPRETATION:

Normal sinus rhythm (NSR) with first degree AV block

IVC delay

LAHB

ST – T abnormality consistent with anterolateral ischemia and/or LVH

Abnormal EKG

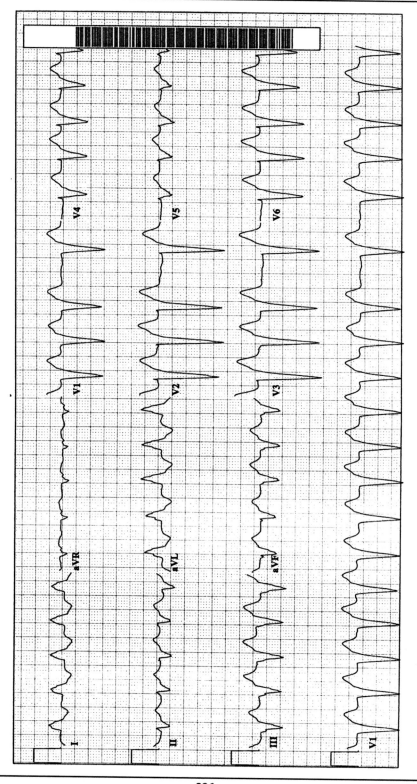

EKG Tracing #20

Heart rate is 111/min. and irregular.

RHYTHM:

QRS complexes are wide, indicating supraventricular rhythm with aberrancy or ventricular rhythm. No P waves are demonstrable in lead AVF or any other lead including the rhythm strip at the bottom of the EKG. R – R is irregular. These findings suggest atrial fibrillation with aberrancy. The morphology of QRS in lead I is consistent with LBBB which explains the cause of aberrant conduction. Hence, the diagnosis is atrial fibrillation with LBBB and rapid ventricular rate.

QRS Axis:

Lead AVF is negative and there is no biphasic lead. Since, the QRS axis is going to be with the minus sign (negative field of lead AVF), start with lead II. Lead II indicates that the QRS axis is more than –30 degrees. Next is lead AVR (–60). This lead indicates that the QRS axis is less than –60 degrees. Therefore, the QRS axis is between –30 and –60 degrees, i.e. –45 degrees.

QRS = 0.16 sec., Q – Tc = 0.543 sec.

SCANNING:

ST – T abnormality secondary to wide QRS. Loss of R wave in leads V1 – 3 is consistent with LBBB, but there is poor R in V4 – 6. Therefore, possible anterolateral M.I. cannot be excluded.

INTERPRETATION:

Atrial fibrillation with rapid ventricular rate

LBBB

LAD (QRS axis of –30 degrees or greater, in the presence of LBBB is interpreted as LAD; not LAHB)

Possible anterolateral M.I., ? Age, cannot be excluded

Prolonged Q – T

Abnormal EKG

EKG Tracing # 21

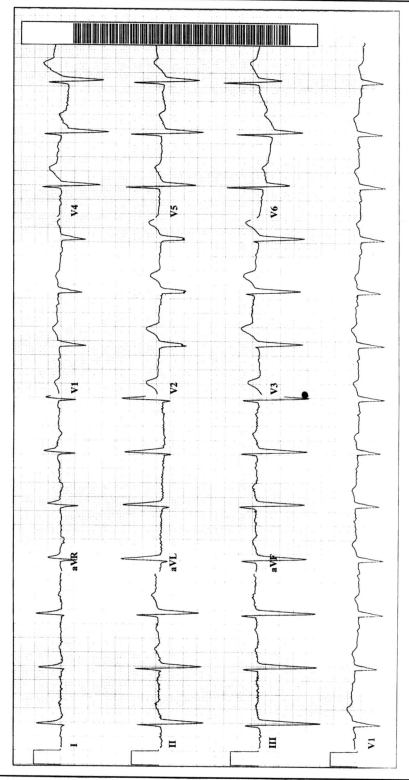

EKG Tracing #21

Heart rate is 78/min. and regular.

RHYTHM:
QRS is wide (0.11 second), indicating supraventricular rhythm with aberrancy or a ventricular rhythm. The rate and the shape of the P wave in lead AVF indicates normal sinus rhythm activating the atria @ 78/min., PR is constant and normal, suggesting normal antegrade AV conduction. Therefore, it is normal sinus rhythm with aberrancy. There is no evidence of RBBB or LBBB. Therefore, it is normal sinus rhythm (NSR) with IVC delay.

QRS Axis:
LEAD AVF is negative and lead AVR is closest to being isoelectric, but a little more positive area than negative. Therefore, the QRS axis is –65 degrees, suggesting LAHB.

PR = 0.12 sec., QRS – o.11 sec., Q – Tc = 0.447 sec.

SCANNING:
Loss of R wave in V2 suggesting anteroseptal M.I., ? Age.

INTERPRETATION:
Normal sinus rhythm

LAHB

IVC delay

Possible ASMI, ? Age, masked by LAHB cannot be excluded

(Note: LAHB can be responsible for the loss of R in V2 as the interventricular septum is activated from right to left; the left ventricle lies posteriorly, whereas lead V2 is anterior).

Abnormal EKG

EKG Tracing # 22

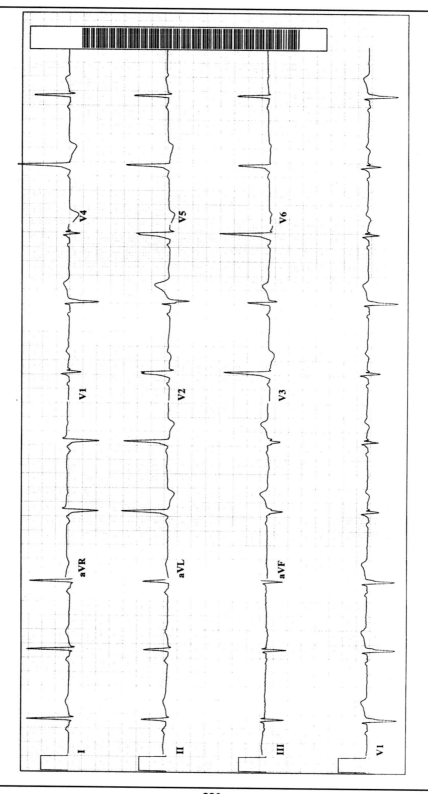

EKG Tracing #22

Heart rate is 60/min. and regular.

RHYTHM:

QRS complexes in leads I,IIand III are narrow, indicating supraventricular rhythm with normal infranodal conduction. The rate and the shape of the P wave in lead AVF is consistent with normal sinus rhythm activating the atria. PR in leads I, II and III is constant and normal, indicating normal antegrade AV conduction. These findings suggest normal sinus rhythm.

QRS Axis:

Lead AVF is negative and none of the limb leads is closest to being isoelectric. Therefore start with the lead associated with the smallest minus number as the QRS axis is going to be negative. This would be lead II associated with the number –30 if it were isoelectric. In the above tracing, lead II is mostly positive, indicating that the QRS axis, according to Anand rule, is a lot less than –30 degrees, i.e. it is 30 – 20 = – 10 degrees.

PR = 0.14 sec., QRS = 0.09 sec., Q – Tc = 0.40 sec.

SCANNING:

In the rhythm strip at the bottom of the tracing, starting from the left, the 4th, 5th, 6th,8th and 9th QRS complexes have similar morphology but different from the morphology of other QRS complexes in the strip. The first three QRS complexes are normal because the corresponding QRS complexes above in leads I, II and III appear to be normal. Therefore, the other QRS complexes with different morphology must be abnormal. If you trace these abnormal QRS complexes upwards into unipolar limb leads, you will note that the QRS complexes are wide and corresponding PR interval is shorter than the PR interval in leads I, II and III. There is also a delta wave at the beginning of the abnormal QRS complexes. This combination of short PR, wide QRS, and delta wave signifies Wolf Parkinson White Syndrome (WPW syndrome). Since these complexes are present only intermittently, it is called intermittent WPW syndrome. T wave inversion in these complexes is secondary to the wide QRS.

INTERPRETATION:

Normal sinus rhythm with intermittent WPW pattern.

Abnormal EKG

EKG Tracing # 23

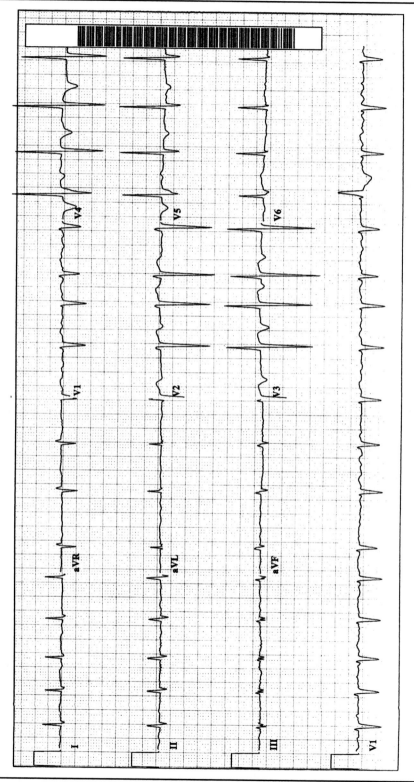

EKG Tracing #23

Heart rate is 102/min. and irregular.

RHYTHM:

QRS complexes are narrow, indicating supraventricular rhythm with normal infranodal conduction. No P waves are demonstrable in lead AVF and serpentine movement with varying morphology is present in the rhythm strip, indicating atrial fibrillation. Irregular R – R supports this diagnosis. The 4th QRS complex from the right, in the rhythm strip, shows RBBB morphology and is preceded by a sequence of short, long, short R – R intervals. This is called Ashman phenomenon in atrial fibrillation.

QRS Axis:

Lead AVF is isoelectric. Therefore, QRS axis is zero degree.

QRS = 0.08 sec., Q – Tc = 0.41 sec.

SCANNING:

T wave inversion in V3 – 5 suggestive of ischemia.

INTERPRETATION:

Atrial fibrillation with rapid heart rate and Ashman phenomenon

T wave abnormality consistent with anterolateral ischemia

Low QRS voltage

Abnormal EKG

EKG Tracing # 24

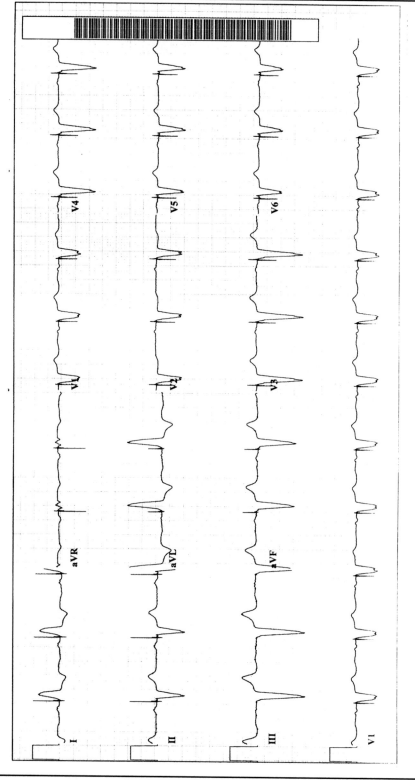

EKG Tracing #24

Heart rate is 66/min. and regular.

RHYTHM:
QRS complexes are wide and accompanied by an electronic artifact at the start of each QRS complex, indicating an electronic pacemaker activating the ventricles. Therefore it is an electronic pacemaker capture ventricular rhythm @ 66/min. The rate and the shape of the P wave in lead AVF suggests sinus node activating the atria @ 66/min. PR is constant indicating antegrade AV conduction but the ventricles are being activated by electronic pacemaker. What is happening here is that electronic ventricular pacemaker is sensing the atrial impulse as it is fired by the sinus node and discharges its own impulse after a predetermined interval to activate the ventricles. Thus the PR interval remains constant. This process requires a catheter electrode in the right atrium to sense the sinus discharge of the impulse and then cause the ventricular discharge of the impulse by pacemaker generator after a predetermined interval, which in this case is 0.12 sec. This is called a dual chamber pacemaker with atrial sensing. Since there is Ventricular pacing, Atrial sensing, and electronic artifact triggering the QRS complexes, it is referred to as the pacemaker set in a VAT mode ("V" stands for ventricular pacing, "A" stands for atrial sensing, and "T" stands for trigger i.e. the blip before each QRS).

INTERPRETATION:
Electronic dual chamber pacemaker in VAT mode.

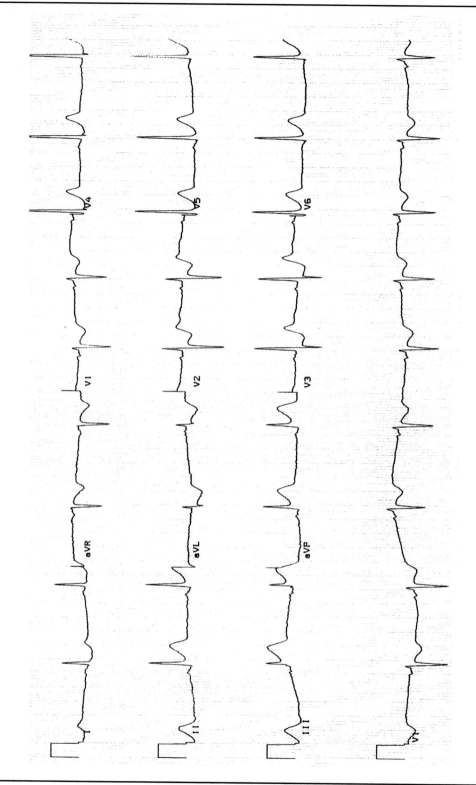

EKG Tracing #25

Heart rate is 54/min. and regular.

RHYTHM:

QRS complexes are narrow, indicating supraventricular rhythm with normal infranodal conduction. The rate and the shape of the P in lead AVF is consistent with sinus bradycardia. PR is constant and normal in duration, suggesting normal antegrade AV conduction. Therefore, the rhythm is sinus bradycardia.

QRS Axis:

Lead AVF is positive and lead AVL is isoelectric. Therefore, the QRS axis is +60 degrees.

PR = 0.14 sec. QRS = 0.09 sec., Q – Tc = 0.402 sec.

SCANNING:

ST elevation in inferior leads (suggesting inferior M.I., acute) with reciprocal ST depression in lead AVL. ST depression in leads V2 – 3 with tall R waves (suggesting acute posterior M.I. with reciprocal changes in anterior leads).

INTERPRETATION:

Sinus bradycardia
Acute inferior and posterior M.I.
Abnormal EKG

EKGs for Practice

Ventricular Rate: 104 BPM
PR interval: 140 ms
QRS interval: 80 ms
QT/QTc: 308/407 ms
QRS axis: +25

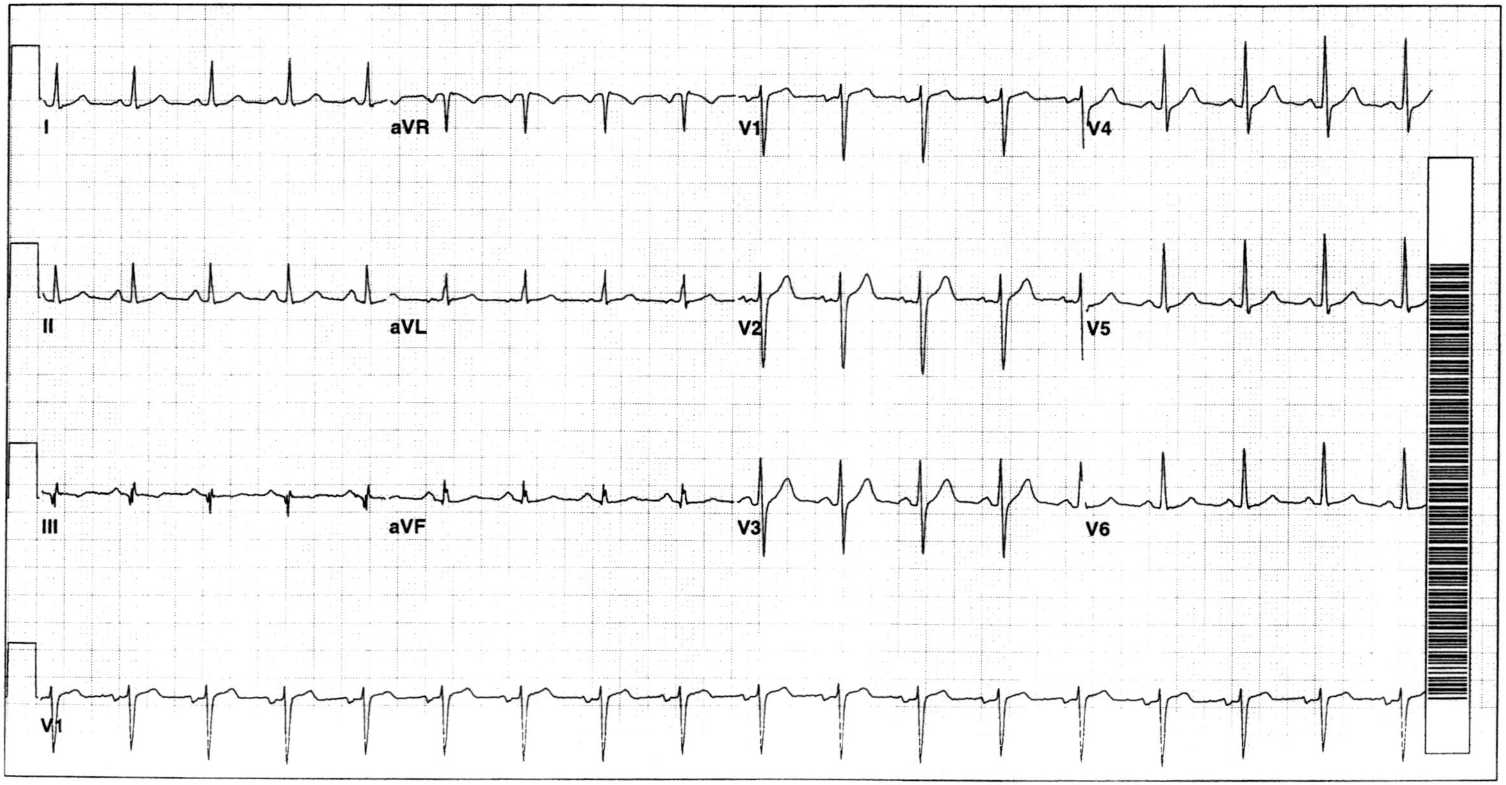

INTERPRETATION: T1
SINUS TACHYCARDIA
OTHERWISE NORMAL EKG

Ventricular Rate: 54 BPM INTERPRETATION: T2
PR interval: 194 ms SINUS BRADYCARDIA WITH SINUS ARRHYTHMIA
QRS interval: 94 ms OTHERWISE NORMAL EKG
QT/QTc: 456/424 ms
QRS axis: +8

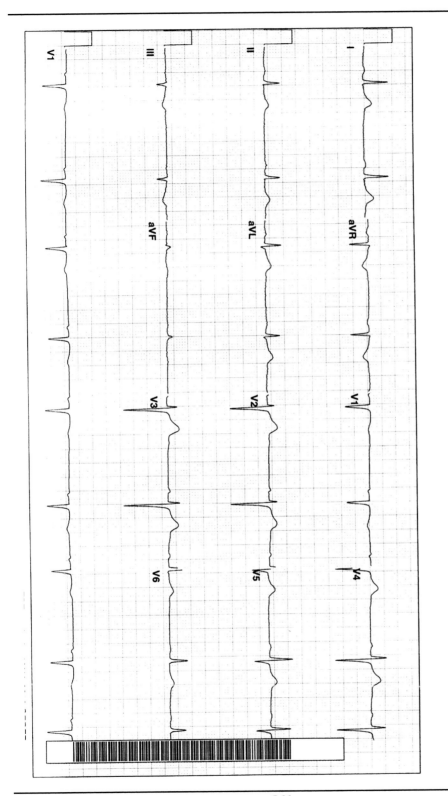

Ventricular Rate:	61 BPM	INTERPRETATION: T3
PR interval:		ATRIAL FLUTTER WITH 4:1 AV CONDUCTION
QRS interval:	90 ms	INDETERMINATE QRS AXIS
QT/QTc:	434/436 ms	INFERIOR INFARCT, ? AGE
QRS axis:	Indeterminate	ABNORMAL EKG

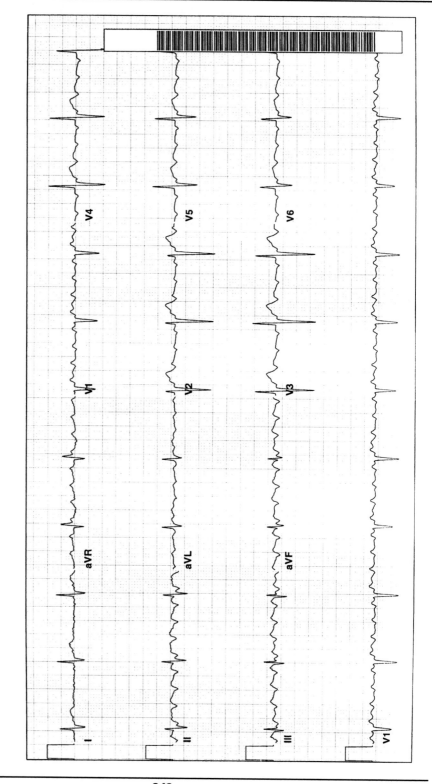

Ventricular Rate: 89 BPM INTERPRETATION: T4
PR interval: ATRIAL FLUTTER WITH VARYING AV BLOCK
QRS interval: 82 ms ABNORMAL EKG
QT/QTc: 396/481 ms
QRS axis: −28

343

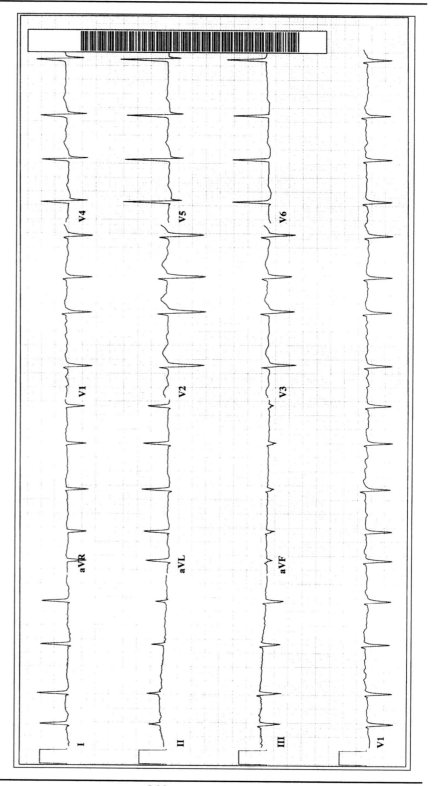

Ventricular Rate: 102 BPM

PR interval:

QRS interval: 100 ms

QT/QTc: 354/459 ms

QRS axis: −10

INTERPRETATION: T5

ATRIAL FIBRILLATION WITH RAPID VENTRICULAR RATE

NONSPECIFIC ST-T ABNORMALITY, CONSISTENT WITH

DIGITALIS EFFECT

ABNORMAL EKG

Ventricular Rate: 66 BPM   INTERPRETATION: T6
PR interval: 100 ms   NODAL RHYTHM
QRS interval: 85 ms   ABNORMAL EKG
QT/QTc: 418/427 ms
QRS axis: +70

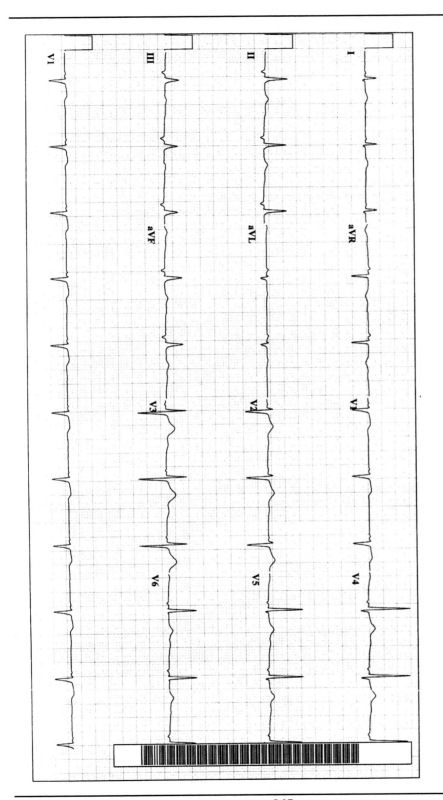

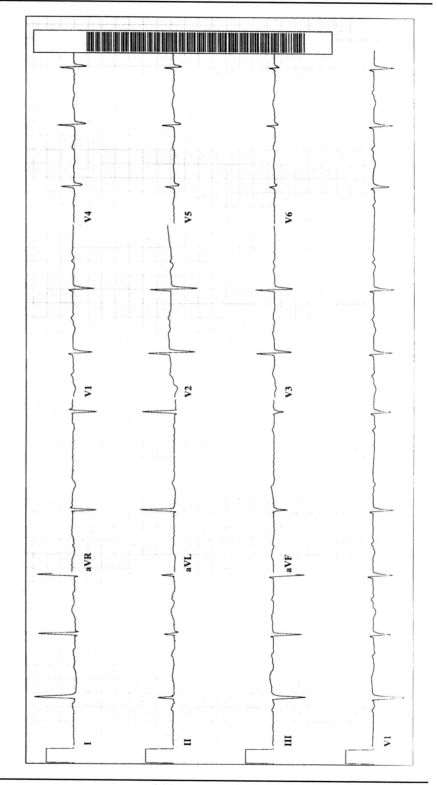

Ventricular Rate: 60 BPM
PR interval:
QRS interval: 90 ms
QT/QTc: 460/460 ms
QRS axis: −12

INTERPRETATION: T7
SINUS RHYTHM WITH 2ND DEGREE AV BLOCK (MOBITZ 1)
NONSPECIFIC ST-T CHANGES
ABNORMAL EKG

Ventricular Rate: 42 BPM
PR interval: 120 ms
QRS interval: 120 ms
QT/QTc: 472/398 ms
QRS axis: +60

INTERPRETATION: T8
SINUS TACHYCARDIA WITH COMPLETE AV BLOCK
AND VENTRICULAR ESCAPE RHYTHM
ABNORMAL EKG

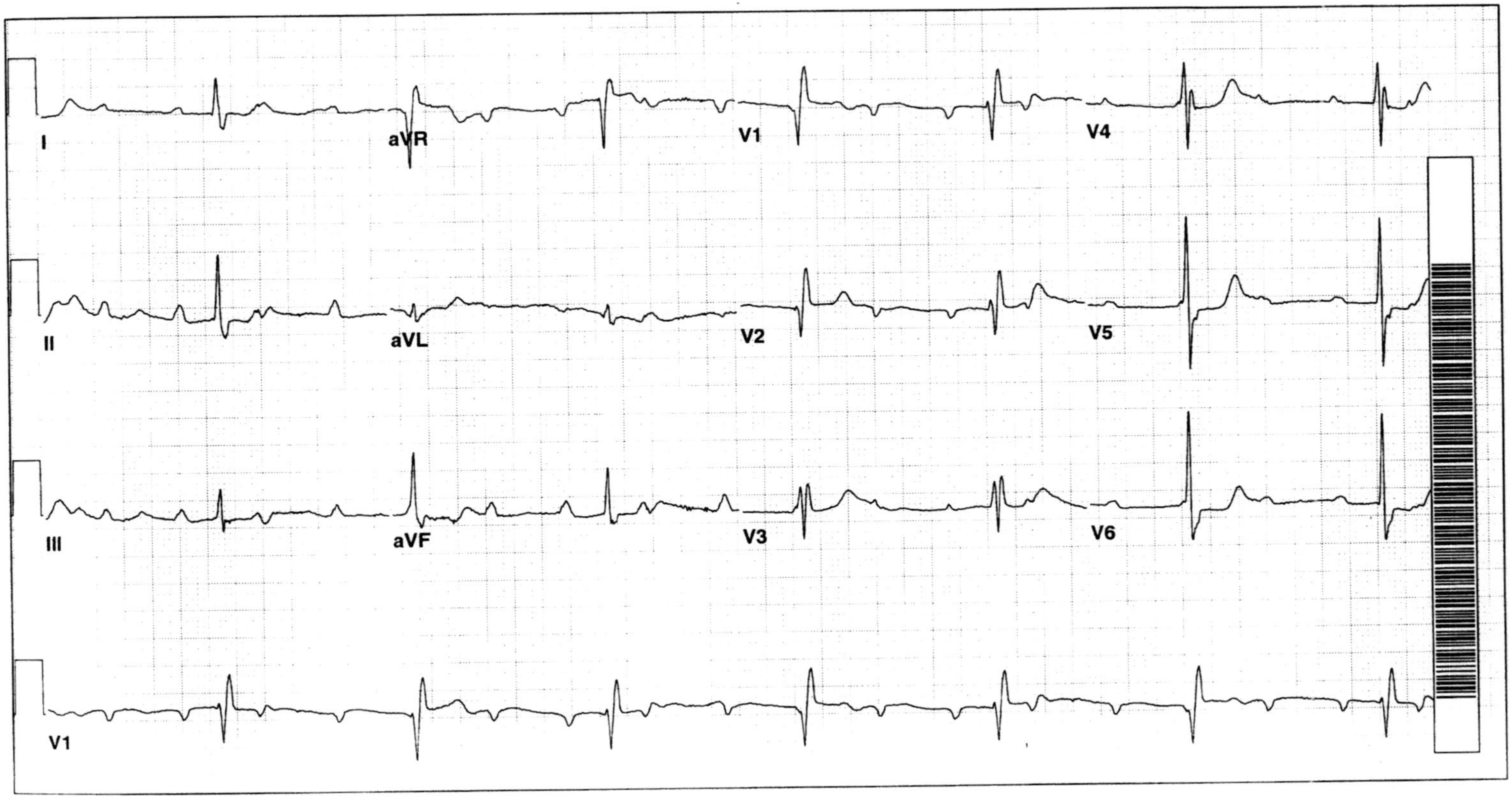

Ventricular Rate:	60 BPM	INTERPRETATION: T9
PR interval:	320 ms	SINUS RHYTHM WITH 1ST DEGREE AV BLOCK
QRS interval:	120 ms	INTRA–VENTRICULAR CONDUCTION DELAY
QT/QTc:	434/436 ms	INFERIOR M.I., ? AGE
QRS axis:	–5	ABNORMAL EKG

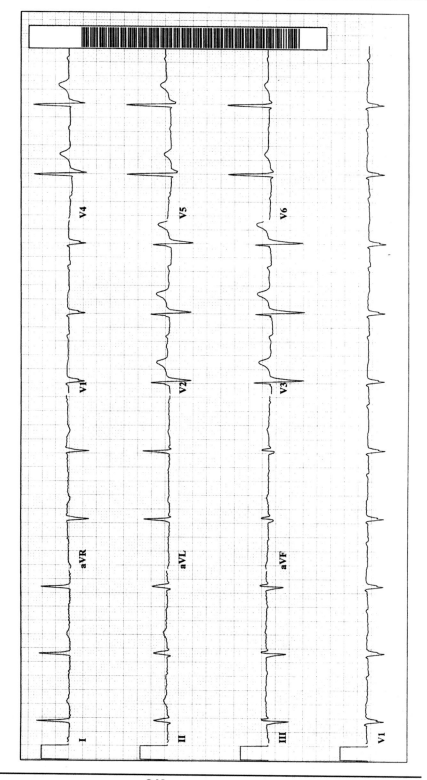

Ventricular Rate: 54 BPM INTERPRETATION: T10
PR interval: 160 ms SINUS BRADYCARDIA
QRS interval: 94 ms POOR R WAVE PROGRESSION IN V1 – 4
QT/QTc: 422/392 ms LAD
QRS axis: –40 ABNORMAL EKG

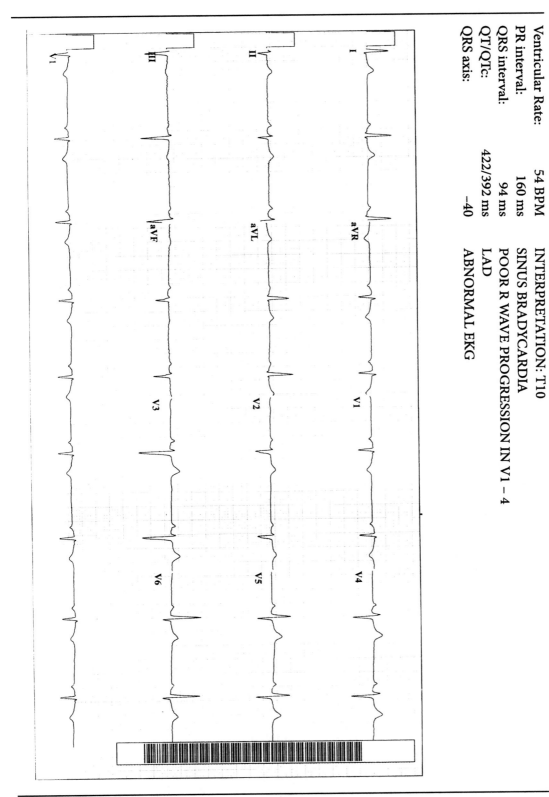

Ventricular Rate:	96 BPM	INTERPRETATION: T11
PR interval:	120 ms	SINUS RHYTHM
QRS interval:	94 ms	RAD
QT/QTc:	346/430 ms	ABNORMAL EKG
QRS axis:	+105	

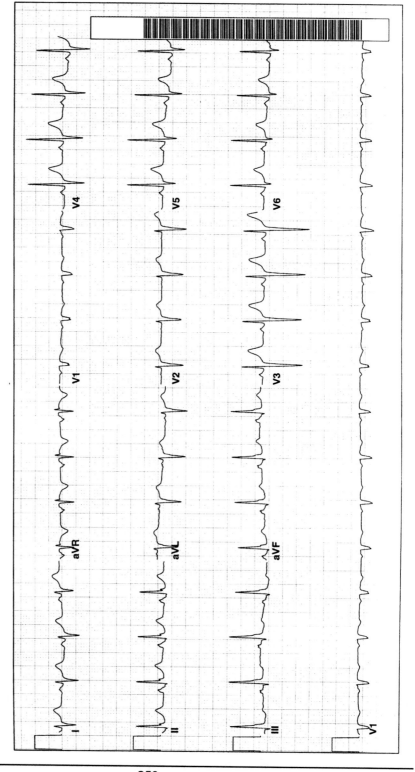

Ventricular Rate: 114 BPM INTERPRETATION: T12
PR interval: ATRIAL FIBRILLATION WITH RAPID VENTRICULAR RATE
QRS interval: 160 ms LBBB
QT/QTc: 328/443 ms LAD
QRS axis: -46 ABNORMAL EKG

351

Ventricular Rate: 84 BPM INTERPRETATION: T13
PR interval: 186 ms SINUS RHYTHM
QRS interval: 86 ms LEFT ANTERIOR HEMIBLOCK
QT/QTc: 382/448 ms ABNORMAL EKG
QRS axis: -48

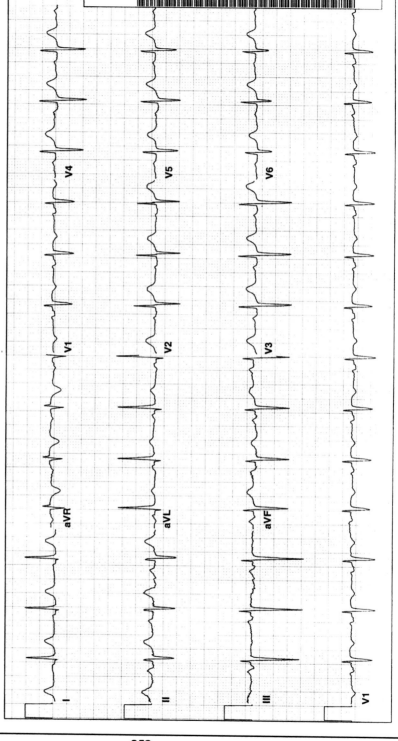

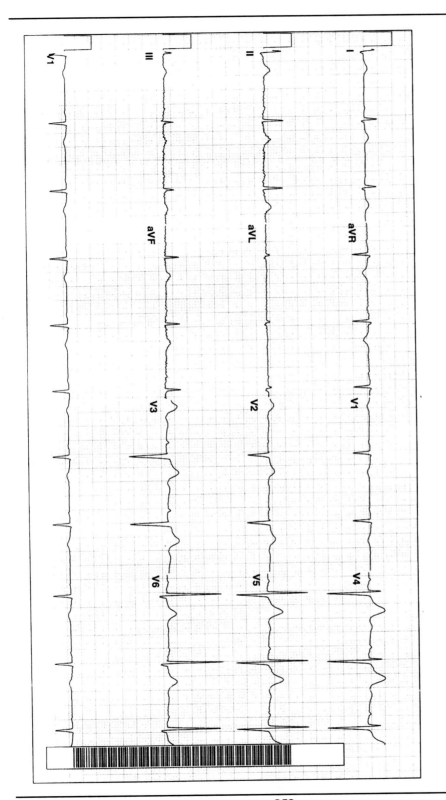

Ventricular Rate: 60 BPM INTERPRETATION: T14

PR interval: 180 ms SINUS RHYTHM

QRS interval: 82 ms ANTERIOR INFARCT, ? AGE

QT/QTc: 422/428 ms ABNORMAL EKG

QRS axis: +60

Ventricular Rate: 54 BPM INTERPRETATION: T15
PR interval: 180 ms SINUS BRADYCARDIA
QRS interval: 100 ms T WAVE INVERSION IN AVL WITH DISCORDANT P WAVE
QT/QTc: 444/424 ms ABNORMAL EKG
QRS axis: +20

Ventricular Rate: 66 BPM
PR interval: 196 ms
QRS interval: 98 ms
QT/QTc: 436/449 ms
QRS axis: -10

INTERPRETATION: T16
SINUS RHYTHM
T WAVE ABNORMALITY IN LATERAL LEADS, SUGGESTIVE OF ISCHEMIA
INFERIOR INFARCT, ? AGE
ANTERIOR INFARCT, ? AGE
ABNORMAL EKG

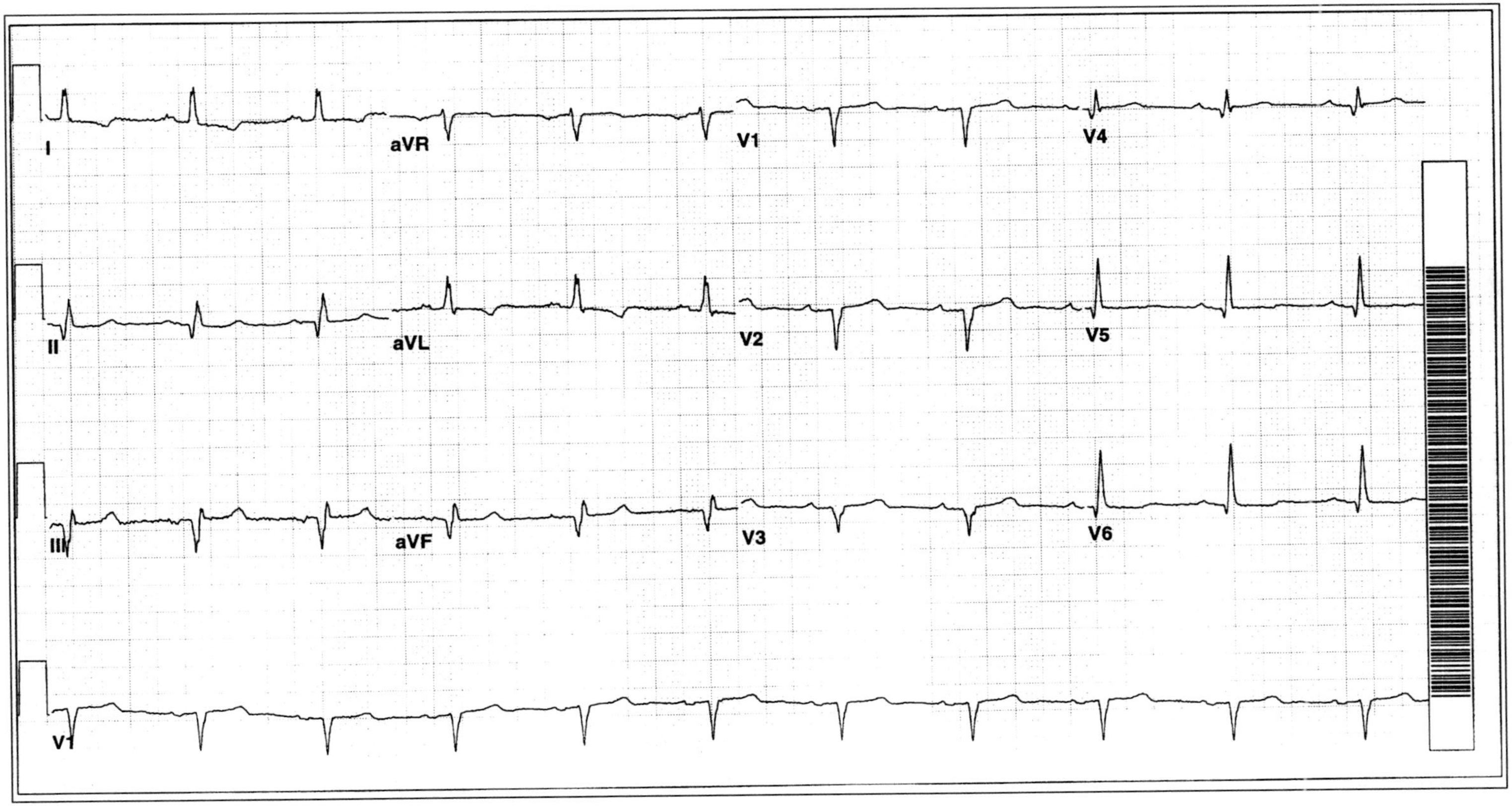

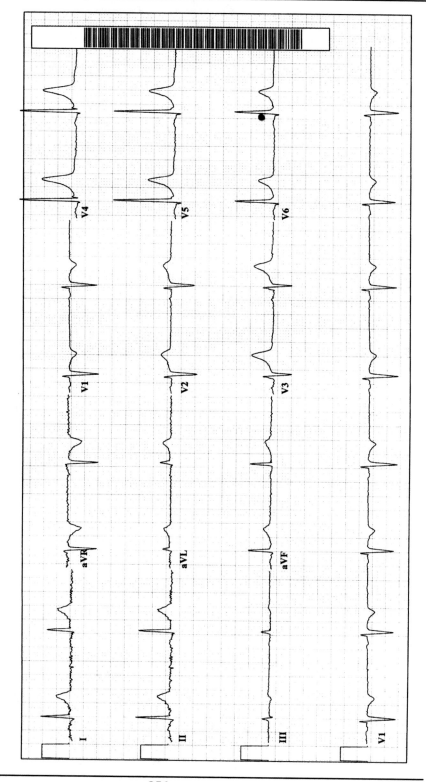

Ventricular Rate:	48 BPM	INTERPRETATION: T17
PR interval:	200 ms	MARKED SINUS BRADYCARDIA
QRS interval:	94 ms	ST ELEVATION IN LATERAL LEADS, CONSISTENT WITH EARLY
QT/QTc:	476/425 ms	REPOLARIZATION
QRS axis:	+40	ABNORMAL EKG

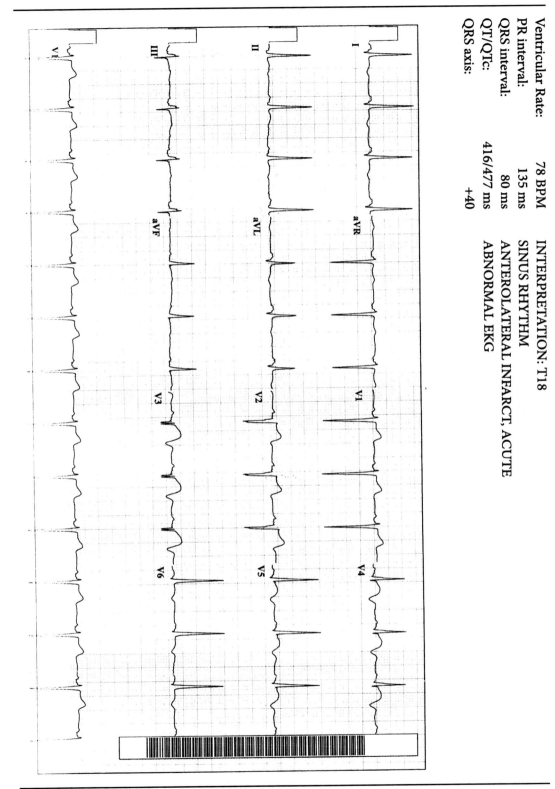

Ventricular Rate: 78 BPM   INTERPRETATION: T18
PR interval: 135 ms   SINUS RHYTHM
QRS interval: 80 ms   ANTEROLATERAL INFARCT, ACUTE
QT/QTc: 416/477 ms   ABNORMAL EKG
QRS axis: +40

Ventricular Rate: 54 BPM
PR interval: 196 ms
QRS interval: 90 ms
QT/QTc: 456/432 ms
QRS axis: +32

INTERPRETATION: T19
SINUS BRADYCARDIA
LVH WITH REPOLARIZATION ABNORMALITY
ABNORMAL EKG

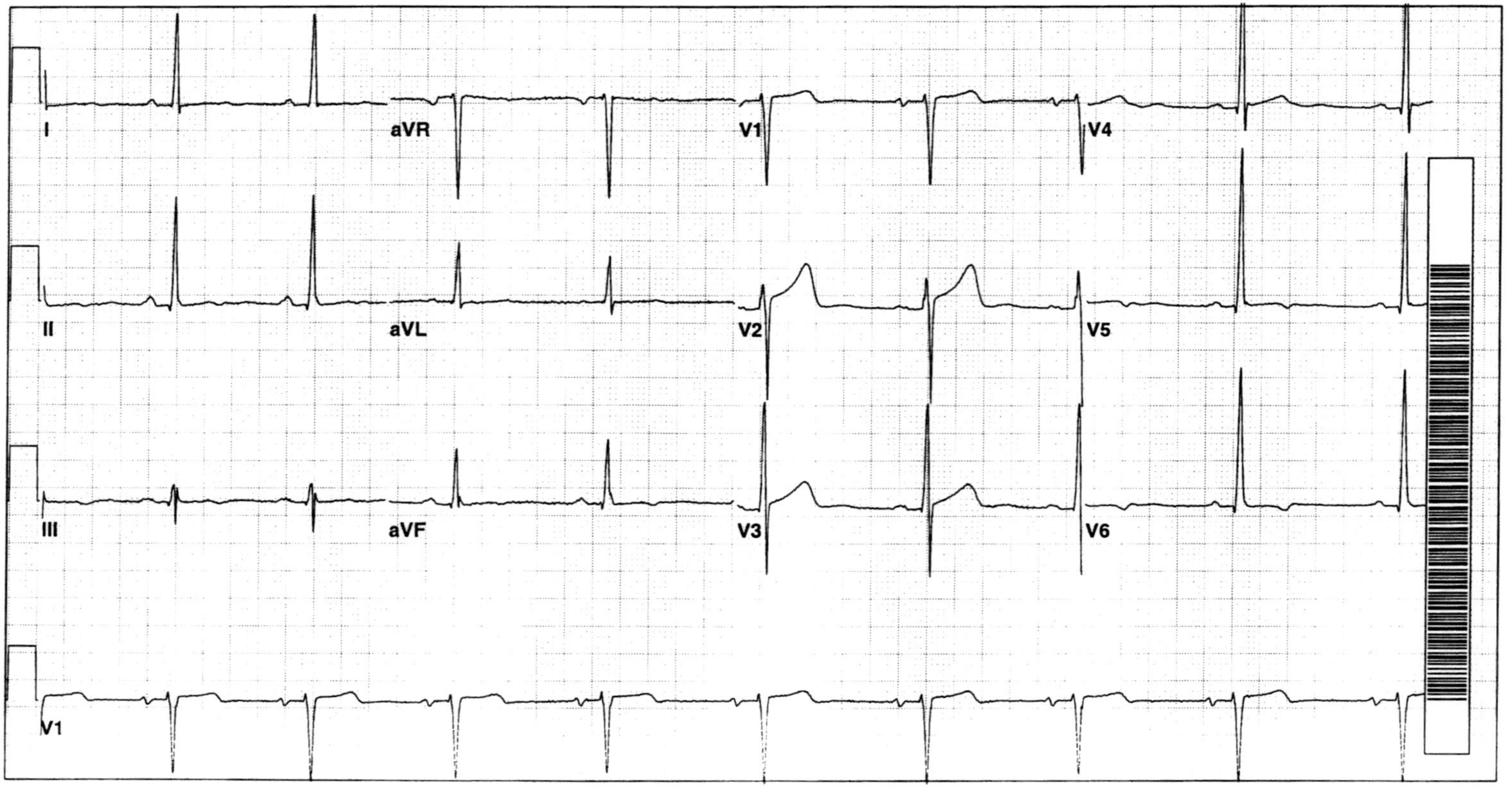

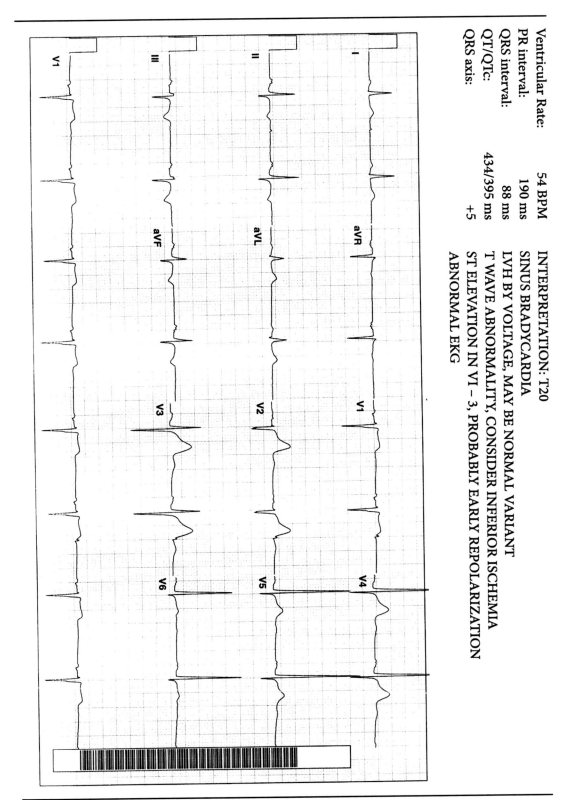

Ventricular Rate: 54 BPM   INTERPRETATION: T20

PR interval: 190 ms   SINUS BRADYCARDIA

QRS interval: 88 ms   LVH BY VOLTAGE, MAY BE NORMAL VARIANT

QT/QTc: 434/395 ms   T WAVE ABNORMALITY, CONSIDER INFERIOR ISCHEMIA

QRS axis: +5   ST ELEVATION IN V1 – 3, PROBABLY EARLY REPOLARIZATION

ABNORMAL EKG

Ventricular Rate: 216 BPM   INTERPRETATION: T21
PR interval: SUPRAVENTRICULAR TACHYCARDIA
QRS interval: 76 ms   ST – T ABNORMALITY, ? ISCHEMIA
QT/QTc: 204/387 ms   ABNORMAL EKG
QRS axis: +70

Ventricular Rate: 132 BPM INTERPRETATION: T22
PR interval: 162 ms SINUS TACHYCARDIA
QRS interval: 66 ms RIGHT AXIS DEVIATION
QT/QTc: 282/419 ms LEFT ATRIAL ENLARGEMENT
QRS axis: +106 ANTERIOR M.I., ? AGE
ABNORMAL EKG

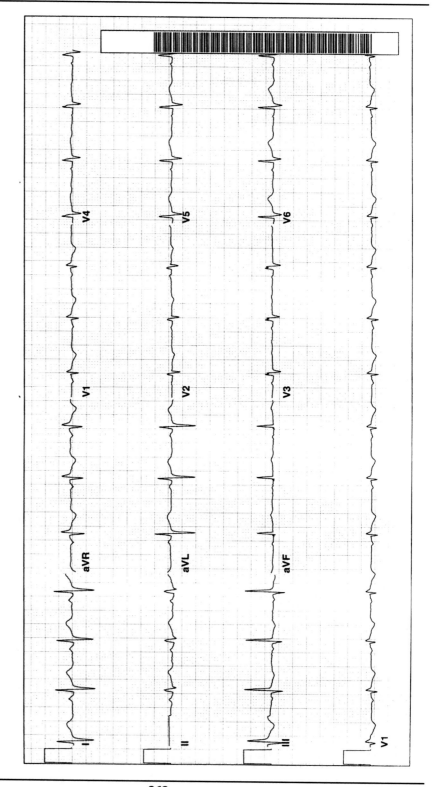

Ventricular Rate: 78 BPM INTERPRETATION: T23

PR interval: 134 ms SINUS RHYTHM

QRS interval: 94 ms INCOMMPLETE RBBB

QT/QTc: 400/458 ms RAD

QRS axis: +110 ABNORMAL EKG

Ventricular Rate: 55 BPM INTERPRETATION: T24
PR interval: 196 ms ARM LEADS ARE INTERCHANGED
QRS interval: 82 ms SINUS BRADYCARDIA
QT/QTc: 496/474 ms PREMATURE VENTRICULAR COMPLEXES AS BIGEMINY
QRS axis: −10 ANTEROSEPTAL M.I., ? AGE
ABNORMAL EKG

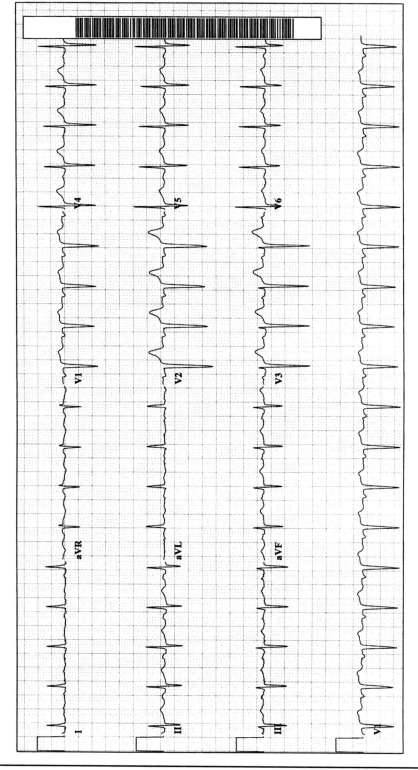

Ventricular Rate:	102 BPM	INTERPRETATION: T25
PR interval:	146 ms	SINUS TACHYCARDIA
QRS interval:	80 ms	ANTEROSEPTAL M.I., ? AGE
QT/QTc:	340/449 ms	ABNORMAL EKG
QRS axis:	–25	

Ventricular Rate: 54 BPM INTERPRETATION: T26
PR interval: 156 ms SINUS BRADYCARDIA
QRS interval: 124 ms LBBB
QT/QTc: 504/477 ms ABNORMAL EKG
QRS axis: +22

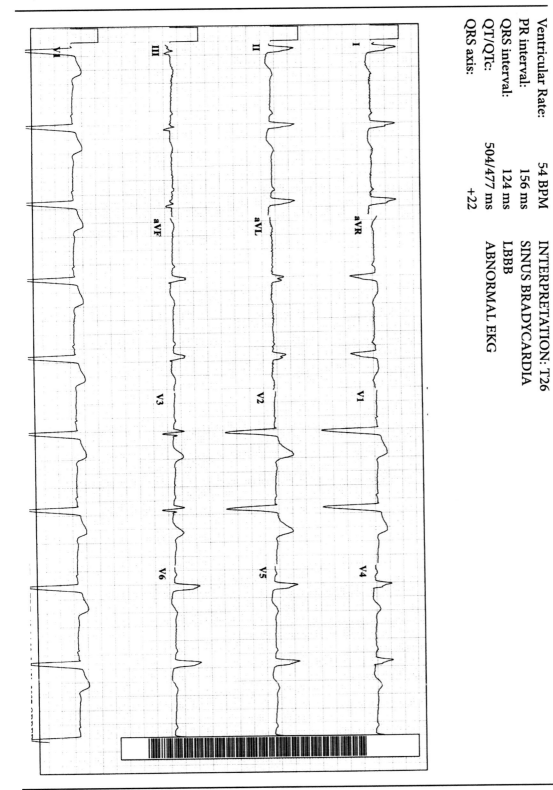

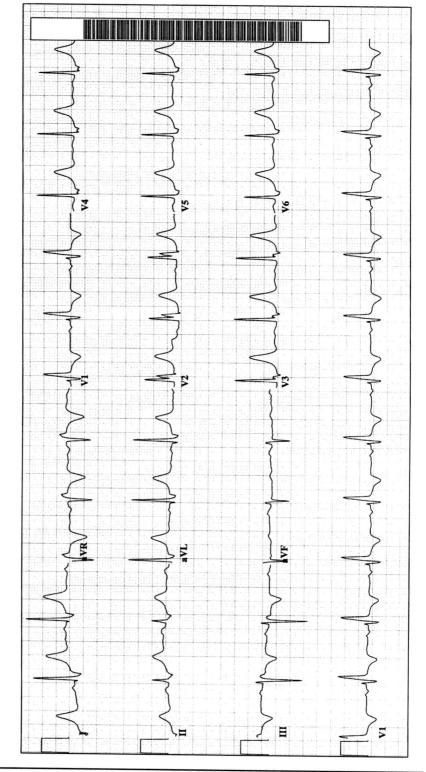

Ventricular Rate: 69 BPM

PR interval: 172 ms

QRS interval: 132 ms

QT/QTc: 474/507 ms

QRS axis: –20

INTERPRETATION: T27

SINUS RHYTHM

RBBB

PROLONGED QT

TALL T WAVES, ? HYPERKALEMIA

ABNORMAL EKG

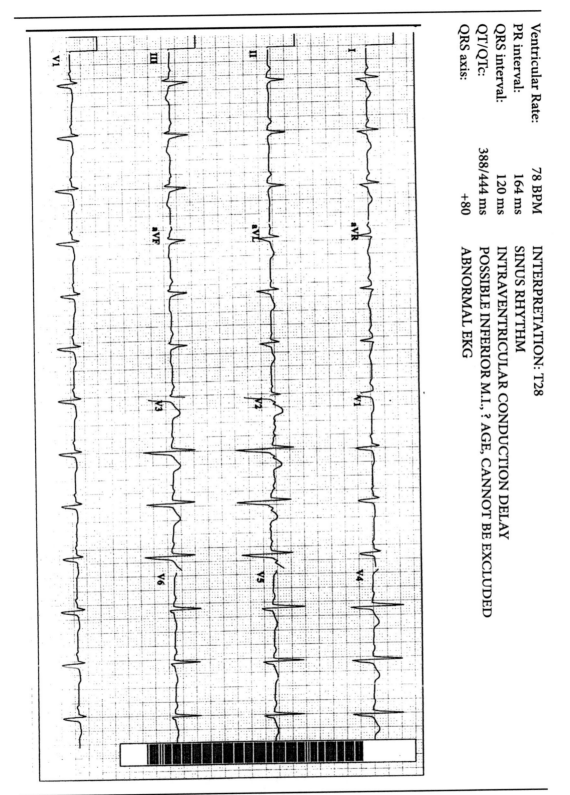

Ventricular Rate: 78 BPM   INTERPRETATION: T28

PR interval: 164 ms   SINUS RHYTHM

QRS interval: 120 ms   INTRAVENTRICULAR CONDUCTION DELAY

QT/QTc: 388/444 ms   POSSIBLE INFERIOR M.I., ? AGE, CANNOT BE EXCLUDED

QRS axis: +80   ABNORMAL EKG

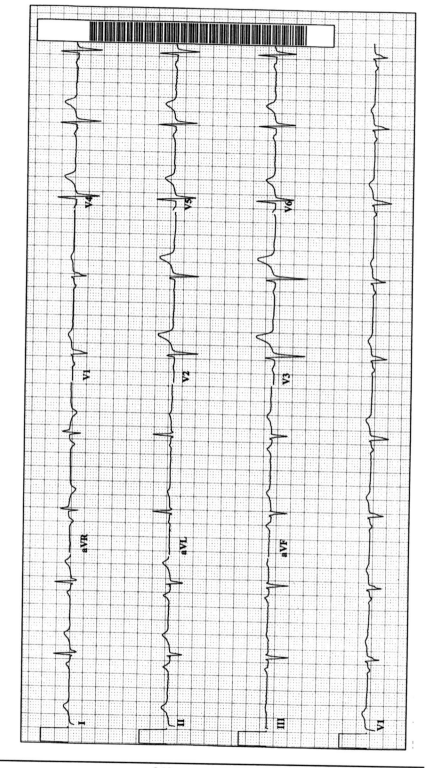

Ventricular Rate: 54 BPM   INTERPRETATION: T29

PR interval: 196 ms   SINUS BRADYCARDIA

QRS interval: 98 ms   LEFT ANTERIOR HEMIBLOCK

QT/QTc: 434/411 ms   ABNORMAL EKG

QRS axis: –52

Ventricular Rate: 66 BPM
PR interval: 122 ms
QRS interval: 86 ms
QT/QTc: 384/408 ms
QRS axis: +16

INTERPRETATION: T30
SINUS RHYTHM
INFERO – POSTERIOR M.I., ? AGE
ABNORMAL EKG

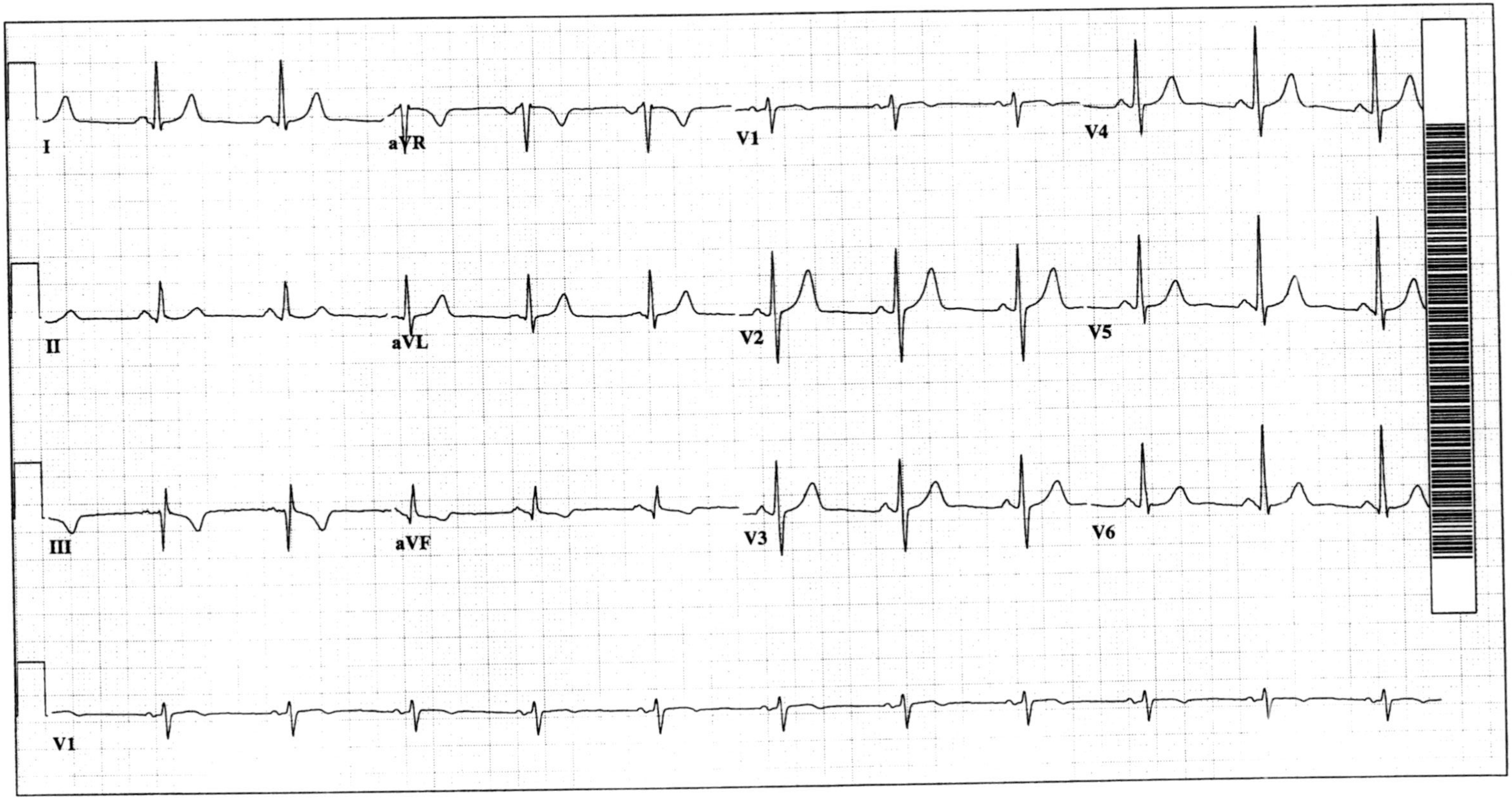

Ventricular Rate:	60 BPM	INTERPRETATION: T31
PR interval:	260 ms	ELECTRONIC ATRIAL PACEMAKER
QRS interval:	108 ms	INFERO M.I., ? AGE
QT/QTc:	436/436 ms	LVH WITH REPOLARIZATION ABNORMALITY
QRS axis:	+15	ABNORMAL EKG

Ventricular Rate: 70 BPM INTERPRETATION: T32
PR interval: 220 ms ELECTRONIC AV SEQUENTIAL PACEMAKER
QRS interval: 160 ms
QT/QTc: 496/535 ms
QRS axis: -72

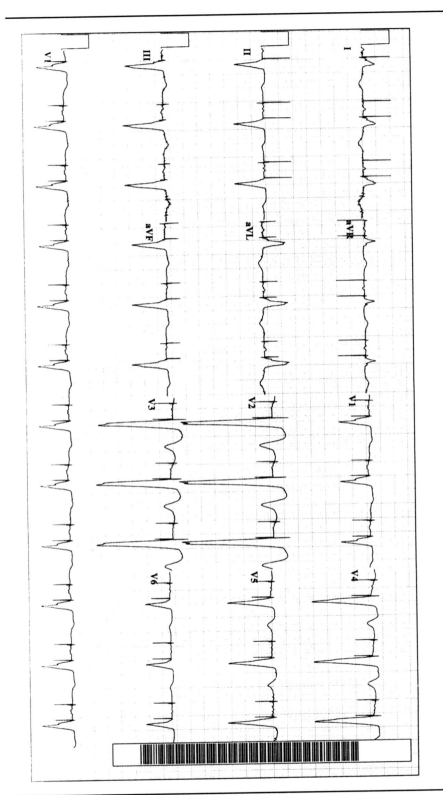

Ventricular Rate:	79 BPM
PR interval:	126 ms
QRS interval:	126 ms
QT/QTc:	426/488 ms
QRS axis:	–72

INTERPRETATION: T33
ELECTRONIC VENTRICULAR PACEMAKER, SENSING P WAVES
(ELECTRONIC DUAL CHAMBER PACEMAKER IN VAT MODE)
ONE PVC

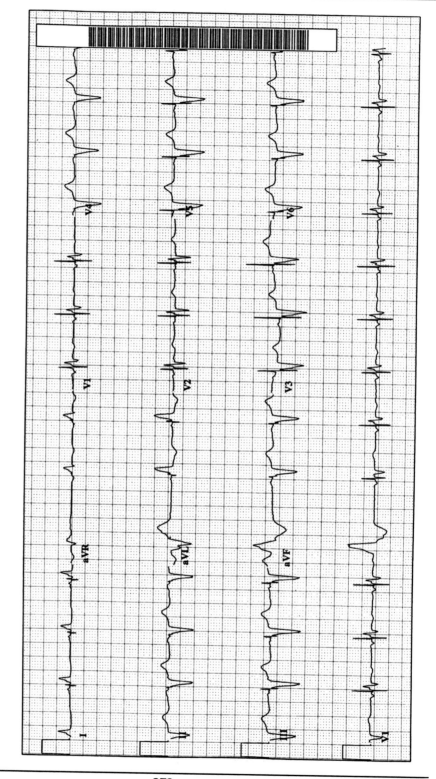

Ventricular Rate: 198 BPM   INTERPRETATION: T34
PR interval: ATRIAL FIBRILLATION WITH RAPID VENTRICULAR RATE
QRS interval: 80 ms   ST ABNORMALITY, CONSIDER LATERAL ISCHEMIA
QT/QTc: 238/431 ms   ABNORMAL EKG
QRS axis: +11

373

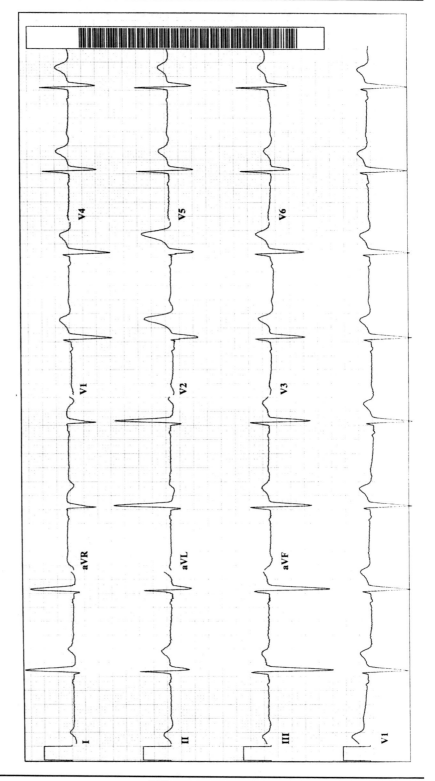

Ventricular Rate: 50 BPM
PR interval: 164 ms
QRS interval: 134 ms
QT/QTc: 454/413 ms
QRS axis: −25

INTERPRETATION: T35
SINUS BRADYCARDIA
LVH WITH REPOLARIZATION ABNORMALITY
IVC DELAY
ANTEROSEPTAL M.I., ? AGE, CANNOT BE EXCLUDED
ABNORMAL EKG

Ventricular Rate:	66 BPM
PR interval:	234 ms
QRS interval:	146 ms
QT/QTc:	474/500 ms
QRS axis:	-30

INTERPRETATION: T36
SINUS RHYTHM WITH FIRST DEGREE AV BLOCK
LAD
LBBB
ABNORMAL EKG

Ventricular Rate:	63 BPM	INTERPRETATION: T37
PR interval:		SINUS RHYTHM WITH ISORHYTHMIC AV DISSOCIATION AND
QRS interval:	120 ms	UNDERLYING VENTRICULAR RHYTHM.
QT/QTc:	408/418 ms	ABNORMAL EKG
QRS axis:	−49	

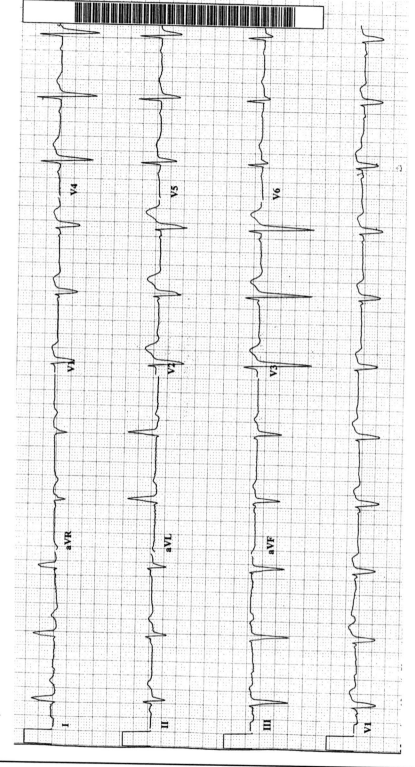

Ventricular Rate: 108 BPM
PR interval:
QRS interval: 84 ms
QT/QTc: 288/387 ms
QRS axis: -8

INTERPRETATION: T38
ARM LEADS ARE INTERCHANGED
ATRIAL FIBRILLATION WITH RAPID VENTRICULAR RATE
ABNORMAL EKG

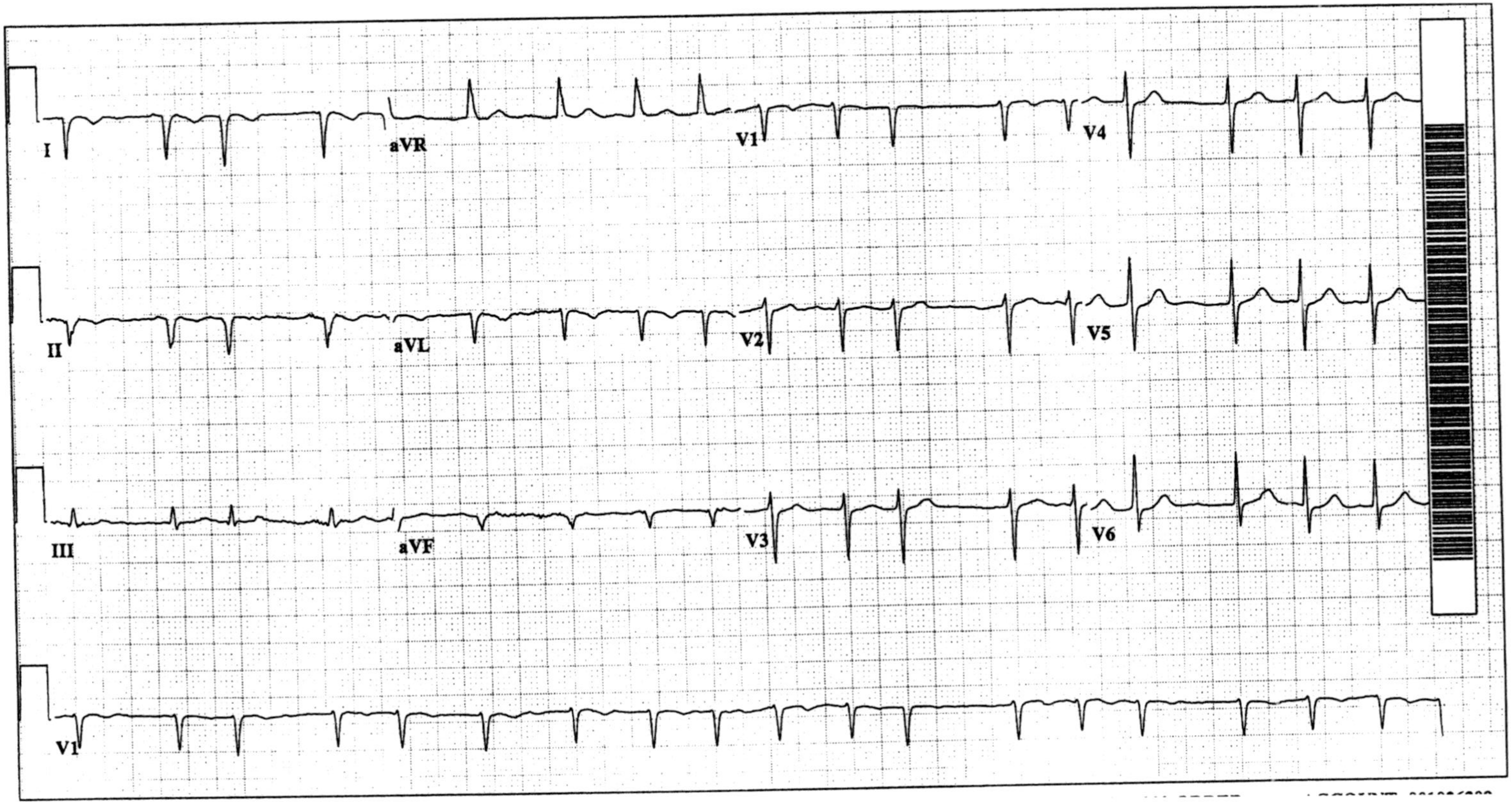

Ventricular Rate: 74 BPM
PR interval: 188 ms
QRS interval: 92 ms
QT/QTc: 388/430 ms
QRS axis: −150

INTERPRETATION: T39
SINUS RHYTHM WITH SINUS ARRHYTHMIA
DEXTROCARDIA
ABNORMAL EKG

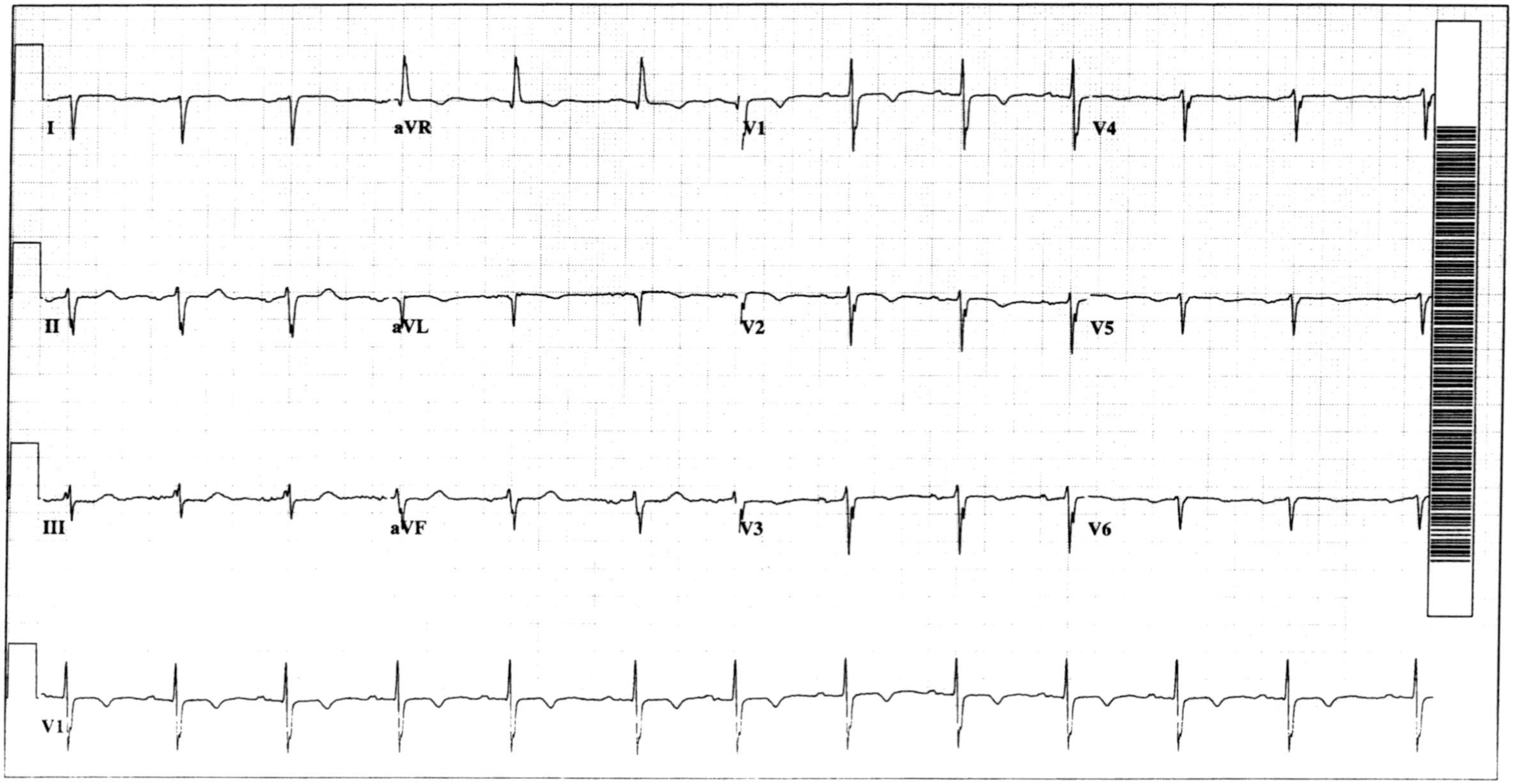

Ventricular Rate: 99 BPM   INTERPRETATION: T40

PR interval: 136 ms   SINUS RHYTHM

QRS interval: 96 ms   LAHB

QT/QTc: 360/462 ms   ANTEROLATERAL INFARCT MASKED BY LAHB CANNOT BE EXCLUDED

QRS axis: −59   ABNORMAL EKG

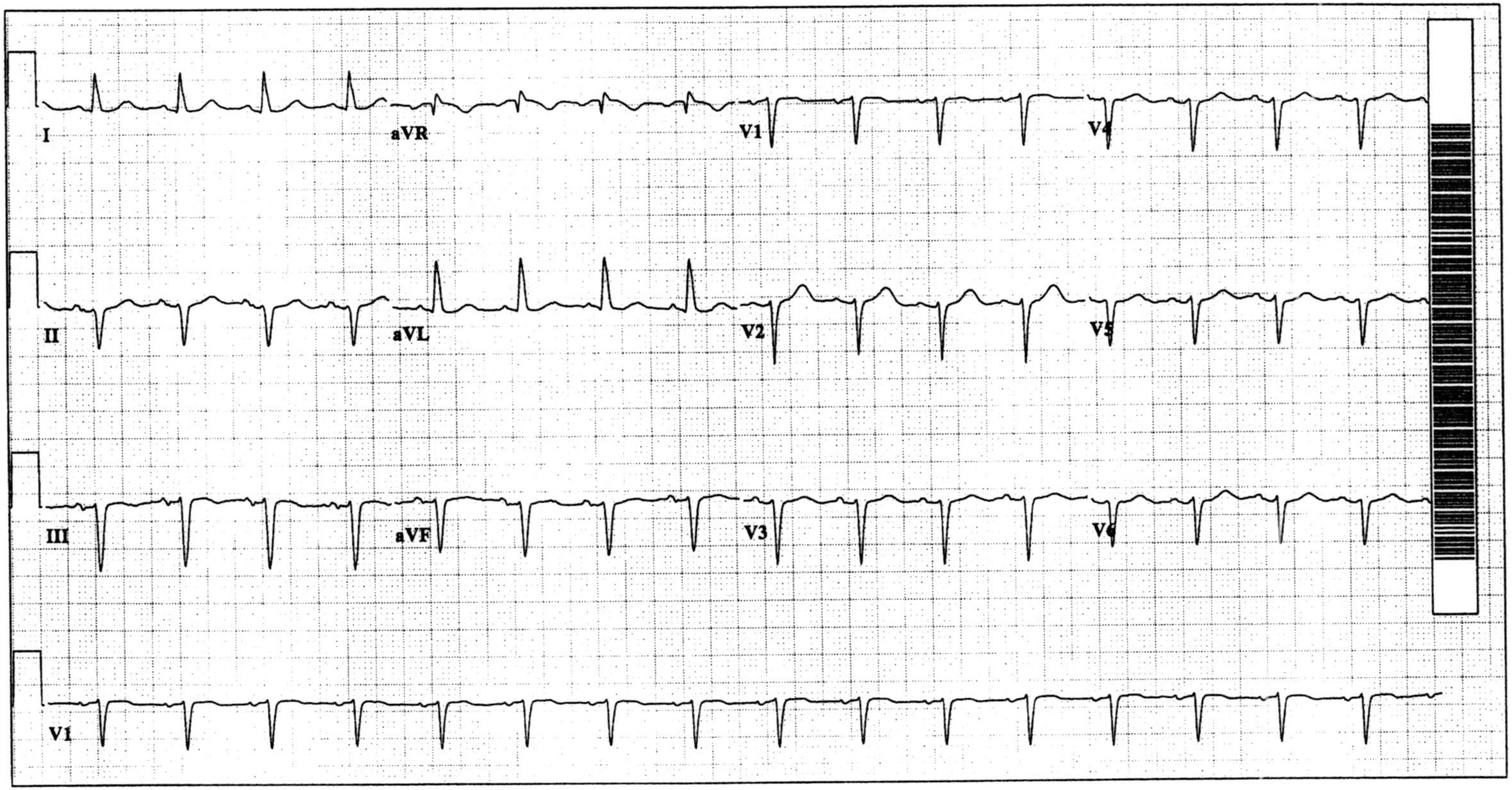

Ventricular Rate:	94–187 BPM	INTERPRETATION: T41
PR interval:		SINUS RHYTHM CONVERTING INTO ATRIAL TACHYCARDIA
QRS interval:	86 ms	LAD
QT/QTc:	282/425 ms	POSSIBLE RIGHT ATRIAL ENLARGEMENT
QRS axis:	–30	ABNORMAL EKG

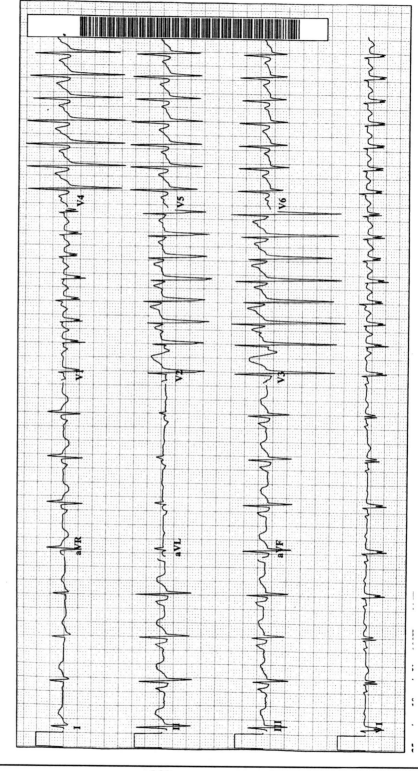

Ventricular Rate: 231 BPM INTERPRETATION: T42

PR interval: VENTRICULAR TACHYCARDIA

QRS interval: 174 ms ABNORMAL EKG

QT/QTc:

QRS axis: 0

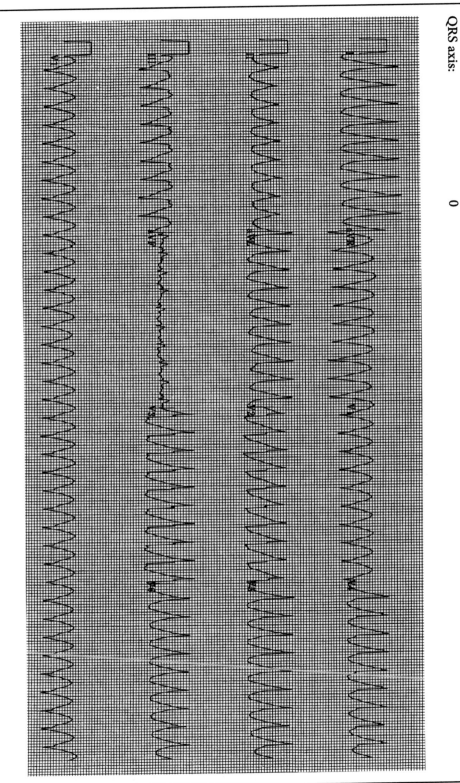

Ventricular Rate:	83 BPM	INTERPRETATION: T43
PR interval:	106 ms	SINUS RHYTHM WITH FREQUENT ISOLATED PACs AND COUPLETS;
QRS interval:	86 ms	OCCASIONALLY WITH ABERRANT CONDUCTION
QT/QTc:	426/500 ms	PROLONGED QT
QRS axis:	+80	ABNORMAL EKG

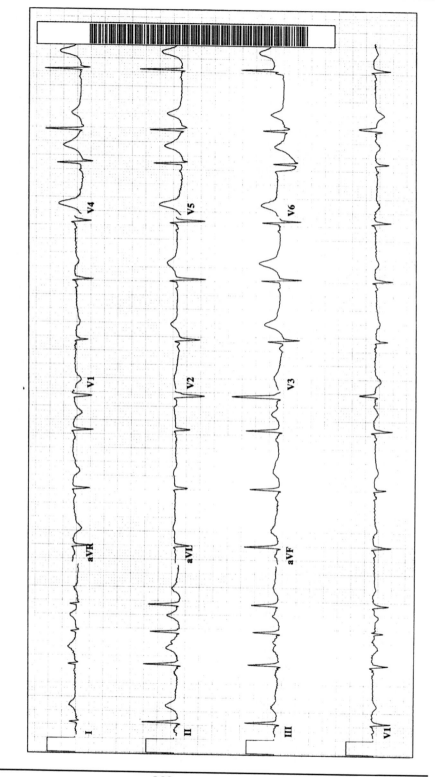

Ventricular Rate: 84 BPM

PR interval:

QRS interval: 76 ms

QT/QTc: 420/493 ms

QRS axis: +40

INTERPRETATION: T44
ATRIAL FIBRILLATION WITH OCCASIONAL ABERRANT CONDUCTION
LOW QRS VOLTAGE
POSSIBLE ANTERIOR M.I., ? AGE
ST–T ABNORMALITY CONSISTENT WITH ISCHEMIA AND/OR
DIGITALIS EFFECT
PROLONGED QT
ABNORMAL EKG

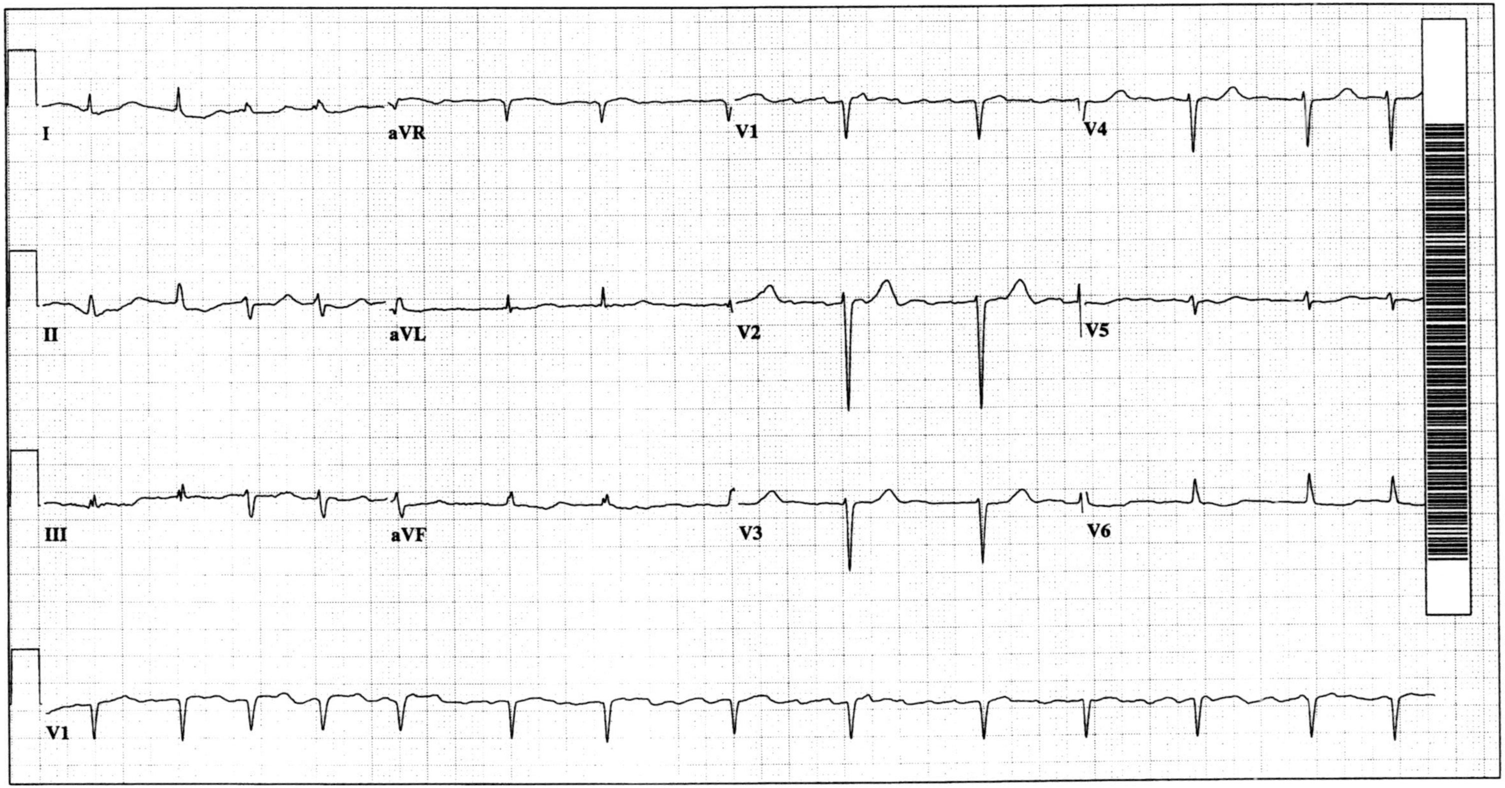

I aVR V1 V4

II aVL V2 V5

III aVF V3 V6

V1

Ventricular Rate:	72 BPM	INTERPRETATION: T45
PR interval:	158 ms	SINUS RHYTHM
QRS interval:	130 ms	LEFT ATRIAL ENLARGEMENT
QT/QTc:	462/505 ms	LAD
QRS axis:	-40	LVH WITH REPOLARIZATION ABNORMALITY
		IVC DELAY
		PROLONGED QT
		POSSIBLE ANTERIOR M.I., ? AGE
		ABNORMAL EKG

Ventricular Rate:	78 BPM
PR interval:	
QRS interval:	128 ms
QT/QTc:	364/430 ms
QRS axis:	-62

INTERPRETATION: T46

PAROXYSMAL ATRIAL TACHYCARDIA WITH VARYING 2ND° AV BLOCK

RBBB
LAHB
ONE PVC
ABNORMAL EKG

NOTE: P waves in lead V1 give the impression of atrial flutter. However, P is upright in inferior leads. The P wave in slow atrial flutter is always inverted in inferior leads. Atrial rate is 200 BPM. An upright P in inferior leads with atrial rate of 150–250 BPM is suggestive of PAT (paroxysmal atrial tachycardia).

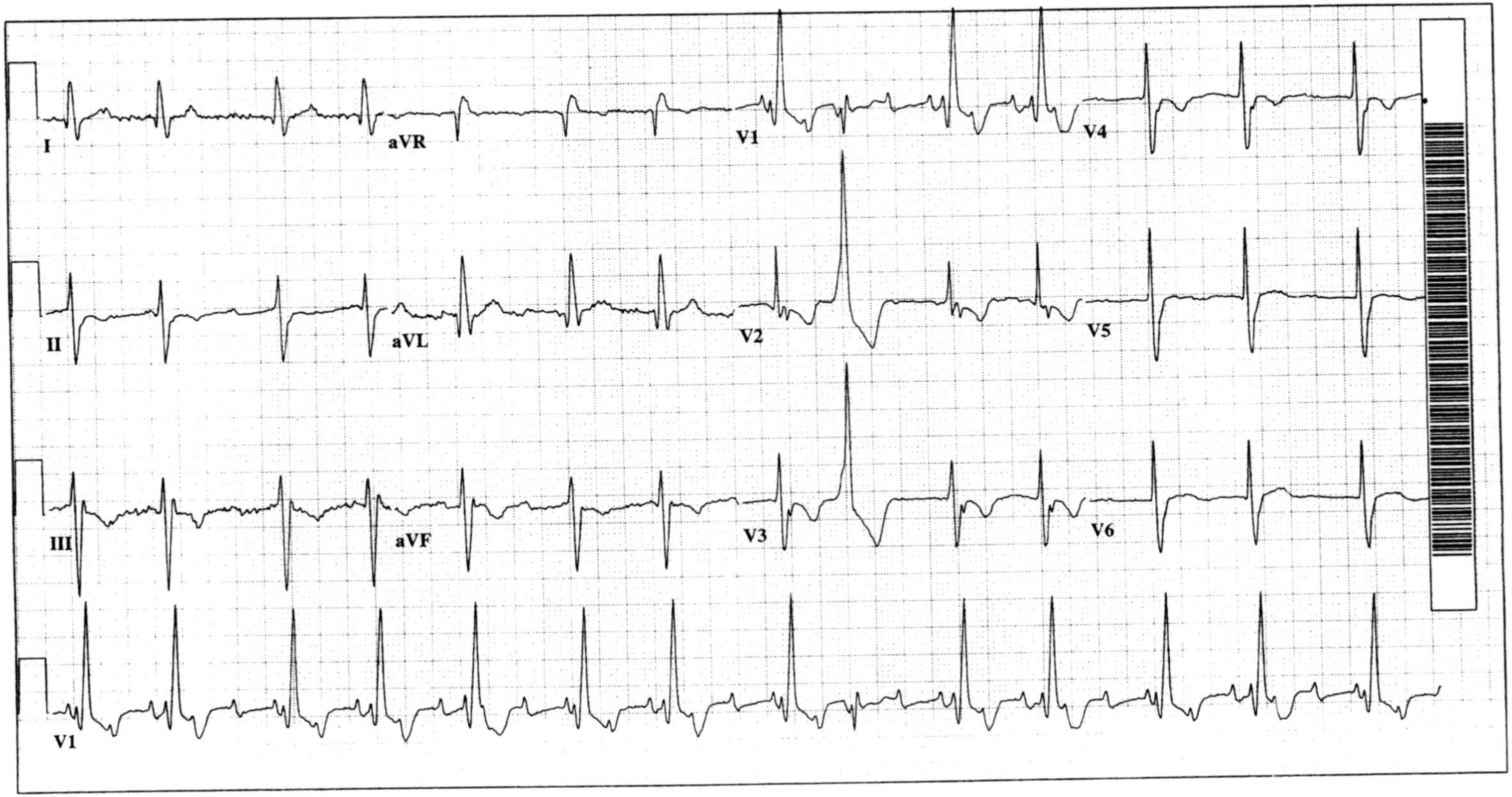

Ventricular Rate: 73 BPM   INTERPRETATION: T47

PR interval: 152 ms   SINUS RHYTHM

QRS interval: 94 ms   FLAT TOP T WAVES (? T + U WAVES COMBINED)

QT/QTc: 548/603 ms   PROLONGED QT (? Q – U INTERVAL)

QRS axis: +70   ? HYPOKALEMIA

ABNORMAL EKG

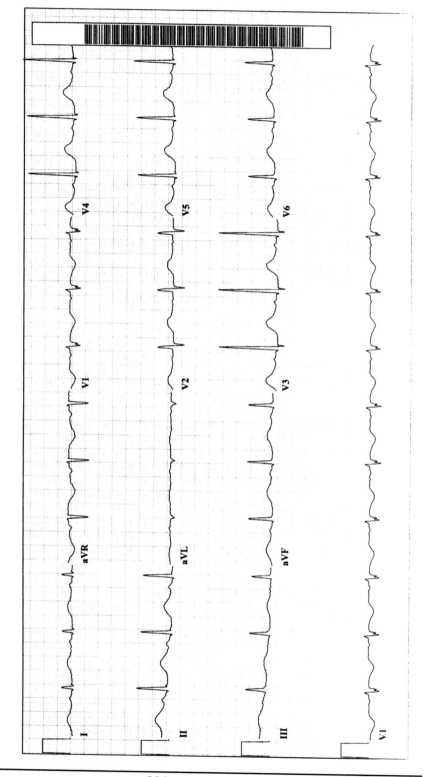

Ventricular Rate: 162 BPM

PR interval:

QRS interval: 128 ms

QT/QTc: 348/571 ms

QRS axis: -82

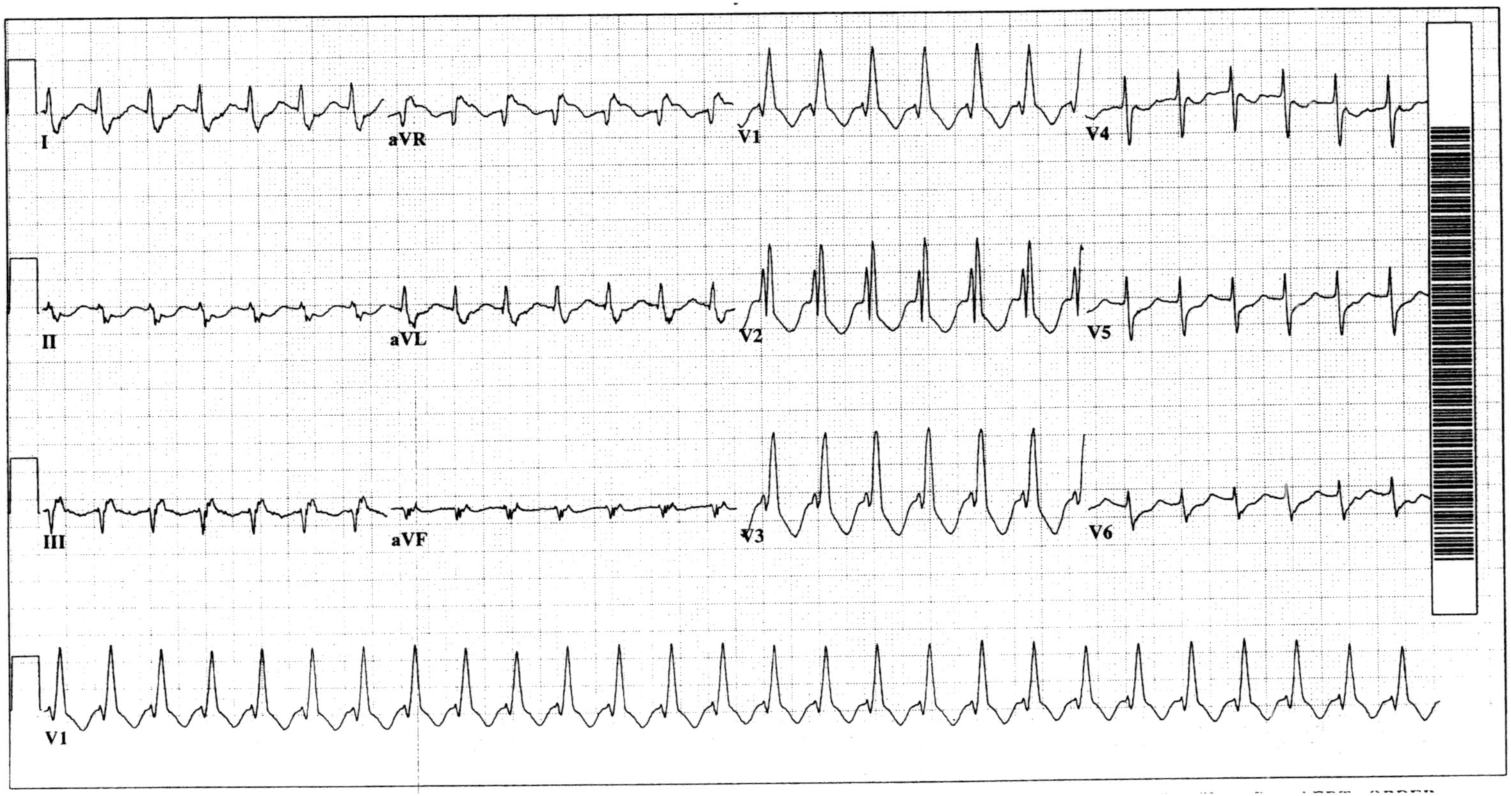

INTERPRETATION: T48
WIDE QRS TACHYCARDIA
ABNORMAL EKG

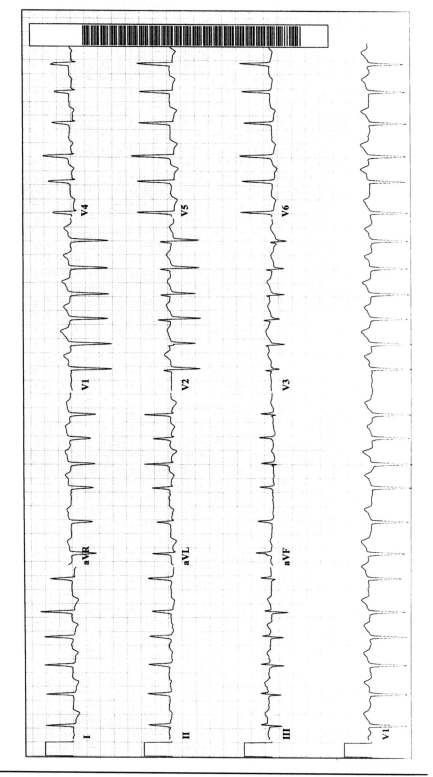

Ventricular Rate:	145 BPM
PR interval:	
QRS interval:	76 ms
QT/QTc:	298/462 ms
QRS axis:	+22

INTERPRETATION: T49
ATRIAL FIBRILLATION WITH RAPID VENTRICULAR RATE
R WAVE REGRESSION IN V3, POSSIBLE LEAD MISPLACEMENT OR OLD
ANTERIOR M.I.
ST–T ABNORMALITY, ? ISCHEMIA AND/OR LVH
ABNORMAL EKG

Ventricular Rate: 60 BPM   INTERPRETATION: T50
PR interval: 200 ms   SINUS RHYTHM
QRS interval: 140 ms   RBBB
QT/QTc: 458/453 ms LAHB
QRS axis: -80   ABNORMAL EKG

Ventricular Rate:	85 BPM
PR interval:	110 ms
QRS interval:	84 ms
QT/QTc:	352/428 ms
QRS axis:	+100

INTERPRETATION: T51

ACCELERATED NODAL RHYTHM WITH OCCASIONAL PACs

RAD

POSSIBLE ANTERIOR M.I., ? AGE

ABNORMAL EKG

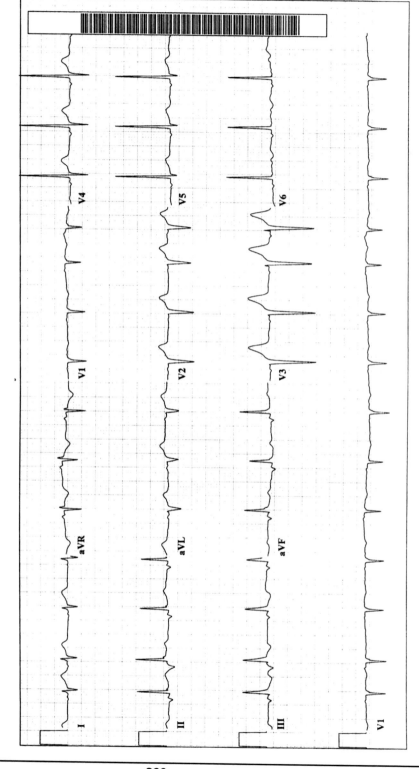

Ventricular Rate:	54 BPM	INTERPRETATION: T52
PR interval:	194 ms	SINUS BRADYCARDIA
QRS interval:	106 ms	RAD
QT/QTc:	434/407 ms	INFERIOR M.I., ? AGE
QRS axis:	+95	ABNORMAL EKG

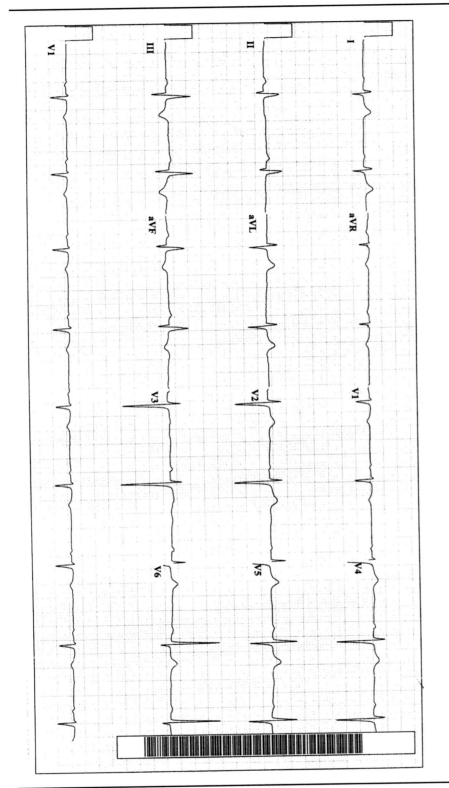

Ventricular Rate: 81 BPM
PR interval: 104 ms
QRS interval: 84 ms
QT/QTc: 372/432 ms
QRS axis: +30

INTERPRETATION: T53
ACCELERATED NODAL RHYTHM
EARLY REPOLARIZATION
ABNORMAL EKG

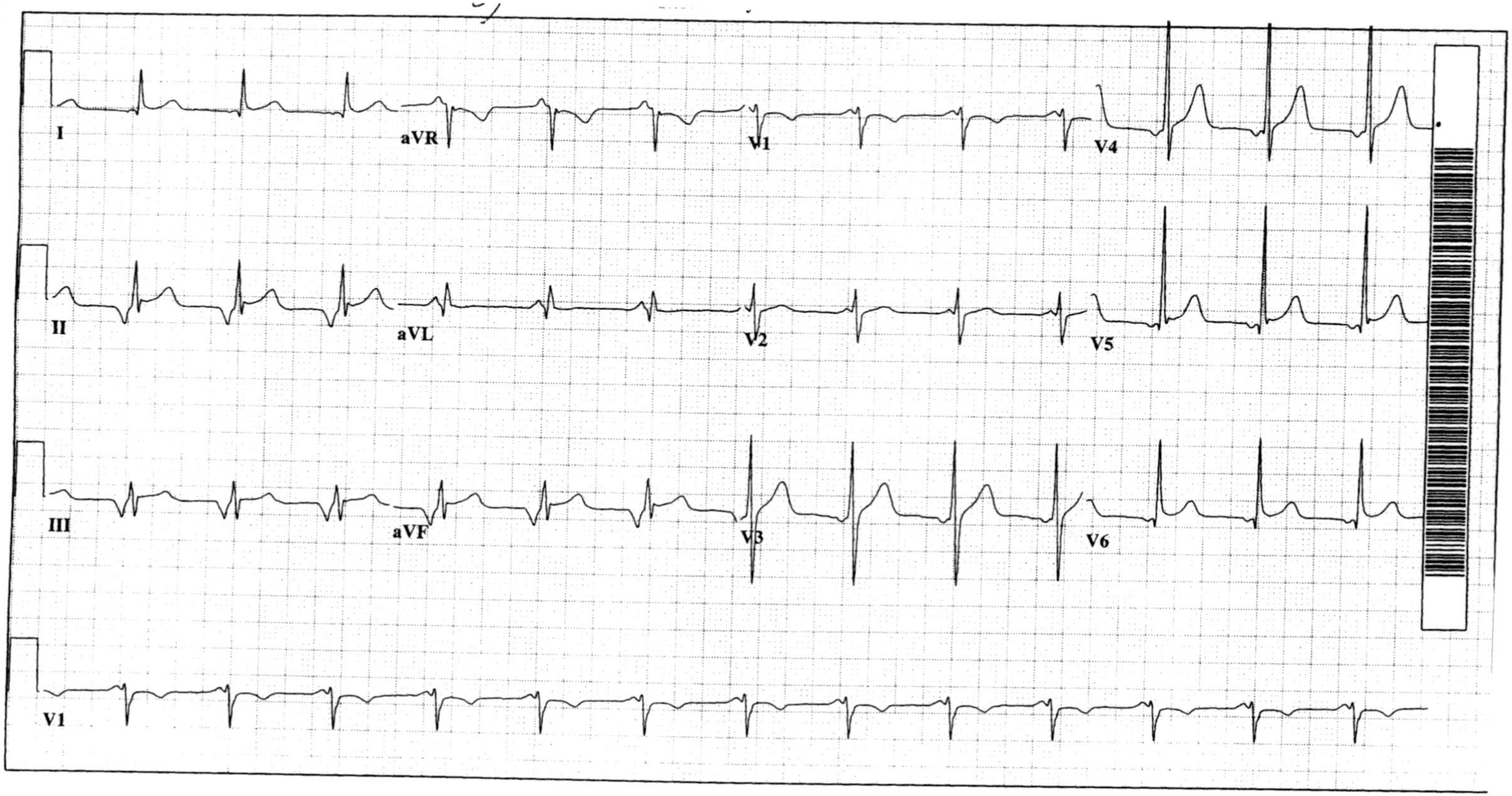

Ventricular Rate: 240 BPM INTERPRETATION: T54

PR interval: ATRIAL TACHYCARDIA WITH 1:1 AV CONDUCTION

QRS interval: 72 ms ABNORMAL EKG

QT/QTc: 162/325 ms

QRS axis: +35

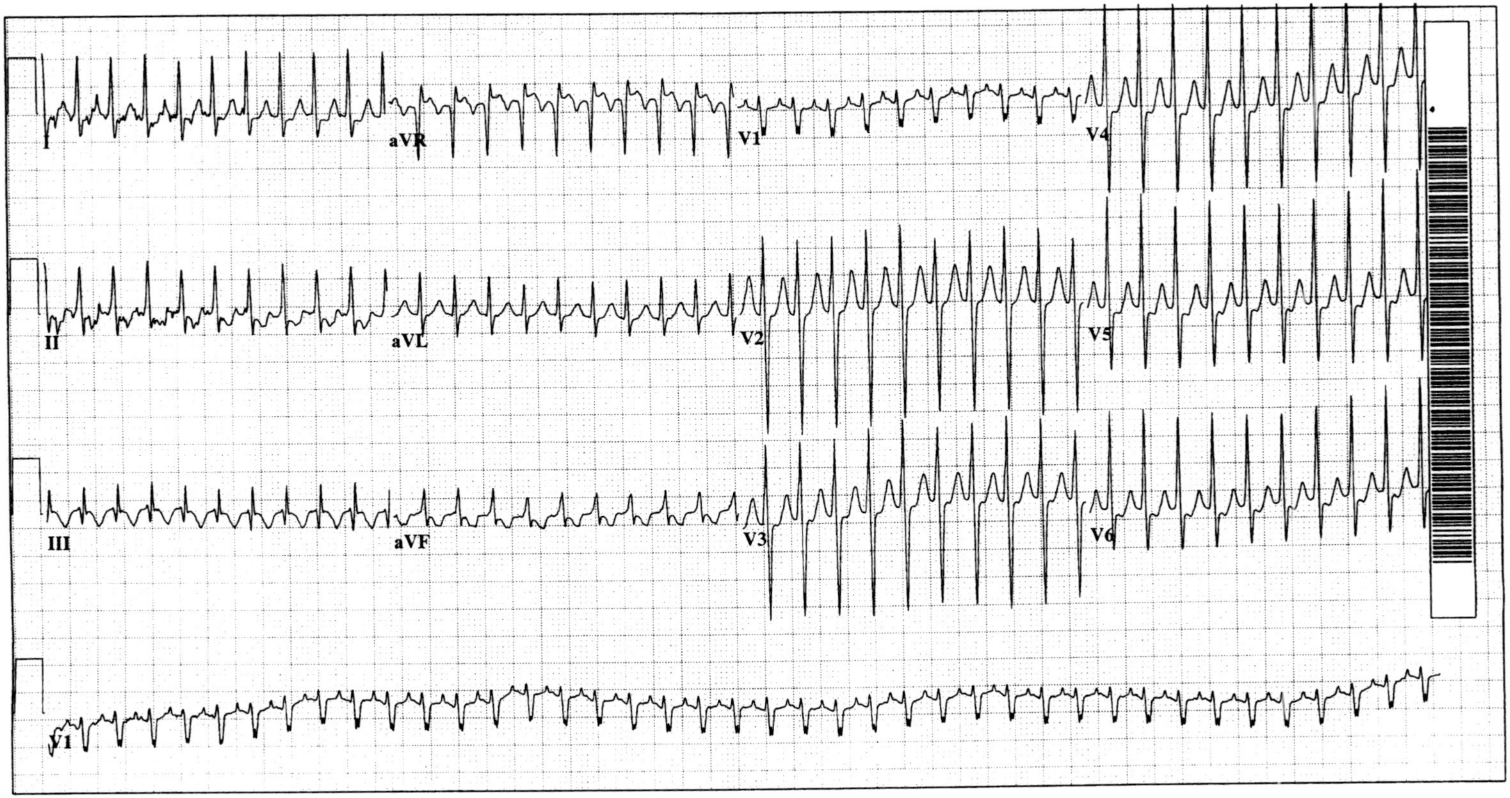

Ventricular Rate: 94 BPM
PR interval: 180 ms
QRS interval: 102 ms
QT/QTc: 388/485 ms
QRS axis: +44

INTERPRETATION: T55
SINUS RHYTHM
ACUTE INFERIOR M.I
ABNORMAL EKG

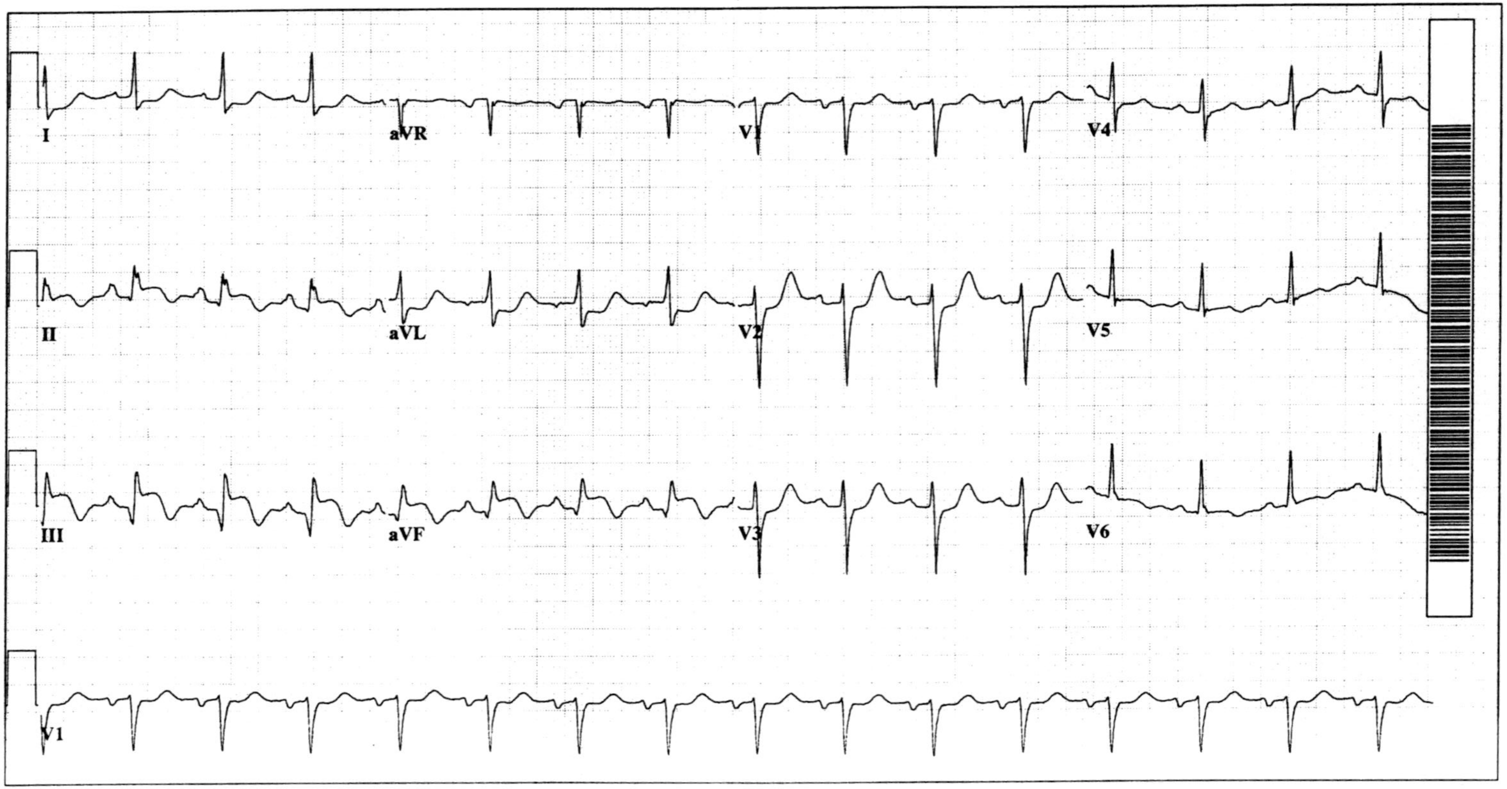

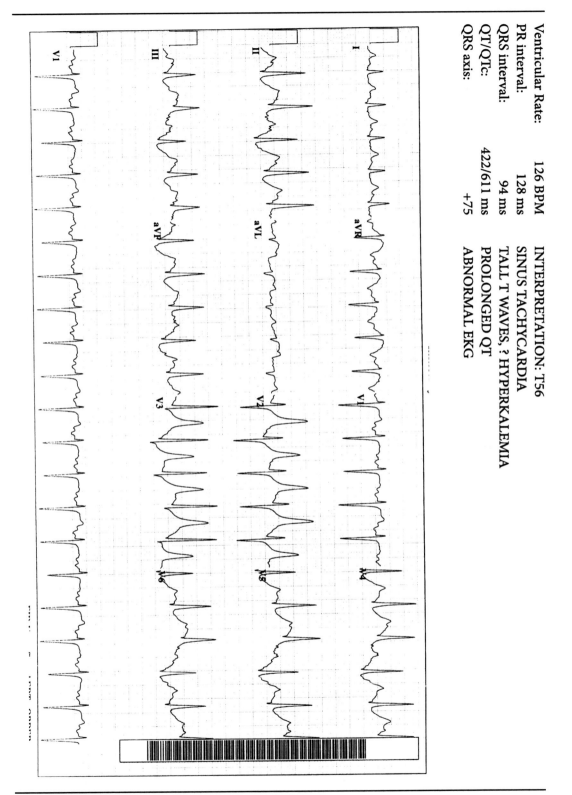

Ventricular Rate: 126 BPM   INTERPRETATION: T56
PR interval: 128 ms   SINUS TACHYCARDIA
QRS interval: 94 ms   TALL T WAVES, ? HYPERKALEMIA
QT/QTc: 422/611 ms PROLONGED QT
QRS axis: +75   ABNORMAL EKG

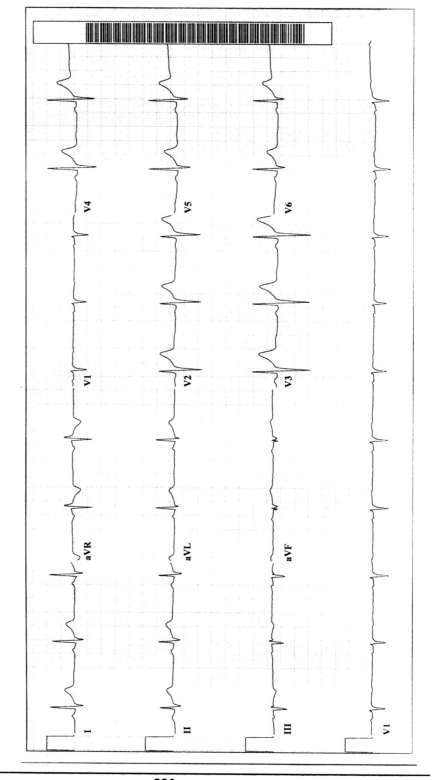

Ventricular Rate: 61 BPM
PR interval: 156 ms
QRS interval: 102 ms
QT/QTc: 380/38 ms
QRS axis: −8

INTERPRETATION: T57
SINUS RHYTHM
INFERIOR M.I., ? AGE, CANNOT BE EXCLUDED
ABNORMAL EKG

NOTE: A "W" pattern QRS morphology in lead AVF suggests
possible inferior M.I.

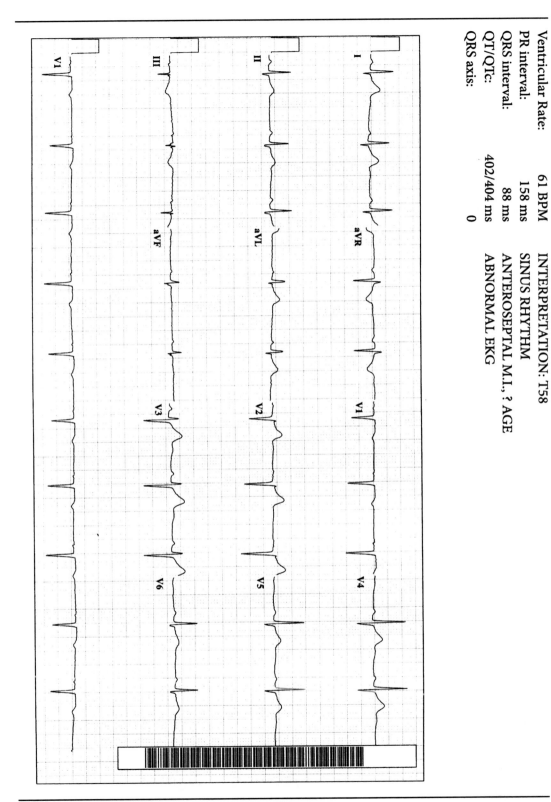

Ventricular Rate: 61 BPM   INTERPRETATION: T58
PR interval: 158 ms   SINUS RHYTHM
QRS interval: 88 ms   ANTEROSEPTAL M.I., ? AGE
QT/QTc: 402/404 ms ABNORMAL EKG
QRS axis: 0

Ventricular Rate:	72 BPM	INTERPRETATION: T59
PR interval:	244 ms	SINUS RHYTHM WITH FIRST DEGREE AV BLOCK
QRS interval:	138 ms	RAD
QT/QTc:	486/539 ms	IVC DELAY
QRS axis:	+110	INFERIOR M.I., ? AGE,
		ANTEROSEPTAL M.I., ? AGE, CANNOT BE EXCLUDED
		PROLONGED QT
		ABNORMAL EKG

Ventricular Rate:	70 BPM
PR interval:	266 ms
QRS interval:	160 ms
QT/QTc:	532/578 ms
QRS axis:	+130

INTERPRETATION: T60
SINUS RHYTHM WITH FIRST DEGREE AV BLOCK
RBBB
RAD
ABNORMAL EKG

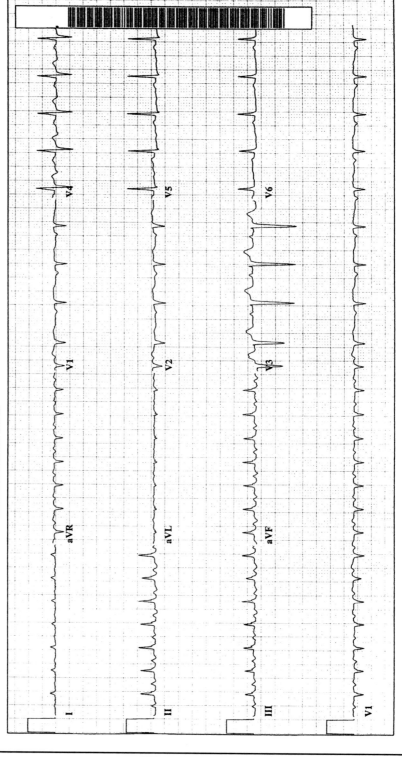

Ventricular Rate: 177 BPM

PR interval:

QRS interval: 78 ms

QT/QTc: 292/420 ms

QRS axis: +75

INTERPRETATION: T61

PAROXYSMAL SUPRAVENTRICULAR TACHYCARDIA CONVERTED

TO SINUS TACHYCARDIA

ANTEROSEPTAL M.I., ? AGE

LOW QRS VOLTAGE

NON-SPECIFIC ST–T ABNORMALITY

ABNORMAL EKG

Ventricular Rate: 64 BPM   INTERPRETATION: T62
PR interval: 260 ms   SINUS RHYTHM WITH FIRST DEGREE AV BLOCK
QRS interval: 130 ms   LAHB
QT/QTc: 454/468 ms   IVC DELAY
QRS axis: -55   ST - T ABNORMALITY, CONSISTENT WITH ISCHEMIA AND/OR LVH
                                  ABNORMAL EKG

Ventricular Rate: 150 BPM   INTERPRETATION: T63
PR interval: ATRIAL FIBRILLATION WITH RAPID VENTRICULAR RESPONSE
QRS interval: 88 ms   AND ASHMAN PHENOMENON
QT/QTc: 346/543 ms   DIFFUSE NON-SPECIFIC ST – T CHANGES
QRS axis: +2   PROLONGED QT
                                   ABNORMAL EKG

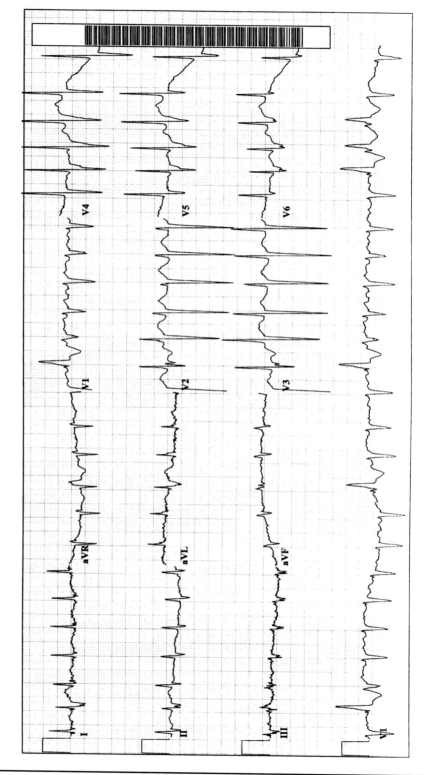

Ventricular Rate: 94 BPM INTERPRETATION: T64

PR interval: ATRIAL FIBRILLATION

QRS interval: 118 ms INCOMPLETE RBBB

QT/QTc: 356/445 ms RAD

QRS axis: +110 ST – T ABNORMALITY, CONSIDER INFERIOR ISCHEMIA

ABNORMAL EKG

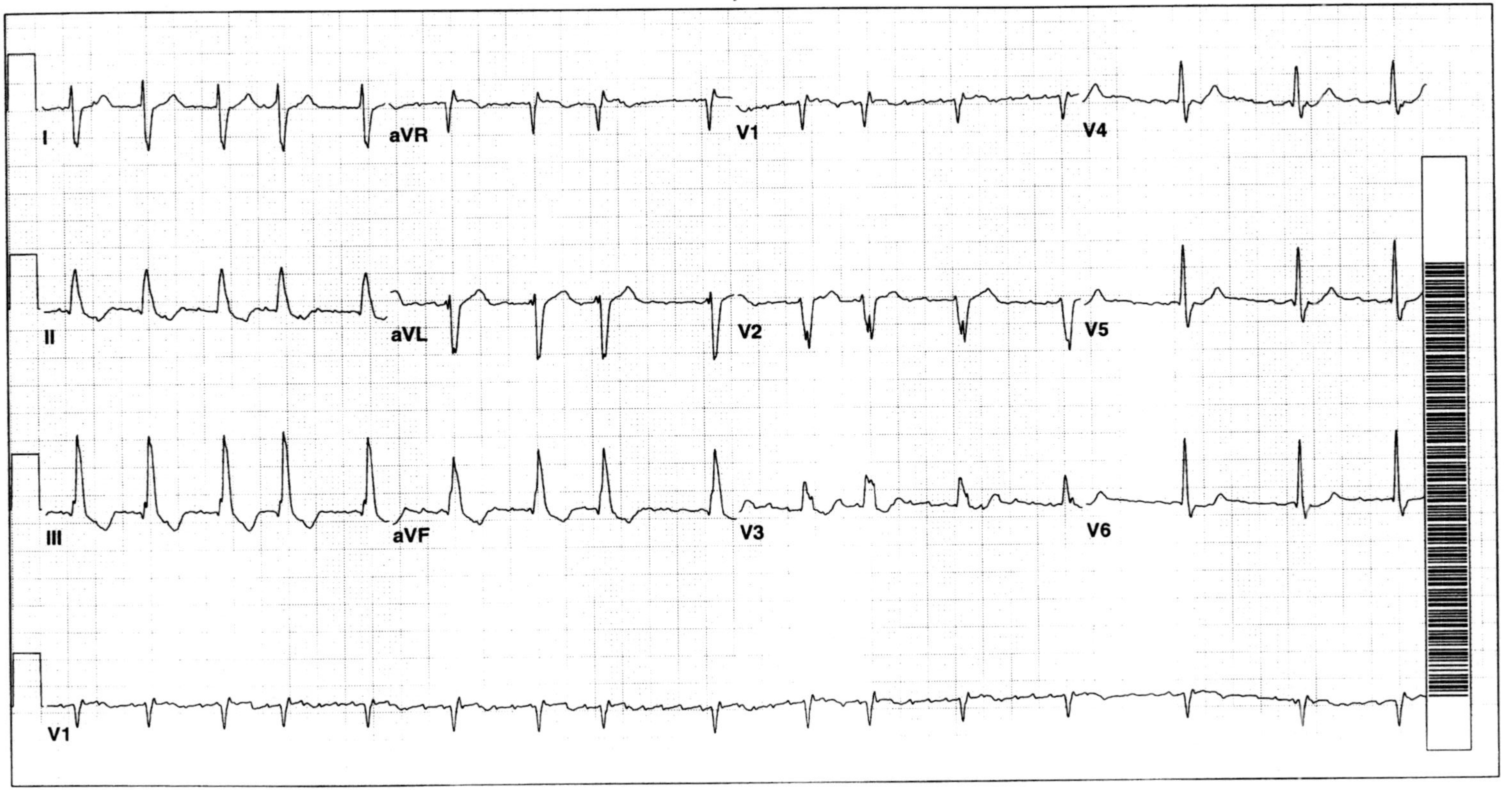

I aVR V1 V4

II aVL V2 V5

III aVF V3 V6

V1

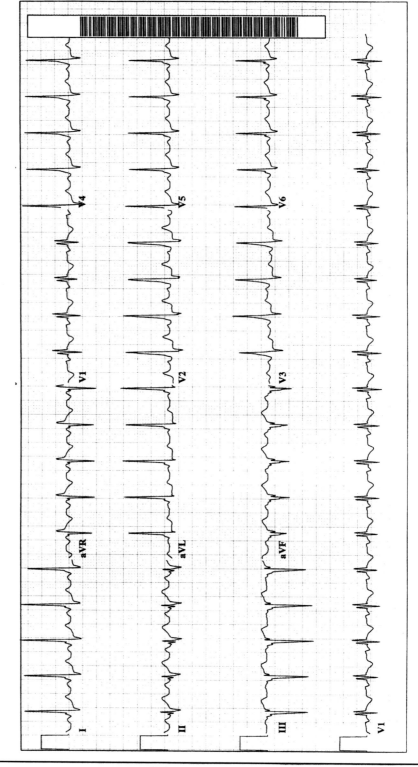

Ventricular Rate: 116 BPM   INTERPRETATION: T65
PR interval: 128 ms   SINUS TACHYCARDIA
QRS interval: 126 ms   WOLF – PARKINSON – WHITE PATTERN
QT/QTc: 352/489 ms   LAD
QRS axis: –35   ABNORMAL EKG

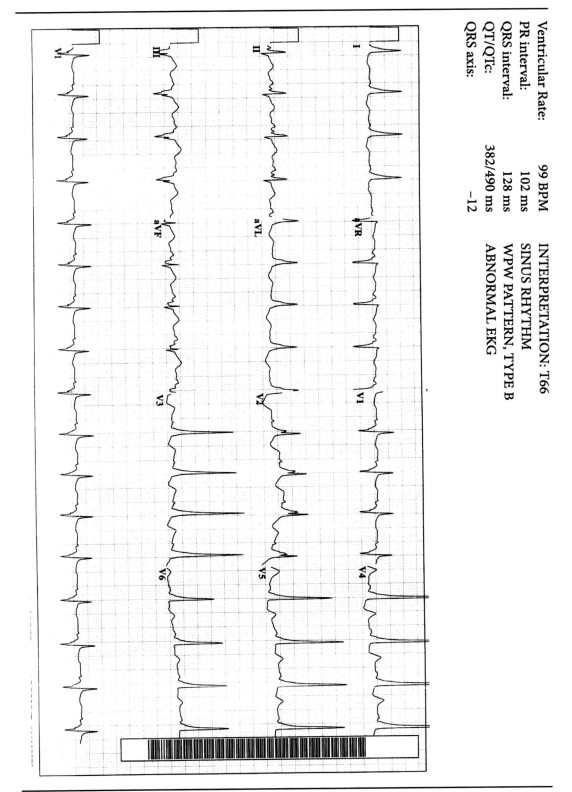

Ventricular Rate: 99 BPM INTERPRETATION: T66

PR interval: 102 ms SINUS RHYTHM

QRS interval: 128 ms WPW PATTERN, TYPE B

QT/QTc: 382/490 ms ABNORMAL EKG

QRS axis: −12

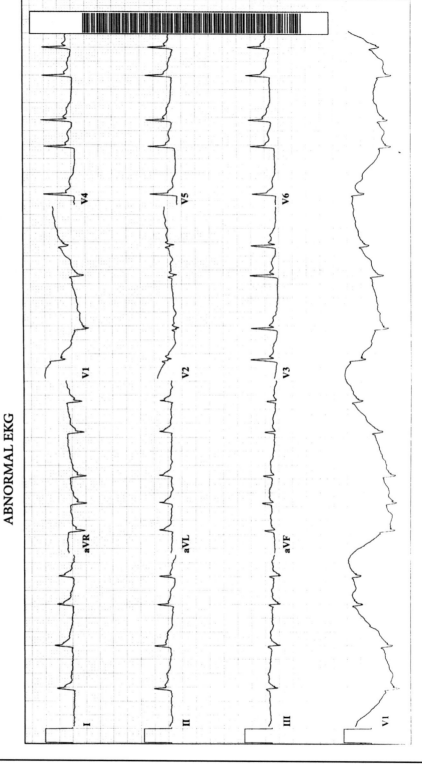

Ventricular Rate: 111 BPM
PR interval:
QRS interval: 80 ms
QT/QTc: 340/462 ms
QRS axis: +12

INTERPRETATION: T67
ATRIAL FIBRILLATION WITH RAPID HEART RATE
OSBORN WAVES (J WAVES) IN ANTEROLATERAL LEADS
DIFFUSE CONCAVE ST ELEVATION WITHOUT RECIPROCAL CHANGES
PR DEPRESSION
THESE FINDINGS ARE CONSISTENT WITH ACUTE PERICARDITIS
ABNORMAL EKG

Ventricular Rate: 60 BPM
PR interval: 194 ms
QRS interval: 108 ms
QT/QTc: 418/418 ms
QRS axis: -48

INTERPRETATION: T68
SINUS RHYTHM
LAHB
IRBBB
J POINT ELEVATION IN V1-3 (2.0MM IN V2-3), WITH SADDLE BACK
ST ELEVATION AND BIPHASIC T WAVE IN V2, SUGGESTIVE OF
BRUGADA SYNDROME
ABNORMAL EKG

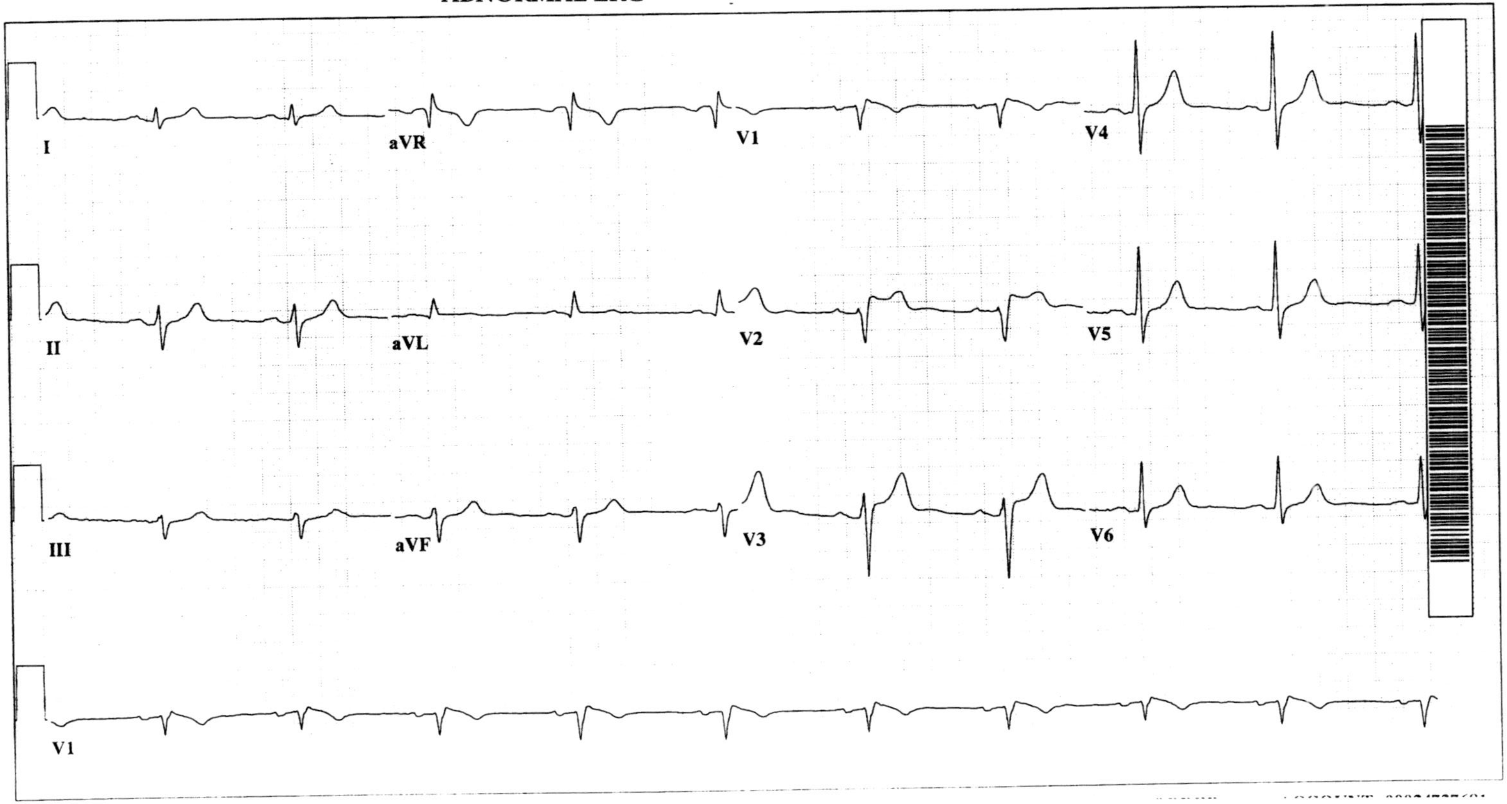

Ventricular Rate: 132 BPM

PR interval:

QRS interval: 92 ms

QT/QTc: 304/453 ms

QRS axis: +4

INTERPRETATION: T69

ECTOPIC ATRIAL TACHYCARDIA WITH VARYING AV BLOCK

ST – T ABNORMALITY, ? LVH AND/OR ISCHEMIA

ABNORMAL EKG

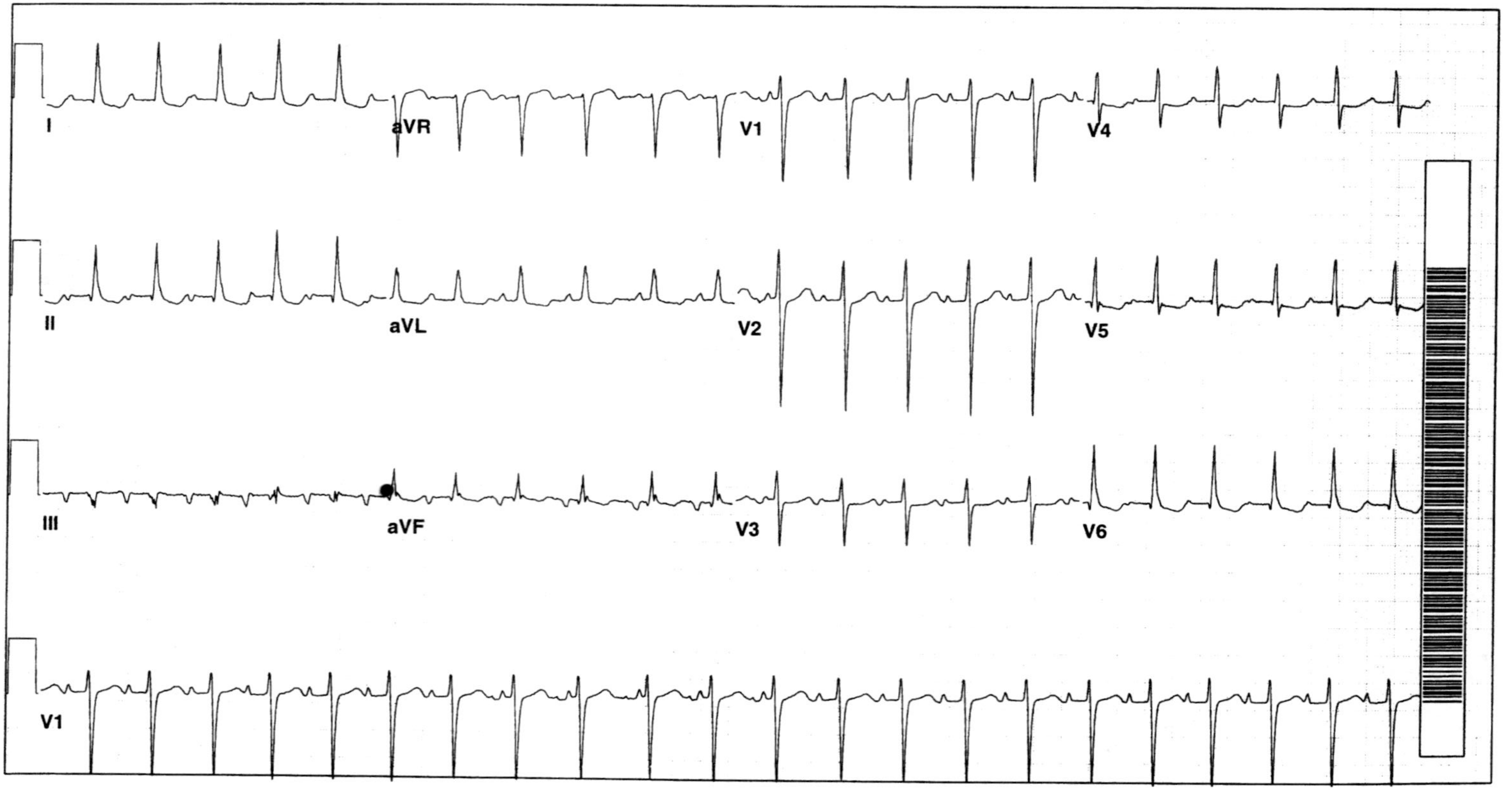

Ventricular Rate: 60 BPM INTERPRETATION: T70
PR interval: 130 ms SINUS RHYTHM
QRS interval: 148 ms RBBB
QT/QTc: 462/476 ms INFERIOR M.I., ? AGE, CANNOT BE EXCLUDED
QRS axis: +30 ABNORMAL EKG

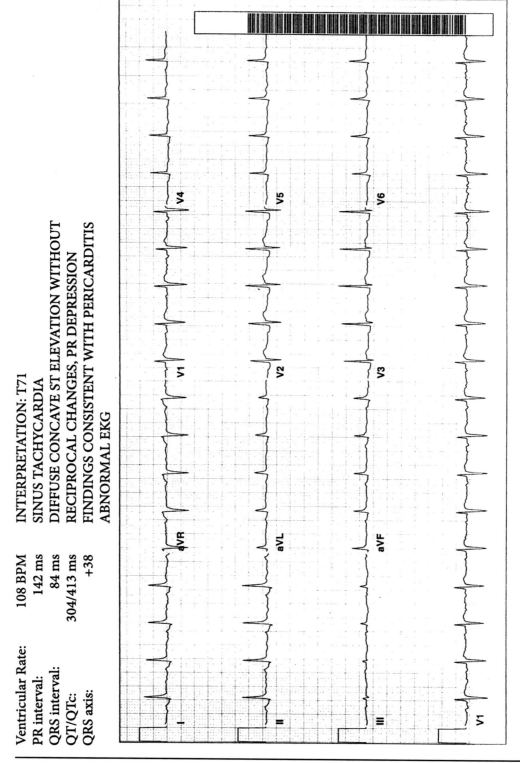

Ventricular Rate: 108 BPM
PR interval: 142 ms
QRS interval: 84 ms
QT/QTc: 304/413 ms
QRS axis: +38

INTERPRETATION: T71
SINUS TACHYCARDIA
DIFFUSE CONCAVE ST ELEVATION WITHOUT
RECIPROCAL CHANGES, PR DEPRESSION
FINDINGS CONSISTENT WITH PERICARDITIS
ABNORMAL EKG

Ventricular Rate: 138 BPM INTERPRETATION: T72
PR interval: 140 ms SINUS TACHYCARDIA
QRS interval: 56 ms RIGHT AXIS DEVIATION
QRS axis: +145 TALL R WAVES IN V1 – 3, SUGGESTING RIGHT VENTRICULAR DOMINANCE
NORMAL EKG FOR A NEWBORN INFANT

CPSIA information can be obtained
at www.ICGtesting.com
Printed in the USA
FFOW03n1847141014
8036FF